OSTEOGENESIS

Edited by **Yunfeng Lin**

Osteogenesis
Edited by Yunfeng Lin

Published by InTech
Janeza Trdine 9, 51000 Rijeka, Croatia

Publishing Process Manager Maja Bozicevic

Technical Editor Teodora Smiljanic

Cover Designer InTech Design Team

Additional hard copies can be obtained from orders@intechopen.com

Osteogenesis, Edited by Yunfeng Lin
p. cm.
ISBN 978-953-51-0030-0

For EU product safety concerns:
IN TECH d.o.o., Prolaz Marije Krucifikse Kozulić 3, 51000 Rijeka, Croatia,
info@intechopen.com or visit our website at intechopen.com.

Meet the editor

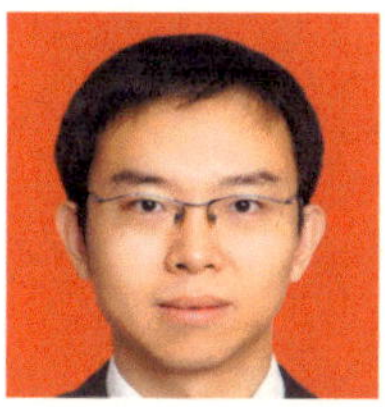

Yunfeng Lin is a full Professor at State Key Laboratory of Oral Diseases and West China School of Stomatology, Sichuan University. He serves as the Vice-Director of State Key Laboratory of Oral Diseases and Assistant Dean of West China School of Stomatology. He received his PhD from Sichuan University in 2006. Dr Lin's research interests include adipose stem cells differentiation and craniofacial regeneration, such as bone, cartilage, tooth, fat tissue regeneration, adipose derived induced pluripotent stem cells, and tissue engineering vascularization. He has published over 60 peer-reviewed papers, reviews and book chapters, and made several seminal contributions to the stem cells fields. He received the ProSPER Net-Scopus Young Scientist Award in the Asia-Pacific region and the Scopus future scientific star in China, New Century Excellent Talents of Chinese Ministry of Education and National Excellent Doctoral Dissertation of China awards.

Contents

Preface

Osteogenesis is the process of formation and development of bony tissue. The exact mechanism by which osteogenesis is triggered remains unclear, because it involves abundant gene, growth factors, cytokines and environmental factors.

This book provides an in-depth overview of current knowledge about the subject of osteogenesis in the human body, including what is known about the molecular mechanisms (eg cytokine and growth-factor-related) via which osteogenesis is triggered. Transcriptional regulators control the expression of target genes by the interaction with cofactors, coactivators, chromatin remodelling complexes and, finally, with the general transcriptional machinery.

As the key factor for osteogenesis, two important types of the scaffolds - doped calcium carbonate-phosphate and fluorocarbon composites modified with rf magnetron sputtering - are discussed in detail. The biological responses of osteoblasts and osteoprogenitors to orthopaedic wear debris are comprehensively reviewed. Prevention strategies and therapies for osteolysis and implant loosening are discussed. These include the development of wear-resistant biomaterials and pharmagolocial modalities for increasing bone formation in the implant.

This book also describes the current knowledge about bone cell biology, application of adipose derived mesenchymal stem cell in osteogenesis, and the way in which bone cells react to mechanical stimuli. Several strategies for improving vascularization are proposed. These include modification of the scaffold design, delivery of angiogenic factors, cells-based techniques, and microsurgery strategies. Another section is devoted to osteogenesis-related diseases, such as osteogenesis imperfecta, and the genetic factors that are responsible for them. .

There are a number of gaps in the knowledge of how osteogenesis occurs. Hopefully, the publication of this book will help researchers in this field to decide where to focus their future efforts. Contributions are therefore sought from anyone who is undertaking research in this area. The book will also provide an overview for surgeons and clinicians who wish to be directed in the developments related to this fascinating subject.

We thanks Dr Xiaoxiao Cai for the English editing of the whole book and for financial support of Natural Science Foundation of China (30801304, 81071273, 31170929), Foundation for Authors of National Excellent Doctoral Dissertation (FANEDD 200977), and Program for the New Century Excellent Talents (NCET-08-0373), Funding for Distinguished Young Scientists in Sichuan (2010JQ0066)

Yunfeng Lin
Professor, State Key Laboratory of Oral Disease
West China School of Stomatology
Sichuan University
P. R. China

1

Transcriptional Control of Osteogenesis

Malgorzata Witkowska-Zimny
Department of Biophysics and Human Physiology, Medical University of Warsaw, Poland

1. Introduction

One of the key issues in studying organogenesis is to understand the mechanisms underlying the differentiation of progenitor cells into more specialized cells of individual tissue. The formation and regeneration of each tissue is associated with a cascade of signals involving a sequential activation of successive genes in response to transcriptional regulators, growth factors, cytokines and hormones. Mediators such as fibroblast growth factor (FGF), transforming growth factor beta (TGF-β), insulin-like growth factors (IGF) and many other proteins influence the early stage of cell and tissue formation. The factors are not tissue-specific and control the proliferation and differentiation of most cell types. The proper tissue formation, maturation and function is controlled by factors unique to particular tissue.

Transcriptional regulation is the most important step controlling the decision which genes will be expressed at a given time, thus affect the fate of cells. The recent progress in molecular biology, animal models and development of the skeletal phenotype induced by genetic mutations in humans, led to a better understanding of the role of transcriptional factors that govern bone formation and are specifically activated during osteogenesis.

The development of the vertebrate skeletal elements may take place through two different mechanisms: osteoblastogenesis and osteochondrogenesis, and relies on the differentiation of the required cell types: osteoblasts and chondrocytes (membranous and endochondral/cartilaginous osteogenesis, respectively), which are derived from common mesenchymal stem cells (Fig. 1.).

Osteoblastogenesis (membranous osteogenesis) takes place in the mesenchymal membrane, where osteoblast progenitor cells differentiate directly from embryonic condensed mesenchyme, mature to osteoblasts and begin to secrete type I collagen, proteoglycans and intercellular substance of the organic component of bone - osteoid. These mechanisms are responsible for the development of skull bones, facial bones and parially colarbone.

Most of the vertebrate skeleton develops through endochondral ossification, whereby a cartilaginous template is initially formed and subsequently mineralized and replaced bone. Endochondral bone formation (cartilaginous osteogenesis) takes place in long bones starting with the condensation of skeletal precursors, proceeding to the formation of a cartilagenous template. Chondrocytes at the condensation centre stop proliferating and become hypertrophic (enlarged). This process induces differentiation of osteoblast precursors in the perichondrium adjacent to the region of hypertrophic cells. Perichondrial cells adjacent to hypertrophic chondrocytes become osteoblasts, forming bone collar. At the subsequent steps hypertrophic chondrocytes secrete a mineralized matrix and die through apoptosis.

Vascular invasion follows, bringing osteoblast progenitors from the bone collar into the centre of the future bone. Chondrocytes continue to proliferate, lengthening the bone. Osteoblasts of primary spongiosa are precursors of eventual trabecular bone; osteoblasts of bone collar become cortical bone. At the end of the bone, the secondary ossification centre forms through cycles of chondrocyte hypertrophy, vascular invasion and osteoblast activity. A bone marrow expands in marrow space along with stromal cells.

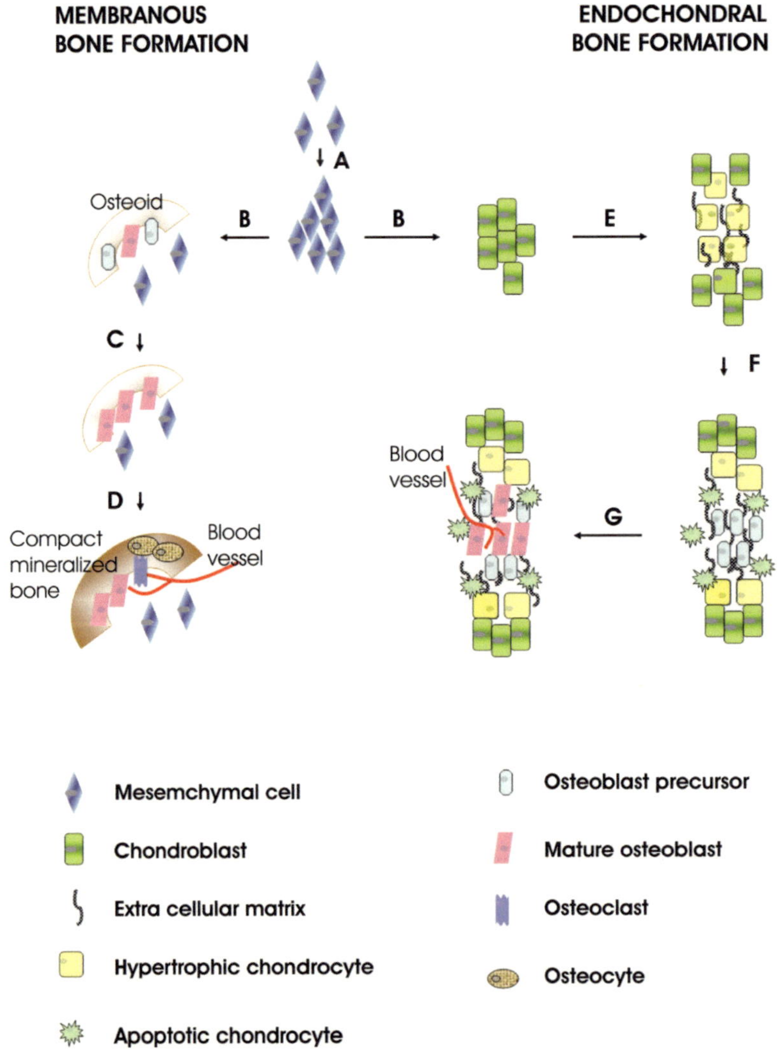

Fig. 1. Schematic representation of membranous and endochondral bone formation. A - mesenchymal cells condensation and proliferation; B – differentiation; C – production of mature osteoblasts; D – osteoblast differente into osteocytes,blood vessels invade and together with osteoblast start to make bone utilize the mineralized matrix; E – synthesis of extracellular matrix and chondrocytes grow to become hypertrophic; F – apoptosis of hypertrophic chondrocytes and osteoblast invasion; G – vascularization of cartilage and osteoblast maturation, secondary ossification center formation are not shown.

All of phenotypic and physiological changes in mesenchymal cells arise as a result of regulatory events at the genetic level. Mutations or deregulation of these processes lead to skeletal malformation, and/or susceptibility to injury. Over the past years on the basis of *in vivo* and *in vitro* studies various transcription factors have been identified that play important roles for skeletal formation being either active in osteoblasts and chondrocytes or in both cell types. The molecular mechanisms controlling the chondrogenic and osteogenic program are becoming elucidated; however, major difficulty in the overall understanding of bone formation is to combine all scattered pieces of information considering the function and importance of individual genes and their products into comprehensive signal network.
This chapter presents recent findings on the role of the most important and unique genetic regulators supporting bone formation.

2. Transcription control of osteoblastogenesis

The specific structure of bone, its function and metabolism are a result of the processes of bone formation, resorption, mineral homeostasis and bone regeneration. Osteoblasts are bone-forming cells that synthesize and mineralize extracellular matrix. In membranous bone formation, they arise from multipotential mesenchymal stem cells under the influence of growth factors, hormones and cytokines. Differentiation of progenitor cells into osteoblast *in vitro* has been induced by the presence of osteogenic supplements in cultured medium (dexamethasone, ascorbic acid, vitamin D3, β-glycerophosphate). The proper maturation and osteoblast function is directly related to the expression of two key transcription factors of osteoblastogenesis: Runx2 and Osterix.

2.1 Runx2 (Runt-related transcription factor 2)

The transcriptional control of the proliferation, growth and differentiation of mesenchymal stem cells into mature bone cells is primarily controlled by Runx2 (also known as CBFA1, AML3 or OSF2). Numerous *in vitro* studies have shown that Runx2 is a positive regulator of gene expression, whose products are bone extracellular matrix proteins, such as type I collagen, osteopontin, bone sialoprotein and osteocalcin (Komori, 2006). Runx2 is frequently described as the master regulator of osteoblastogenesis. Its deficiency in homozygots leads to different types of bone dysplasia, consisting of genetically determined disorders in the structure of the skeleton (Marie, 2008). Runx2 is also involved in processes related to the maturation of cartilage cells (Makita et al., 2008). However, during dentinogenesis, Runx2 expression is downregulated, and Runx2 inhibits the terminal differentiation of odontoblast. Runx2 expression has also been recently demonstrated in non-skeletal tissues such as breast, brain, sperm and T cells (Leong et al., 2009). Therefore, it may play a role in transmitting epigenetic information encoded in DNA. The mechanism for regulating the expression of genetic information by Runx2 has been intensively studied for many years. Runx2 is a DNA-binding transcriptional factor that interacts with the promoters of specific target genes through the Runt domain. Its potential binding site has been identified at target promoters, for example in the promoter region of sialoproteins between position -84 to -79 and -184 to -179 relative to the transcription start point (Paz et al., 2005). Regions recognized by Runx2 demonstrate a consensus sequence (PuACCPuCa) described as an osteoblast specific element (OSE2). Runx2 belongs to the Runt family. It should be noted that the other two regulators of the Runt family, Runx1 and Runx3, also participate in the induction of osteoblastic genes. Amino acid sequence alignments of all main Runt family proteins are shown in Fig. 2.

```
--------------MRIPVDASTSRRFTPPSTALSPG----KMSEALPLGAP--------  34   Runx1
MASNSLFSTVTPCQQNFFWDPSTSRRFSPPSSSLQPG----KMSDVSPVVAAQQQQQQQQ  56   Runx2
--------------MRIPVDPSTSRRFTPPSPAFPCGGGGGKMGENSGALSA--------  38   Runx3
               .:  *.******:***.::  *    **.:     :.

---------------------------DAGAALAGKLRS--GDRSMVEVLADHPGELVRT  65   Runx1
QQQQQQQQQQQQQQQEAAAAAAAAAAAAAAAAAVPRLRPPHDNRTMVEIIADHPAELVRT 116   Runx2
---------------------------QAAVGPGGRARP--EVRSMVDVLADHAGELVRT  69   Runx3
                            *...   : *.     *:**:::***..*****

DSPNFLCSVLPTHWRCNKTLPIAFKVVALGDVPDGTLVTVMAGNDENYSAELRNATAAMK 125   Runx1
DSPNFLCSVLPSHWRCNKTLPVAFKVVALGEVPDGTVVTVMAGNDENYSAELRNASAVMK 176   Runx2
DSPNFLCSVLPSHWRCNKTLPVAFKVVALGDVPDGTVVTVMAGNDENYSAELRNASAVMK 129   Runx3
***********:*********:********:*****:******************:*.**

NQVARFNDLRFVGRSGRGKSFTLTITVFTNPPQVATYHRAIKITVDGPREPRRHRQKLDD 185   Runx1
NQVARFNDLRFVGRSGRGKSFTLTITVFTNPPQVATYHRAIKVTVDGPREPRRHRQKLDD 236   Runx2
NQVARFNDLRFVGRSGRGKSFTLTITVFTNPTQVATYHRAIKVTVDGPREPRRHRQKLED 189   Runx3
*******************************.**********:***************:*

QTKPGSLSFSERLSELEQLRRTAMRVSPHHPAPTPNPRASLNHS-TAFNPQPQSQMQDTR 244   Runx1
-SKPS--LFSDRLSDLGRIPHPSMRVG----VPPQNPRPSLNSAPSPFNPQGQSQITDPR 289   Runx2
QTKP----FPDRFGDLERLR---MRVT----PSTPSPRGSLSTT-SHFSSQPQTPIQG-- 235   Runx3
 :**    *.:*:.:* ::    ***      .. .** **. : : *..* *: : .

QIQPSPPWSYDQSY-QYLGSIASPSVHPATPISPGRASGMTTLS---------------- 287   Runx1
QAQSSPPWSYDQSYPSYLSQMTSPSIHSTTPLSSTRGTGLPAITDVPRRISDDDTATSDF 349   Runx2
------------------------------------------------------------ 235   Runx3

----AELSSR-LSTAPDLTAFSDPRQ----FPALPSISD-----PRMHYP----GAFTYS 329   Runx1
CLWPSTLSKKSQAGASELGPFSDPRQ----FPSISSLTESRFSNPRMHYP----ATFTYT 401   Runx2
--------------TSELNPFSDPRQFDRSFPTLPTLTESRFPDPRMHYPGAMSAAFPYS 281   Runx3
              :.:* .******    **::.::::     ******    .:*.*:

PTPVTSGIG----IGMSAMGSATRYHTYLPPPYPGSSQAQGGPFQASSPSYHLYYGASAG 385   Runx1
P-PVTSGMS----LGMSAT---THYHTYLPPPYPGSSQSQSGPFQTSSTPY-LYYGTSSG 452   Runx2
ATPSGTSISSLSVAGMPATS--RFHHTYLPPPYPGAPQNQSGPFQANPSPYHLYYGTSSG 339   Runx3
. *  :.:.     **.*      :**********:.* *.****:....* ****:*:*

SYQFSMV-----GGERSPPRILPPCTNAST---GSALLNPSLPNQSDVVEAEGSHSNSPT 437   Runx1
SYQFPMVP----GGDRSPSRMLPPCTTTSN---GSTLLNPNLPNQNDGVDADGSHSSSPT 505   Runx2
SYQFSMVAGSSSGGDRSPTRMLASCTSSAASVAAGNLMNPSLGGQSDGVEADGSHSNSPT 399   Runx3
****.**     **:***.*:*..**.::    .. *:**.* .*.* *:*:****.***

NMAPSARLEEAVWRPY 453   Runx1
VLNSSGRMDESVWRPY 521   Runx2
ALSTPGRMDEAVWRPY 415   Runx3
 : ...*::*:*****
```

Fig. 2. Amino acid sequence alignments of human Runt family transcriptional regulators: Runx1, Runx2 and Runx3. Residues conserved are colored in red and marked with a star. The dots indicate amino acids with very similar properties. Green bar below the sequence alignment represents DNA binding motif - Runt domain. Sequence accession numbers: Q01196, Q13950, Q13761, respectively.

Two distinct mechanisms involving osteoblast-mediated membranous and endochondrial ossification have been proposed: Runx1 participates in membranous bone formation which corresponds to the involvement of this protein in the early stages of osteoblastogenesis, while Runx2 plays an exclusive role in both membranous and endochondral bone forming processes that is in the process of osteoblast maturation. Runx3 is engaged in the differentiation of chondrocytes in cartilaginous ossification. The Runt family regulators are proteins that have transcription isoforms. Three isoforms of Runx2 protein are a result of complex process of alternative splicing (Li & Xiao, 2007). However, the specific molecular mechanism involved in the potential isoform functions in bone formation are not well understood. Positive transcription regulators of Runx2 were identified earlier (bone morphogenetic proteins, homeodomain proteins), while the first reports of proteins that inhibit Runx2 gene expression were published in 2009, when the Nieto group showed Snail1 to be a transcriptional repressor at the Runx promoters. Snail1 is a protein involved in the transformation of epithelial cells in the development of embryonic mesenchymal cells (EMT, called the epithelial mesenchymal transition) (De Frutos et al., 2009). Another repressor of Runx2 is Twist - basic helix-loop-helix transcription factor that regulates differentiation of multiple cell types. Twist inhibits osteoblastogenesis by interaction with Runx2-DNA binding domain and in this way prevents its ability to bind DNA (Bialek et al., 2004). Expression of Runx2 is controlled by Foxo1 which can also directly interact with this transcription factors. Teixeira and coworkers suggested that Foxo1 is an early molecular regulator during mesenchymal cell differentiation into osteoblast exerting its effects through regulation and interaction with Runx2 (Teixeira et al., 2010).

Several studies have indicated that Runx2 is a context-dependent transcriptional activator and repressor and may interact with other regulatory proteins, suggesting a complex mechanism of osteoblastogenesis control by this factor. So far coactivators of a Runx2-dependent transcription include p300 and CBP (CREB-binding protein), which function as transcriptional adapters in interactions with other proteins in multiprotein regulatory complexes. Through direct interaction with Runx2, they up-regulate Runx2-dependent transcription. Runx2 corepressors are components of multiprotein complexes that mediate histone deacetylation and condensation of chromatin, such as the TLE (transducin-like enhancer), mSin3A and HDAC3/4/6. Runx2 interacts with many transcription factors, such as Smad1 and Smad5, Twist, Dlx family, Zfp521. The nature of this cooperation is of great interest to many research teams.

The functional activity of Runx2 is particularly sensitive to posttranslational modification of the protein (e.g. phosphorylation, acetylation, methylation). It seems that the preferred interaction of Runx2 with specific cofactors depends on its post-translational modifications (Bae & Lee, 2006). Although Runx2 and its impact on osteoblast differentiation has been widely accepted, our knowledge on the mechanism underlying the process and factors influencing Runx2 expression or activity still require further studies.

2.2 Osterix

Osterix (SP7, OSX) is another transcriptional regulator, essential for differentiation of progenitor cells into osteoblasts, and hence for bone formation. This protein belongs to the Sp/XKLF family of transcriptional factors. The common feature of these regulators is the presence of a DNA binding domain, consisting of Cys2His2 zinc fingers. The OSX protein is comprised of 431 amino acids and contains three zinc finger motifs located in the C-terminal part. It is also possible to distinguish a proline- and serine-rich activation domain between 141 and 210 amino acids. Osterix transcription is positively regulated by Runx2, and in Runx2 null mutants, Osterix expression does not occur (Nakashima et al., 2002). It is an osteoblast-specific regulator and its activity has not yet been demonstrated in other cell types. The expression of early markers of osteoblast differentiation (e.g. osteopontin, alkaline phosphatase) in the human osteosarcoma cell line MG63 is not dependent on Osterix (Hatta et al., 2006). In contrast, the activation of late genes, such as osteocalcin, is correlated with the presence of this regulator; thus, it appears that Osterix is a factor required to progress the differentiation of preosteoblasts into mature osteoblasts. Despite its involvement in osteoblast differentiation, Osterix regulatory mechanism is not fully understood yet. Osterix activation region is known to interact with many regulatory proteins, including NFAT (nuclear factor of activated T cell) and primary transcription factor - TF-IIB, or Brg1 - chromatin-remodeling factor. Using matrix-assisted laser desorption ionization time-of-flight mass spectrometry, novel Osterix-interacting factors have been identified, such as RNA helicase A (RHA) (Amorim et al., 2007). Immunoprecipitation and Western blot analysis has shown Osterix to directly associate with RNA helicase A. Hence, RNA helicase A may act as a component in Osterix regulation of osteoblast differentiation. Osterix activity is regulated by various post-translational modifications including phosphorylation and glycosylation (Chu & Ferro, 2005). It has been shown that calcineurin, a protein phosphatase, affects the function of Osterix through direct interaction and altering its posttranslational phosphorylation form. The application of calcineurin inhibitor resulted in an increasing level of phosphorylated form of Osterix. Nevertheless, it remains unclear how the phosphorylation of Osterix occurs and modulates its function.

3. Transcriptional control of osteochondrogenesis

In mammals, most skeletal elements are formed through endochondral bone formation, which is characterized by the initial formation of cartilage molds from mesenchymal condensations and their subsequent replacement by bones. Two groups of transcription factors that control the key steps of chondrocyte differentiation have been identified: Sox (sex reversal Y-related high-mobility group box protein) and Runt families.

Natural chondrogenesis is initiated by Indian hedgehog signaling and associated with the expression of the major transcription factor Sox9 that controls downstream genes involved in chondrogenesis, and promoting cells to produce cartilage-specific extracellular matrix including collagen type X, collagen type II alpha 1, cartilage oligomeric matrix protein and proteoglycans. In chondrogenesis, Sox9 requires the activity of two other Sox family members: Sox6 and the large isoform of Sox5. Runt family members has also ability to drive chondrocyte differentiation. The stages of chondrocyte differentiation are regulated by a complex series of signaling molecules and transcription factors but also by paracrine factors such as TGF-β, BMPs, FGFs, and Wnts.

3.1 Sox protein and chondrocyte commitment

Sox9 is considered the master protein that control chondrogenic lineage commitment. Role of Sox9 in chondrogenesis was first demonstrated in a human genetic disease campomelic dysplasia. This disease is caused by heterozygous inactivating mutations in and around the Sox9 gene and is characterized by hypoplasia of all endochondral skeletal elements.

Sox9 belongs to a large family of SRY (sex-determination factors) transcriptional regulators which are characterized by a high mobility group DNA-binding domain (HMG-box). This domain preferentially binds CA/TTTGA/TA/T sequence *in vitro* (Han & Lefebvre, 2008).

Sox9 binds to DNA within the minor groove of double helix. Chondrocyte-specific genes (i.e.: collagen type II alpha1-Col2a1, collagen type XI alpha2-Col11a2) contain Sox9-binding sites, mutations in this DNA region abolished DNA binding of Sox9 inactivated these gene *in vivo* and *in vitro*. Sox9 is required during sequential steps of the chondrocyte differentiation pathway. In skeletal development, Sox9 is expressed during the formation of mature cartilage and mesenchymal condensation in endochondrial ossification except hypertrophic chondrocytes. Abnormal expression of Sox9 leads to severe skeletal disorders like skeletal dysmorphology syndrome or campomelic dysplasia. It was shown in experiments in mouse chimeras using Sox9-double null embryonic stem cells that development of cartilages gene is not carried out without active Sox9. On the other hand, forced expression of Sox9 in non-chondrogenic cells leads to the expression of chondrogenic markers, such as collagen type II alpha1 (Col2a1), aggrecan (Acan) and cartilage oligomeric matrix protein (Comp). Interestingly, overexpression of Sox9 in the cartilage causes a decrease in chondrocyte proliferation and a delay in bone development. This decrease in proliferation may result from binding of Sox9 to β-catenin, the essential component of the canonical Wnt signaling pathway. Along with the observation, overactivation or deletion of β-catenin in chondrocytes resulted in severe skeletal dysplasias. The expression and function of Sox9 is not restricted to chondrogenesis, suggesting that this regulator may cooperate with other factors in various/different cellular processes. The activity of Sox9 is regulated by a number of intracellular factors. The function of Sox9 may be modulated by phosphorylation cAMP-dependent protein kinase A by parathyroid hormone-related peptide signaling pathway (PTHrP). It is, therefore, possible that Sox9 mediates part of PTHrP action to regulate hypertrophic differentiation (Zhao et al., 2009).

Other Sox genes necessary for cartilage formation include Sox5 and Sox6. They are expressed downstream of Sox9 from the prechondrocyte stage and later remain coexpressed with Sox9. Sox5 gene is highly similar to Sox6, and the two proteins share 50% homology with Sox9 in the Sox domain but not in remaining domains. The expression of Sox5 and Sox6 requires Sox9. Roles of Sox5 and Sox6 in chondrogenic differentiation were demonstrated in genetically manipulated mice. Single Sox5 or Sox6 knock-out mice mutants are born with relatively small skeletal defects, whereas double Sox5/Sox6 mutants exhibit a lack of cartilage and endochondral bone formation, becouse Sox5, Sox6, with Sox9 form a trio of transcription factors needed and sufficient for chondrogenesis. Sox5 and Sox6 may form homo- and heterodimers with each other, which bind much more efficiently to pairs of HMG-box binding sites than to single binding sites. Sox5 and Sox6 do not contain any domain that allows for transactivation or -repression of genes transcription and may thus act only to facilitate the organization of transcriptional complexes. Yu Han and Veronique Lefebvre data suggest a new model for the chondrogenic action of the Sox trio: "mesenchymal cells and prechondrocytes express chondrocyte markers at low or undetectable levels because Sox9 has a limited ability to bind to the cartilage enhancers of these genes in the absence of Sox5/Sox6. By inducing Sox5 and Sox6 expression in overtly differentiating chondrocytes, Sox9 gives itself the potential to upregulate its own activity as Sox5/Sox6 now binds to distinct sites on the enhancers and thereby secures Sox9 binding to its recognition site" (Han & Lefebvre, 2008). Only combination of all factors: Sox5, Sox6, and Sox9 successfully induce chondrogenic differentiation *in vivo*. Chondrogenic system *in vitro* via the changes in combination of the three Sox protein levels provide a new chondrogenic differentiation model, which may help us to better understand the mechanism of this process, but also adds a powerful tool to cartilage and bone regenerative medicine.

3.2 Role of Runt family members in osteochondrogenesis

The Runt family of DNA-binding transcription factors regulates cell fate determination in a number of tissues and has been shown to play an essential role in the differentiation of osteoblasts. They play a major role at the late stage of chondrocyte differentiation: in hypertrophic and maturating chondrocytes. In addition to osteoblasts, Runx2 is expressed in the lateral mesoderm, mesenchymal condensations, and chondrocytes. Runx3, which is another Runt family transcription factor, is engaged in the terminal differentiation of chondrocytes (Komori, 2005). Chondrocytes divide and produce a characteristic matrix but then stop dividing, change the matrix they synthesize, and become quite large (hypertrophic). Runx2 and, to a lesser extent, Runx3, are the major transcription factors controlling the crucial steps of osteochondrogenesis. Mice missing Runx2 show a defect in chondrocyte maturation, with lack of hypertrophic chondrocytes in many bones, and mice missing both Runx2 and Runx3 completely lack chondrocytes. The activity of Runx2 and Runx3 is modulated through the interactions with other factors. During chondrogenesis, expression of Runx2, is abolished in cells with heterozygous mutations in and around Sox9 (Akiyama et al., 2005). Dlx5 and Dlx6 proteins cooperate with Runx2 in activation of hypertrophic gene expression as they can physically interact with Runx2 and control chondrocyte hypertrophy *in vivo* and *in vitro* (Chin et al., 2007). Karsenty group results suggest that Runx2, in addition to promoting hypertrophy through its expression in chondrocytes, negatively regulates hyperthrophy by acting in the perichondrium thereby providing an additional level of control in order to coordinate chondrocyte maturation and osteoblastogenesis (Hinoi et al., 2006). By using small interfering RNA-mediated knock-down of Bapx1 (also know as Nkx3.2) in cultured chondrocytes an increase in Runx2 expression was shown, what indicate that Bapx1 act as a negative regulator of chondrocyte maturation (Hartman, 2009).

3.3 c-Maf protein

Chondrocyte differentiation in the growth plate is an important process for the longitudinal growth of endochondral bones. Sox9 and Runx2 are the most often-studied transcriptional regulators of the chondrocyte differentiation processes, but the importance of additional factors is also becoming apparent. One such factor is c-Maf. It belongs to a subfamily of the basic ZIP (bZIP) transcription factor superfamily, which act as key regulators of tissue-specific gene expression and terminal differentiation in many tissues. This regulator is low expressed in immature proliferating chondrocytes but high expressed in late hypertrophic and terminal chondrocytes, making it a candidate for controlling terminal differentiation. There is increasing evidence that c-Maf and its splicing variant Lc-Maf play a role in chondrocyte differentiation in a temporal-spatial manner. Various types of abnormalities in endochodrnal ossification or chondrocytic differentiation are caused by abnormalities concerning target genes regulated by c-Maf and Lc-Maf as well as lack of c-Maf itself (as phenotype of mice lacking c-Maf show) (Hong et al., 2011). Although the differential expression patterns of c-Maf and Lc-Maf during chondrogenesis were described, the functional differences between them are still unknown.

c-Maf can form homodimers as well as heterodimers with other transcription factors. c-Maf binding site was identified: two 13- and 14-base pair palindrome sequences, TGCTGACTCAGCA and TGCTGACGTCAGCA (Kataoka et al., 1994).

Studies of the roles of Maf proteins in chondrocyte differentiation and cartilage are under way, as is the identification of genes directly regulated by c-Maf. A causative role for c-Maf will require more hard evidence from direct experiments.

4. Tissue-nonspecific factors for bone formation

During the development of multicellular organisms, cell fate specification is followed by the sorting of different cell types into distinct domains where the different tissues and organs are formed. It has been shown that the formation and differentiation of tissues and organs during embryogenesis is regulated by the activation of a number of factors, which cannot be considered skeletal specific, although they are thought to play a key role in the differentiation and maturation of the osteoblast phenotype, and were observed in tissues that undergo both membranous and endochondral ossification. Alterations in functions of various other non-bone-specific transcription factors have been also demonstrated to affect osteoblastic differentiation and function. Among the many factors essential for organogenesis, and required for skeletal development are: bone morphogenetic proteins (BMPs), Wingless-type (WNT), homeobox genes HOX/HOM, DLX, MSX, ZPA (regulating the activity of tissue polarity, zone polarizing activity), FGF (fibroblast growth factor), Sonic and Indian Hedgehog (Shh and Ihh, respectively) (Witkowska-Zimny et al., 2010).

4.1 Bone morphogenetic proteins

Bone Morphogenetic Proteins (BMPs) belonging to the superfamily of transforming growth factors β (TGF-β) are important regulators involved in the differentiation process of forming tissues and organs during embryogenesis, including growth and differentiation of mesenchymal stem cells into osteogenic cells (Phimphilai et al., 2006). BMPs also play a key role in tissue regeneration in the post-embryonic period. Several proteins belonging to the group of BMPs have been described, of which BMP2, BMP4, BMP7 are acknowledged as osteogenic BMPs since they have been demonstrated to induce osteoblast differentiation in a variety of cell types. BMPs, which function by activating intracellular SMAD proteins and kinase signaling cascades (MAP, ERK PI3-K/AKT) are involved in the expression of multiple target genes (Osyczka et al., 2005). BMPs signals directly correspond to the early embryogenesis proteins containing homeodomain (called homeodomain proteins) involved in the development of the skeleton (HoxA10, Dlx3) (Hassan et al., 2006). Furthermore, the transcription factor of early ostoblastogenesis, Runx2, is induced in response to the presence of BMP2, by a SMAD-dependent signal transduction pathway (Phimphilai et al., 2006). Leong and colleagues demonstrated that palmitoylation was involved in the BMP2-dependent pathway. The inhibition of palmitoylation reduce osteoblast differentiation and mineralization, but had no effect on cell proliferation (Leong et al., 2009). This study was the first one to show that protein palmitoylation plays an important role in osteoblast differentiation and function.

BMPs also play a role in many stages of chondrogenic differentiation, initiating chondroprogenitor cell determination and differentiation of precursors into chondrocytes, and also at the stage of chondrocyte maturation and terminal differentiation (Pizette & Niswander, 2000; Retting et al., 2009). In addition, signalling through the BMP receptors is required for the maintenance of the articular cartilage in postnatal organisms (Rountree et al., 2004). Moreover, BMPs promote cell death and apoptosis of chondrocytes (Zou & Niswander, 1996).

Despite numerous studies, the regulatory pathway dependent on BMP is still not fully understood. Although the molecular mechanisms of signal transduction by BMPs are not known, recombinant human BMP2 and BMP7 have been successfully used in clinical applications as a factor assisting the regeneration of bone tissue (Bessa et al., 2008).

4.2 WNTs

WNTs are secreted glycoproteins involved in the regulation of embryonic development, as well as in the proliferation and differentiation of many tissues, including bone. WNT signal transmission in the cell occurs via various WNT-dependent pathways, which are always activated by binding WNT proteins to the endothelial Frizzled receptor (Fzd) and its coreceptor (Mbalaviele et al., 2005). Activation of a specific pathway depends on the type of WNT ligand and the current conditions within the cell. Gain- or loss-of-function studies in mice have revealed the function of various component of the pathway. To date 19 WNT ligands and 10 different subtypes of Fzd receptors have been detected. The many players in the WNT cascade hamper the precise elucidation of the mechanism by which WNT signaling specificity is achieved. By far the best characterized cascade is the canonical signaling pathway. It has been reported that binding the WNT to the endothelial Fzd receptor and LRP-5/6 protein (lipoprotein-related protein 5 and 6) on the surface of osteoblast progenitor cells, involves the stabilization of the central player in the canonical WNT pathway - β-catenin, and regulation of multiple transcription factors. The level of β-catenin increases in the cytoplasm, which results in its transport to the nucleus and activation ofosteoblast differentiation genes expression. This process is mediated by transcriptional factors, including Runx2 and Osterix. An appropriate level of the canonical Wnt signalling is crucial for chondrogenesis, demonstrated by the abnormal growth plate phenotype in mice harbouring inactivated β-catenin in chondrocytes (Ryu et al., 2002). β-catenin is highly expressed in mesenchymal cells committed to the chondrocytic lineage but down-regulated at the stage of early chondrogenic differentiation, upon up-regulation of Sox9 (Akiyama et al., 2004). Sox9 interacts with β-catenin and enhances its phosphorylation and subsequent degradation. Wnt signalling is again up-regulated during hypertrophy and promotes chondrocyte hypertrophy and endochondral ossification (Hill et al., 2005). WNT/β-catenin signaling is also important for mechanotransduction and fracture healing (Westendorf et al., 2004; Chen et al., 2007).

4.3 HOX – homeobox proteins

HOX protein family, encoded by a subclass of homebox genes, belongs to the regulators controlling the process of embryogenesis in vertebrates. These homeobox transcriptional factors are capable of binding to specific nucleotide sequences on DNA where they either activate or repress genes. The expression of the HOX genes in the developing area is temporally and spatially dynamic. They are critical for proper formation of skeletal tissue. HoxA and HoxD serve in a dose-dependent manner to regulate the size of specific cartilage elements. A surprising finding was that loss of these genes does not interfere the chondrocyte proliferation and differentation, but the growth of the individual elements is not established properly. Therefore, in controlling osteochondrogenesis they act later to regulate longitudinal growth of skeletal elements (Boulet & Capecchi, 2004).

HoxA10 and other homeobox genes responsible *inter alia* for osteoblastogenesis also participate in the regulation of cell proliferation, differentiation and maturation of osteoblasts in the process of modeling and regeneration of bone tissue in adult organism (Zakany et al., 2007). Research conducted in the last two years has shown the dependence of Runx2 gene expression and Runx2-dependent genes (encoding osteocalcin, alkaline phosphatase, bone sialoprotein) on HoxA10. It also showed that HoxA10, both directly and independently of Runx2, regulates the transcription of certain genes during osteoblastogenesis. Two mechanisms of HoxA10 action have been proposed: as a component of the BMP2 signaling cascade, prior to Runx2 involvement in the induction of genes as a factor osteoblastogenesis, and as a chromatin modifier in the promoter regions of genes specific to bone tissue. Combinatory mechanisms are operative for a regulated transcription of osteoblast genes through the diversification of sequence-specific activators and repressors that contribute to patterns of gene expression and the multistep process of programming involved in bone formation.

4.4 DLX – Distal-less homeodomain proteins

DLX is a family of transcription regulators containing the homeobox domain, which are activated by a BMP2 signal. Dlx3 expression is synchronized with the stages of osteoblast growth and induced by BMP2 (Hassan et al., 2006). An overexpression of Dlx3 in osteoblast progenitor cells changes the expression of the differentiation markers: type I collagen, osteocalcin and alkaline phosphatase. It has been demonstrated that two members of this family, Dlx3 and Dlx5, up-regulate the endogenous expression of Runx2. Like HoxA10, Dlx3 and Dlx5 may participate in ostoblastogenesis through the activation of Runx gene expression, but also directly through other genes, independently of Runx2. It has been demonstrated that Dlx3 and Dlx5 regulate the synthesis of Runx2, but at different stages of the osteoblast differentiation process: Dlx3 in the early stages of osteoblastogenesis, while Dlx5 in mature osteoblasts (Hassan et al., 2009). DLX proteins may bind to Runx2 promoter region, but only after the removal of another homeobox protein, MSX (mesh-less homeodomain), which acts as a repressor. Dlx3 and Dlx5 binding sites next to Runx2 binding site have been identified in the promoter region of alkaline phosphatase and osteocalcin genes. However, it has been shown that the process of bone tissue differentiation occurs in mutants without the Dlx5 gene. This suggests that the Dlx5 protein acts as a regulator of expression in the multiprotein activation complex and not as the main transcription activator of genes involved in the differentiation of the osteogenic lineage (Samee et al., 2008). The specific regulation mechanism of Runt gene expression, alongside with other Runx2-dependent genes with the participation of several classes of homeotic genes, has been suggested in a few works by Jane B. Lian team (Hassan et al., 2006, 2009).

4.5 MSX proteins

Vertebrate Msx are homeobox-containing genes that bear homology to the *Drosophila* muscle segment homeobox gene. The mammalian Msx gene family consists of three members, named Msx1, Msx2, and Msx3. Msx3 is expressed only in the dorsal neural tube, whereas Msx1 and Msx2 are widely expressed in many organs during embryonic development. Msx proteins interact with other homeodomain proteins to regulate transcription. Heterodimers formed between Msx and other homeodomain proteins such as Dlx2, Dlx5, Lhx2 and Pax3 result in mutual functional antagonism *in vitro*. Msx1 and Msx2 are among the critical factors involved in osteoblastogenesis. Null mutation of Msx2 leads to a number of defects in the construction of the skeleton especially in craniofacial region. Loss-of-function and gain-of-function studies show that in mice as in humans Msx1 and Msx2 are required for normal craniofacial morphogenesis (Alappat et al., 2003). They play a role in crucial processes during limb morphogenesis. Mice homozygous for a null mutation in either Msx1 or Msx2 do not display abnormalities in limb development. By contrast, Msx1; Msx2 double mutants exhibit a severe limb phenotype. A number of data have shown that Msx genes are downstream targets of BMP signaling in the limb. At early stages, Msx1 and Msx2 are expressed in nearly identical patterns that overlap significantly with BMP2, BMP4 and BMP7.

An antagonistic role of Msx2 has been demonstrated in relation to Dlx5 during osteoblast proliferation and differentiation. Dlx5 is activated in the later stages of osteoblastogenesis, which correlate with increasing levels of proteins characteristic of terminally differentiated osteoblasts, such as osteocalcin, while Msx2 adversely affect these processes. On the basis of these studies, it has been suggested that Msx2 stimulates the process of cell proliferation and inhibits cell differentiation. Several models for the Msx2 and Dlx5 relationship have been proposed. In the first model, Runx2-Msx2 forms a complex that deactivates expression of Runx2 and Runx2-dependent genes. With the increasing levels of Dlx5, a Dlx5-Msx2 complex is formed and free Runx2 protein can in consequence activate specific genes. In the second model for Dlx5 and Msx2 interaction, proteins compete for binding to common binding sites in the promoter region of specific genes and they also regulate each other at the transcriptional level. In both cases a balance between the levels of Msx2 and Dlx5 may be critical for osteoprogenitor cell proliferation and differentiation (Lallemand et al., 2005). It is certain that, Msx with other morphogenes and transcription factors build a complex cellular network that control the development and behavior of cells. It would be of great interest to identify the direct target genes of Msx proteins in *vivo* and their associated cellular processes including proliferation, apoptosis, cell adhesion and migration during organogenesis.

4.6 Hedgehog proteins

Hedgehog (Hh) is evolutionarily conserved family in vertebrates, which include Sonic (Shh), Indian (Ihh), and Desert (Dhh) hedgehogs that control numerous aspects of development: cell growth, survival, and differentiation, and pattern almost every aspect of the vertebrate body plan. Dhh expression is largely restricted to gonads. Ihh is specifically expressed in a limited number of tissues, including primitive endoderm, gut and prehypertrophic chondrocytes in the growth plates of bones. Shh is the most broadly expressed mammalian Hh signaling molecule. During early vertebrate embryogenesis, Shh expressed in midline tissues affects skeletal development and most epithelial tissues. The use of a single morphogen for such a wide variety of functions is possible because cellular responses to Hh depend on the type of responding cell, the amount of Hh received, and the time cells are exposed to it (Varjosalo & Taipale, 2008). During skeletogenesis, Shh and Ihh provide positional information and initiate or maintain cellular differentiation programs regulating the formation of cartilage and bone. Malfunction of the Hh signaling network can cause severe skeletal disorders.

4.6.1 Sonic hedgehog

Shh signaling acts to initiate an osteogenic program of mesenchymal cells. The human Shh has three exons that encodes a 462 amino acid polypeptide. The protein is synthesized as a precursor molecule that undergoes cleavage of a signal peptide and then autoproteolytic cleavage. This reaction mediated by cholesterol leads to a 19 kDa N-terminal product (Shh-N) with the signalling domain and a C-terminal product of 25 kDa (Shh-C) possessing the cleavage domain closely associated with cholesterol transferase activity. The Shh is highly conserved among vertebrates. For example, there is 92.4% identity between human and mouse Shh proteins. Increased Hh signaling promotes osteogenesis in various bone-forming cells *in vitro*. The stimulatory action of Shh on osteogenic differentiation was already reported in few studies, suggesting a close interaction between Shh and BMP-2 or parathyroid hormone-related peptide (Yuasa et al., 2002.) Shh has been shown to play a key role in patterning of the limb, i.e. misregulation of Shh results in severe limb abnormalities. Hence, Shh is required for proper ZPA (regulating the activity of tissue polarity, zone polarizing activity) signaling and anterior/posterior limb formation (Hill, 2007; Towers et al., 2008, James et al., 2010).

4.6.2 Indian hedgehog

Growth and differentiation of the endochondral skeleton relies on a complex interplay among different signaling factors to regulate the orderly morphogenesis of the skeleton. Among these, Ihh appears to play a central role in coordinating chondrocyte proliferation, chondrocyte differentiation and osteoblast differentiation. During endochondral bone development, Ihh is synthesized by chondrocytes leaving the proliferative pool (prehypertrophic chondrocytes) and by early hypertrophic chondrocytes. Ihh is a master regulator of both chondrocyte and osteoblast differentiation during endochondral bone formation.

Ihh mutants show: (i) reduced chondrocyte proliferation; (ii) initially delayed, then abnormal chondrocyte maturation, and (iii) absence of mature osteoblasts. St-Jacques and coworkers suggest a model in which Ihh coordinates diverse aspects of skeletal morphogenesis through parathyroid hormone-related peptide dependent and independent processes (St-Jacques et al., 1999). Mouse Ihh cDNA encodes a 411 amino acids polypeptide with a predicted 27 amino acids signal peptide. After the post-translational modification arises a 19 kDa lipid-modified protein. At the cell surface, Ihh activity is mediated by binding to the transmembrane receptor, and signaling through the transmembrane G-protein coupled receptor. Hedgehogs, including Ihh are important signaling molecules during embryonic development and are highly conserved within and across species. Mouse and human Ihh share 100% amino acid identity of the signaling domain.

4.7 Zinc finger protein: PLZF and Zfp521

Zinc finger proteins are believed to be one of the most common classes of proteins in humans (approx. 3-4% of human genes encode proteins containing zinc finger domains). One of previously described osteoblastogenesis factor - Osterix also belong to this protein type.

Promyelocytic leukaemia zinc finger protein (Zinc finger protein 145, PLZF) belongs to the family of Krüppel-like zinc finger proteins. It is a transcriptional repressor involved in cell cycle control and has been implicated in limb development, differentiation of myeloid cells, and spermatogenesis. So far little is known about the regulation of PLZF expression.

PLZF is one of the highly expressed genes during *in vitro* osteoblastic differentiation in many human cell types. Small interfering RNA-mediated gene silencing of PLZF results in a reduction of osteoblast-specific genes expression such as alkaline phosphatase, collagen type 1, osteocalcin and even Runx2 genes. These findings indicate that PLZF plays important roles in early osteoblastic differentiation as an upstream regulator of Runx2. Because the expression of PLZF was unaffected by the addition of bone morphogenetic protein 2 *in vitro*, it may indicate that PLZF acts independently of the BMP signaling pathway (Ikeda et al., 2005). The molecular pathways by which PLZF exerts its function in bone formation are still under investigation.

Another regulator from Kruppel-like zinc finger protein family associated with osteogenesis is Zfp521. Zfp521 is expressed in osteoblast precursors, osteoblasts and osteocytes, as well as chondrocytes. Forced expression of Zfp521 in osteoblasts *in vivo* increases bone formation and bone mass. In contrast, overexpression of Zfp521 *in vitro* antagonizes, while knockdown favors, osteoblast differentiation and nodule formation. Zfp521 binds to Runx2, repressing its transcriptional activity (Wu et al., 2009). The balance between Zfp521 and Runx2 may therefore contribute to the regulation of osteoblast differentiation and bone formation.

5. MicroRNAs in skeletal development

One of the first steps in understanding of cell determination requires ascertaining which particular genes are activated in a particular cell, either temporarily or continuously. Microarrays technology are used as a tool for quantitative expression analysis of many gene transcripts in parallel as well as study expression of small non-coding microRNAs that repress mRNA translation and thereby regulate differentiation and development. Post-transcriptional regulation by non-coding RNA molecules has been discovered to be an important mechanism to control cellular differentiation, also during bone formation. An increasing number of miRNAs have been identified to regulate osteoblast differentiation. They promote bone formation by targeting negative regulators of osteogenesis or negatively regulate osteoblastogenesis by targeting important osteogenic factors.

Among many miRNA negatively regulating osteogenesis are Runx2-targeting miRNAs: miR-23a, miR-30c, miR-34c, miR-133a, miR-135a, miR-137, miR-204, miR-205, miR-217, and miR-338 (Zhang et al., 2011a, 2011b). They significantly impede osteoblast differentiation, and their effects can be reversed by the corresponding anti-miRNAs.

Only a few miRNAs have been identified to specifically regulate chondrogenesis and cartilage homeostasis: miR-140 and miR-199 as negative regulators and miR-675 as a positive regulator (Miyaki *et al.*, 2009; 2010;). miR-675, whose expression is upregulated by Sox9, positively regulates chondrocyte specific gene i.e. Col2a1, and in this way promotes chondrogenesis (Dudek *et al.*, 2010; Lin *et al.*, 2009).

6. Conclusion

Bone is a highly dynamic tissue, which is regulated by tissue-specific transcription factors, as well as by the number of homeotic genes, active both during the organization of tissue and organs in the embryonic period as well as in mature bone. The most important factors for osteogenesis are compiled and briefly overview in the Table 1.

Transcriptional regulators control the expression of target genes by the interaction with cofactors, coactivators, chromatin remodelling complexes and finally with the general transcriptional machinery. Their participation in the regulation of bone formation process is complex and require further experimental work to provide understanding of their role and elucidate interactions with other factors of signal cascades. Cellular balance between various regulatory proteins is extremely important. Many studies have been conducted using murine or human cell lines, which are often tumor cell lines e.g. MG63 - human osteosarcoma line. The regulatory pathways and routes of signal transduction in these experimental systems may not correspond to those occurring in healthy human bone cells. Therefore, it is important to enhance our knowledge about proliferation, differentiation and regeneration of bone based on *in vitro* and *in vivo* studies of normal human cells in the context of natural tissue. From a biomedical point of view, identifying an important regulators of bone formation and regeneration in humans has raised the possibility that manipulating its expression, function, or signalling pathway could have a major therapeutic impact in identifying new targets and opening new avenues for the treatment of bone diseases, such as osteoporosis.

Protein (Synonym) **Full recommended name**	**Length (aa)**	**DNA binding motif (position)**	**Accession number UniProtKB/ Swiss-Prot**	**Gene locus**	**Number of isoforms**
Runx1 (AML1, CBFA2) **Runt-related transcription factor 1**	453	Runt domain (50-178 aa)	Q01196	21q22.3	11
Runx2 (AML3, CBFA1, OSF2, PEBP2A) **Runt-related transcription factor 2**	521	Runt domain (101-229 aa)	Q13950	6p21	3
Runx3 (AML2, CBFA3, PEBP2A3) **Runt-related transcription factor 3**	415	Runt domain (54-182 aa)	Q13761	1p36	2
Osterix (SP7, OSX) **Transcription factor Sp7**	431	Three C2H2-type zinc fingers (294-318 aa; 324-348 aa; 354 – 376 aa)	Q8TDD2	12q13.13	1
Sox9 (SRY-box9) **Transcription factor SOX-9**	509	HMG box DNA-binding domain (105-173 aa)	P48436	17q23	1
Sox5 **Transcription factor SOX-5**	763	HMG box DNA-binding domain. (556-624 aa)	P35711	12p12.1	4
Sox6 **Transcription factor SOX-6**	828	HMG box DNA-binding domain (621-689 aa)	P35712	11p15.3	4
c-Maf **Transcription factor Maf**	373	Leucine-zipper (316-337 aa)	O75444	16q22-q23	2

Table 1. Summary of human main bone tissue-specific transcriptional regulators.

7. Acknowledgment

Studies in the laboratory of the author are supported by grants no. N N302157037 from the Polish funds for scientific research in 2009-2012.

8. References

Akiyama, H., Lyons, J. P., Mori-Akiyama, Y., Yang, X., Zhang, R., Zhang, Z., Deng, J. M., Taketo, M. M., Nakamura, T., Behringer, R. R., McCrea P. D. & de Crombrugghe, B. (2004) Interactions between Sox9 and beta-catenin control chondrocyte differentiation. *Genes Dev,* Vol.18, No.9 (May 2004), pp. 1072-1087

Akiyama, H., Kim, J. E., Nakashima, K., Balmes, G., Iwai, N., Deng, J. M., Zhang, Z.; Martin, J. F., Behringer, R. R., Nakamura, T. & de Crombrugghe B. (2005) Osteo-chondroprogenitor cells are derived from Sox9 expressing precursors. *Proc Natl Acad Sci U S A,* Vol.102, No.41, (October 2005) pp. 14665-14670

Alappat, S., Zhang, Z. Y. & Chen, Y. P. (2003) Msx homeobox gene family and craniofacial development. *Cell Res,* Vol.13, No.6, (December 2003), pp. 429-442

Amorim, B. R., Okamura, H., Yoshida, K., Qiu, L., Morimoto H. & T. Haneji, T. (2007) The transcriptional factor Osterix directly interacts with RNA helicase A. *Biochem Biophys Res Commun,* Vol.355, No.2, (April 2007), pp. 347-351

Bae, S. C. & Lee, Y. H. (2006) Phosphorylation, acetylation and ubiquitination: the molecular basis of RUNX regulation. *Gene,* Vol.366, No.1, (January 2006), pp. 58-66

Bessa, P. C., Casal, M. & Reis, R. L. (2008) Bone morphogenetic proteins in tissue engineering: the road from laboratory to clinic, part II (BMP delivery). *J Tissue Eng Regen Med,* Vol.2, No.2, (March-April 2008), pp. 81-96

Bialek, P., Kern, B., Yang, X., Schrock, M., Sosic, D., Hong, N., Wu, H., Yu, K., Ornitz, D. M., Olson, E. N., Justice, M. J. & Karsenty, G. (2004) A twist code determines the onset of osteoblast differentiation. *Dev Cell,* Vol.6, No.3, (March 2004) pp. 423-435

Boulet, A. M. & Capecchi, M. R. (2004) Multiple roles of Hoxa11 and Hoxd11 in the formation of the mammalian forelimb zeugopod. *Development,* Vol.131, No.2, (January 2004), pp. 299-309

Chen, Y., Whetstone, H. C., Lin, A. C., Nadesan, P., Wei, Q., Poon, R. & Alman, B. A. (2007) Beta-catenin signaling plays a disparate role in different phases of fracture repair: implications for therapy to improve bone healing. *PLoS Med,* Vol.4, No.7, (July 2007), pp. e249

Chin, H. J., Fisher, M. C., Li, Y., Ferrari, D., Wang, C. K., Lichtler, A. C., Dealy, C. N. & Kosher, R. A. (2007) Studies on the role of Dlx5 in regulation of chondrocyte differentiation during endochondral ossification in the developing mouse limb. *Dev Growth Differ,* Vol.49, No. 6, (August 2007), pp. 515-521

Chu, S. & Ferro, T. J. (2005) Sp1: regulation of gene expression by phosphorylation. *Gene,* Vol.348, (March 2005) pp. 1-11

de Frutos, C. A., Dacquin, R., Vega, S., Jurdic, P., Machuca-Gayet, I. & Nieto, M. A. (2009) Snail1 controls bone mass by regulating Runx2 and VDR expression during osteoblast differentiation. *EMBO J,* Vol.28, No.6, (March 2009), pp. 686-696

Dudek, K. A., Lafont, J. E., Martinez-Sanchez, A. & Murphy, C. L. (2010) Type II collagen expression is regulated by tissue-specific miR-675 in human articular chondrocytes. *J Biol Chem,* Vol.285, No.32, (August 2010), pp. 24381-24387

Han, Y. & Lefebvre, V. (2008) L-Sox5 and Sox6 drive expression of the aggrecan gene in cartilage by securing binding of Sox9 to a far-upstream enhancer. *Mol Cell Biol,* Vol.28, No. 16, (August 2008), pp. 4999-5013

Hartmann, C. (2009) Transcriptional networks controlling skeletal development. *Curr Opin Genet Dev,* Vol.19, No.5, (October 2009), pp. 437-443

Hassan, M. Q., Tare, R. S., Lee, S. H., Mandeville, M., Morasso, M. I., Javed, A., van Wijnen, J., Stein, J. L., Stein, G. S. & Lian, J. B. (2006) BMP2 commitment to the osteogenic lineage involves activation of Runx2 by DLX3 and a homeodomain transcriptional network. *J Biol Chem,* Vol.281, No. 52, (December 2006), pp. 40515-40526

Hassan, M. Q., Saini, S., Gordon, J. A., van Wijnen, A. J., Montecino, M., Stein, J. L., Stein, G. S. & Lian, J. B. (2009) Molecular switches involving homeodomain proteins, HOXA10 and RUNX2 regulate osteoblastogenesis. *Cells Tissues Organs,* Vol.189, No. 1-4, pp. 122-125

Hatta, M., Yoshimura, Y., Deyama, Y., Fukamizu, A. & Suzuki, K. (2006) Molecular characterization of the zinc finger transcription factor, Osterix. *Int J Mol Med,* Vol.17, No.3, (March 2006), pp. 425-430

Hill, R. E. (2007) How to make a zone of polarizing activity: insights into limb development via the abnormality preaxial polydactyly. *Dev Growth Differ,* Vol.49, No.6, (August 2007), pp. 439-448

Hill, T. P., Spater, D., Taketo, M. M., Birchmeier, W. & Hartmann, C. (2005) Canonical Wnt/beta-catenin signaling prevents osteoblasts from differentiating into chondrocytes. *Dev Cell,* Vol.8, No.5, (May 2005), pp. 727-738

Hinoi, E., Bialek, P., Chen, Y. T., Rached, M. T., Groner, Y., Behringer, R. R., Ornitz, D. M. & Karsenty, G. (2006) Runx2 inhibits chondrocyte proliferation and hypertrophy through its expression in the perichondrium. *Genes Dev,* Vol.20, No.21, (November 2006), pp. 2937-2942

Hong, E., Di Cesare, P. & Haudenschild, D. E (2011) Role of c-Maf in Chondrocyte Differentiation. *Cartilage* Vol. 2 No.1 (January 2011), pp. 27-35

Ikeda, R., Yoshida, K., Tsukahara, S., Sakamoto, Y., Tanaka, H., Furukawa, K. & Inoue, I. (2005) The promyelotic leukemia zinc finger promotes osteoblastic differentiation of human mesenchymal stem cells as an upstream regulator of CBFA1. *J Biol Chem,* Vol.280, No.9, (March 2005), pp. 8523

James, A. W., Leucht, P., Levi, B., Carre, A. L., Xu, Y., Helms, J. A. & Longaker, M. T. (2010) Sonic Hedgehog influences the balance of osteogenesis and adipogenesis in mouse adipose-derived stromal cells. *Tissue Eng Part A,* Vol.16, No.8, (August 2010), pp. 2605-2616

Kataoka, K., Noda, M. & Nishizawa, M. (1994) Maf nuclear oncoprotein recognizes sequences related to an AP-1 site and forms heterodimers with both Fos and Jun. *Mol Cell Biol,* Vol.14, No. 1, (January 1994), pp. 700-712

Komori, T. (2005) Regulation of skeletal development by the Runx family of transcription factors. *J Cell Biochem,* Vol.95, No.3, (June 2005), pp. 445-453

Lallemand, Y., Nicola, M. A., Ramos, C., Bach, A., Cloment, C. S. & Robert, B. (2005) Analysis of Msx1; Msx2 double mutants reveals multiple roles for Msx genes in limb development. *Development,* Vol.132, No.13, (July 2005), pp. 3003-3014

Leong, W. F., Zhou, T., Lim, G. L. & Li, B. (2009) Protein palmitoylation regulates osteoblast differentiation through BMP-induced osterix expression. *PLoS ONE,* Vol.4, No.1, (January 2009), e4135

Li, Y. L. & Xiao, Z. S. (2007) Advances in Runx2 regulation and its isoforms. *Med Hypotheses,* Vol.68, No.1, (January 2007), pp. 169-175

Lin, E. A., Kong, L., Bai, X. H., Luan, Y. & Liu, C. J. (2009) miR-199a, a bone morphogenic protein 2-responsive MicroRNA, regulates chondrogenesis via direct targeting to Smad1. *J Biol Chem,* Vol.284, No. 17, (April 2009), pp. 11326-11335

Makita, N., Suzuki, M., Asami, S., Takahata, R., Kohzaki, D., Kobayashi, S., Hakamazuka, T. & Hozumi, N. (2008) Two of four alternatively spliced isoforms of RUNX2 control osteocalcin gene expression in human osteoblast cells. *Gene,* Vol.413, No.1-2, (April 2008), pp. 8-17

Marie, P. J. (2008) Transcription factors controlling osteoblastogenesis. *Arch Biochem Biophys,* Vol.473, No.2, (May 2008), pp. 98-105

Mbalaviele, G., Sheikh, S., Stains, J. P., Salazar, V. S., Cheng, S. L., Chen, D. & Civitelli, R. (2005) Beta-catenin and BMP-2 synergize to promote osteoblast differentiation and new bone formation. *J Cell Biochem,* Vol.94, No.2, (February 2005), pp. 403-418

Miyaki, S., Nakasa, T., Otsuki, S., Grogan, S. P., Higashiyama, R., Inoue, A., Kato, Y., Sato, T., Lotz, M. K. & Asahara, H. (2009) MicroRNA-140 is expressed in differentiated human articular chondrocytes and modulates interleukin-1 responses. *Arthritis Rheum,* Vol.60, No.9, (September 2009), pp. 2723-2730

Miyaki, S., Sato, T., Inoue, A., Otsuki, S., Ito, Y., Yokoyama, S., Kato, Y., Takemoto, F., Nakasa, T., Yamashita, S., Takada, S., Lotz, M. K., Ueno-Kudo, H. & Asahara, H. (2010) MicroRNA-140 plays dual roles in both cartilage development and homeostasis. *Genes Dev,* Vol.24, No.11, (June 2010), pp. 1173-1185

Nakashima, K., Zhou, X., Kunkel, G., Zhang, Z., Deng, J. M., Behringer, R. R. & de Crombrugghe, B. (2002) The novel zinc finger-containing transcription factor osterix is required for osteoblast differentiation and bone formation. *Cell,* Vol.108, No.1, (January 2002), pp. 17-29

Osyczka, A. M. & Leboy, P. S. (2005) Bone morphogenetic protein regulation of early osteoblast genes in human marrow stromal cells is mediated by extracellular signal-regulated kinase and phosphatidylinositol 3-kinase signaling. *Endocrinology,* Vol.146, No. 8, (August 2005), pp. 3428-3437

Paz, J., Wade, K., Kiyoshima, T., Sodek, J., Tang, J., Tu, Q., Yamauchi, M. & Chen, J. (2005) Tissue- and bone cell-specific expression of bone sialoprotein is directed by a 9.0 kb promoter in transgenic mice. *Matrix Biol,* Vol.24, No.5, (August 2005), pp. 341-352

Phimphilai, M., Zhao, Z., Boules, H., Roca, H. & Franceschi, R. T. (2006) BMP signaling is required for RUNX2-dependent induction of the osteoblast phenotype. *J Bone Miner Res,* Vol.21, No.4, (April 2006), pp. 637-646

Pizette, S. & Niswander, L. (2000) BMPs are required at two steps of limb chondrogenesis: formation of prechondrogenic condensations and their differentiation into chondrocytes. *Dev Biol,* Vol.219, No.2, (March 2000), pp. 237-249

Retting, K. N., Song, B., Yoon, B. S. & Lyons, K. M. (2009) BMP canonical Smad signaling through Smad1 and Smad5 is required for endochondral bone formation. *Development,* Vol.136, No.7, (April 2009), pp. 1093-1104

Rountree, R. B., Schoor, M., Chen, H., Marks, M. E., Harley, V., Mishina, Y. & Kingsley, D. M. (2004) BMP receptor signaling is required for postnatal maintenance of articular cartilage. *PLoS Biol,* Vol.2, No.11, (November 2004), e355.

Ryu, J. H., Kim, S. J., Kim, S. H., Oh, C. D., Hwang, S. G., Chun, C. H., Oh, S. H., Seong, J. K., Huh, T. L. & Chun, J. S. (2002) Regulation of the chondrocyte phenotype by beta-catenin. *Development,* Vol.129, No.23, (December 2002), pp. 5541-5550

Samee, N., Geoffroy, V., Marty, C., Schiltz, C., Vieux-Rochas, M., Levi, G. & de Vernejoul, M. C. (2008) Dlx5, a positive regulator of osteoblastogenesis, is essential for osteoblast-osteoclast coupling. *Am J Pathol,* Vol.173, No. 3 (September 2008), pp. 773-780

St-Jacques, B., Hammerschmidt, M. & McMahon, A. P. (1999) Indian hedgehog signaling regulates proliferation and differentiation of chondrocytes and is essential for bone formation. *Genes Dev,* Vol.13, No. 16, (August 1999), pp. 2072-2086

Teixeira, C. C., Liu, Y., Thant, L. M., Pang, J., Palmer, G. & Alikhani, M. (2010) Foxo1, a novel regulator of osteoblast differentiation and skeletogenesis. *J Biol Chem,* Vol.285, No. 40, (October 2010), pp. 31055-31065

Towers, M., Mahood, R., Yin, Y. & Tickle, C. (2008) Integration of growth and specification in chick wing digit-patterning. *Nature,* Vol.452, No. 7189, (April 2008), pp. 882-886

Varjosalo, M. & Taipale, J. (2008) Hedgehog: functions and mechanisms. *Genes Dev,* Vol.22, No.18, (September 2008), pp. 2454-2472

Westendorf, J. J., Kahler, R. A. & Schroeder, T. M. (2004) Wnt signaling in osteoblasts and bone diseases. *Gene,* Vol.341, (October 2004), pp. 19-39

Witkowska-Zimny, M., Wrobel, E. & Przybylski, J. (2010) The most importan trancsroptional factors of osteoblastogenesis. *Advances in cell biology,* Vol.2, No.1, (January 2010), pp. 17-28

Wu, M., Hesse, E., Morvan, F., Zhang, J. P., Correa, D., Rowe, G. C., Kiviranta, R., Neff, L., Philbrick, W. M., Horne, W. C. & Baron, R. (2009) Zfp521 antagonizes Runx2, delays osteoblast differentiation in vitro, and promotes bone formation in vivo. *Bone,* Vol.44, No.4, (April 2009), pp. 528-536

Yuasa, T., Kataoka, H., Kinto, N., Iwamoto, M., Enomoto-Iwamoto, M., Iemura, S., Ueno, N., Shibata, Y., Kurosawa, H. & Yamaguchi, A. (2002) Sonic hedgehog is involved in osteoblast differentiation by cooperating with BMP-2. *J Cell Physiol,* Vol.193, No.2, (November 2002), pp. 225-232

Zakany, J. & Duboule, D. (2007) The role of Hox genes during vertebrate limb development. *Curr Opin Genet Dev,* Vol.17, No.4, (August 2007), pp. 359-366

Zhang, Y., Xie, R. L., Croce, C. M., Stein, J. L., Lian, J. B., van Wijnen, A. J. & Stein, G. S. (2011a) A program of microRNAs controls osteogenic lineage progression by targeting transcription factor Runx2. *Proc Natl Acad Sci U S A,* Vol.108, No.24, (June 2011), pp. 9863-9868

Zhang, J. F., Fu, W. M., He, M. L., Xie, W. D., Lv, Q., Wan, G., Li, G., Wang, H., Lu, G., Hu, X., Jiang, S., Li, J. N., Lin, M. C., Zhang, Y. O. & Kung, H. (2011b) MiRNA-20a promotes osteogenic differentiation of human mesenchymal stem cells by co-regulating BMP signaling. *RNA Biol,* Vol.8, No. 5, (September 2011), pp. 829-838

Zhao, L., Li, G. & Zhou, G. Q. (2009) SOX9 directly binds CREB as a novel synergism with the PKA pathway in BMP-2-induced osteochondrogenic differentiation. *J Bone Miner Res,* Vol.24, No.5, (May 2009), pp. 826-836

Zou, H. & Niswander, L. (1996) Requirement for BMP signaling in interdigital apoptosis and scale formation. *Science,* Vol.272, No. 5263 (May 1996), pp. 738-741

2

Genes and Molecular Pathways of the Osteogenic Process

Wanda Lattanzi and Camilla Bernardini
Institute of Anatomy and Cell Biology, Catholic University – Faculty of Medicine, Rome, Italy

1. Introduction

Bone tissue represents a specialized connective tissue, comprising metabolically active cells within a mineralized extracellular matrix, that are vital to the performance of its structural, mechanical and metabolic roles (Milat & Ng, 2009). The first descriptions of the bone formation process date back to two centuries ago and since then much effort has been spent by the scientific community to depict the complete scenario of the cellular and molecular events leading to ossification (Howship, 1815; Zaidi et al., 2007). Bone is formed through a complex process named osteogenesis, involving the proliferation of mesenchymal precursors, condensation of cells in closely interacting groups, differentiation and functional activation of bone cells, which finally leads to the deposition of an organic matrix and subsequent mineralization. Most bones are formed through the progressive growing and differentiation of condensed groups of mesenchymal cells into round chondrocytes that proliferate and secrete extracellular matrix (ECM): a cartilage mold is being formed. Thereafter, these cells stop proliferating, enlarge, modifiy the ECM composition by changing the type of collagen they secrete, and finally direct the mineralization of the new formed tissue. These hyperthrophic chondrocytes (HC) signal to adjacent perichondrial cells to stimulate their osteogenic differentiation and to promote vascular invasion. In this way, the primitive bone tissue, the primary "spongiosa", is formed starting from the center of the cartilage mold and proceeding to surrounding cells, following a longitudinal direction in long bones. Subsequently, osteoclasts derived from hematopoietic precursors of the bone marrow enter the cartilage mold and digest the ECM synthesized by the HC. These shortly undergo apoptosis at the border between cartilage and primary spongiosa, while HC at the extremities of the mold continue proliferating. Through the progressive proliferation and hypertrophy of growing numbers of chondrocytes, secondary sites of ossification are formed, and the process persist to engine the bone lengthening during post-natal life. Flat bones of the skull, conversely, undergo a direct "intramembranous" ossification process, as in this case mesenchymal cells directly differentiate into osteoblasts that start producing bone matrix.

The whole process requires a careful coordination of signals within cells, to drive proliferation, migration and differentiation in a chronologically and spatially organized fashion. It is therefore not so surprising that a wide number of molecules and cross-talking pathways drive this coordinated mechanisms through a complex network of interactions which is at least partially known. The best known signaling pathways that orchestrate the osteogenic process involve molecules belonging to the wingless-int (WNT), the bone morphogenetic protein (BMP), the hedgehog (HH) and the fibroblast growth factor (FGF) families. During the last decades, new details on the control of bone mass remodeling and regeneration has been achieved, mainly thank to the rapidly growing body of knowledge regarding the genome structure, control and functioning. This chapter will provide an up-to-date depiction of the molecular networks involved in the osteogenic process, focusing on main genes and signaling pathways (schematically represented in Figure 1), whose integrity is required for the correct skeletal morphogenesis and patterning and for maintaining bone homeostasis. Particular attention will be devoted to list and dissect the human syndromes and disorders associated to genes belonging to the main osteogenic pathways, with regard to the skeletal phenotype.

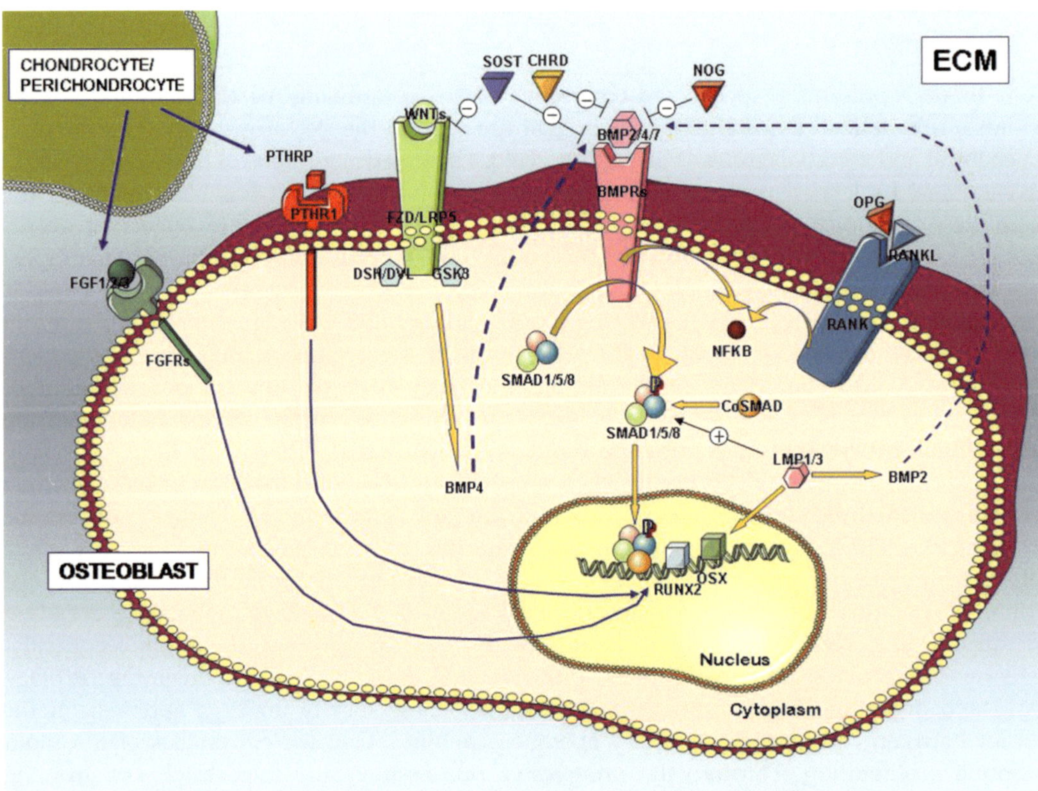

Fig. 1. The osteogenic network. The figure stigmatizes the main signaling pathways and reciprocal cross-talks acting during osteoblast differentiation. See text for details.

2. Osteogenic genes and pathways

2.1 The Transforming Growth Factor- ß (TGF-ß) superfamily

The Transforming Growth Factor- β (TGF-β) superfamily incorporate over 30 multifunctional growth factors implicated in the regulation of a wide variety of biological functions, such as proliferation, differentiation, migration, and apoptosis. The role of TGF-β ligands is context-dependent, being affected by diverse environmental features, including tissue and cell type, cell differentiation stage and level of expression of interacting genes. Also, the quantity and the quality, in terms of type of isoform, of the growth factor itself, along with its paracrine or autocrine effect, influence the downstream cascade. TGF-β superfamily members are grouped into 3 families, on the basis of sequence homologies and functional activities exploited through the activation of a specific signaling pathway: 1. the TGF-β/activin/nodal family; 2. the bone morphogenetic protein (BMP); 3. the growth differentiation factor (GDF)/Muellerian inhibiting substance (MIS) family. As a rule, all the molecules acting in the TGF-β signaling pathway are extremely conserved across species during evolution (Miyazono, 2000).

A fine regulation of the spatio-temporal expression and function of TGF-β pathway players occurs during embryonic development, leading to an astounding heterogeneity of cellular responses (Ripamonti et al, 2006). Signaling is initiated when binding of the ligand induces the assembly of a heteromeric complex of type I and type II serine/threonine kinase receptors (Cohen, 2006; Miyazono, 2000). The constitutively active type II receptor recruits and activates a type I receptor (also known as activin receptor-like kinase; ALK) by phosphorylating its cytoplasmic domain, inducing the assembly of two type I, and two type II receptors. This, in turn, results in the phosphorylation and activation of specific intracellular proteins, belonging to the SMAD (mothers against decapentaplegic (MAD) homologs) family, by the type I receptor (receptor-regulated Smads, R-Smads: Smad1–3, 5, and 8). The consequent activation of the Smad signaling cascade implies the formation of heterodimeric complexes with the common partner Smad (Co-Smad, Smad4), which translocates to the nucleus and recruits distinct transcription factors to regulate transcription. The transcriptional targets of this signaling pathway are represented by over 500 genes, which are regulated in a cell-specific, ligand dose–dependent manner (Cohen, 2006; Miyazono, 2000). Generally, Smad-2 and -3 transduce cellular responses downstream of the TGF- β and activin receptors, while Smad-1, -5 and -8 primarily mediate BMP signals (as further discussed). Signaling by the TGF- β family is carefully regulated at several levels, through either of the TGF-β ligand agonists and antagonists, which compete for receptor binding, or capture the ligand in the extracellular compartment. In addition, the different downstream effects of TGF-β signalling activation are due to the different combinations of receptors (seven type I receptors and five type II receptors are classified), leading to alternative ligand-specific composition of the receptor complex. Finally, diverse biological response to the same signaling pathway are also obtained through the recruitment of different accessory proteins (Kanaan RA & Kanaan LA, 2006). The vast majority of TGF-β superfamily members actively involved in bone formation belong to the most numerous family, represented by the bone morphogenetic proteins.

2.2 Bone morphogenetic proteins (BMPs)

Bone morphogenetic proteins (BMPs) were originally identified and named after their ability to induce ectopic bone formation (Urist, 1965). The BMP family comprises over 20 distinct highly conserved secreted proteins, further categorized into multiple subgroups according to functional and/or structural features (Miyazono et al., 2005; X. Wu et al., 2007). BMP functions cover several aspects of the cell differentiation program. In particular they induce the osteoblastic commitment of mesenchymal cells, inhibit their differentiation along the myoblastic and adipogenic lineage and increase osteoclastogenesis (Katagiri et al., 1994;

Okamoto et al., 2006; Pham et al., 2011; X. Wu et al., 2007). On the whole, BMPs play a pivotal role in skeletogenesis during all processes associated with limb development. Nonetheless, the biological activities of BMPs are not identical among members. In fact, despite their name, not all members of the BMP family are directly involved in skeletogenesis; they display distinct spatio-temporal expression patterns, with consequent diversified roles in the morphogenesis of even non-skeletal structures during embryo development (H. Chen et al., 2004; Cheng et al., 2003; Dudley et al., 1995; Jena et al., 1997; Luo et al., 1995; Mcpherron et al., 1999; Solloway et al., 1998; Zhao et al., 1996).

BMP2, BMP4 and BMP7 (also known as osteogenic protein-1, OP-1, see Figure 1) are the most extensively studied osteogenic BMPs, being involved in basic skeletal body patterning mechanisms (Bahamonde et al., 2001; Gimble et al., 1995; Ozkainak et al., 1990). *In vitro*, BMP-2, BMP-4, and BMP-7 can induce the differentiation of multipotent mesenchymal cells into both osteochondrogenic lineage cells and osteoblast precursor cells, suggesting their essential contribute to both direct and indirect ossification mechanisms occurring in vertebrates (Balint et al., 2003; Canalis et al., 2003; Yamaguchi et al., 2000). BMP2 and BMP4 are essential during embryonic development; mice deficient in BMP2 are not viable because of amnio-chorial defects and severe impairment of cardiac development. The BMP4-null mutation is lethal between 6.5 and 9.5 days of gestation because of the lack of mesodermal differentiation and patterning defects (X. Wu et al., 2007). During skeletal development, BMP2/4 are involved in the molecular regulation of condensation, the pivotal stage during which previously dispersed mesenchymal progenitors proliferate, migrate and aggregate to form a growing cell mass (Hall et al., 1995). The molecular basis of BMP osteogenic properties have been extensively studied *in vitro*, studying the osteoblastic differentiation process and *in vivo* using transgenic and knockout mice along with animals and humans with naturally occurring mutations in the corresponding genes (D. Chen et al., 2004). Disruption of BMP7, leads to multiple skeletal defects, lack of eye and glomerular development, and subsequent renal failure and neonatal death (Jena et al., 1997). A wide number of preclinical studies have been demonstrating that these small molecules are capable of inducing ectopic bone formation upon intramuscular implantation and efficient bone healing/regeneration, when delivered in the appropriate concentration and on the appropriate scaffold into a bone defect site (Boden, 2005; Evans, 2011; Lattanzi et al., 2005). The use of recombinant human BMP2 and BMP7 has been approved both in Europe and the United States for selected clinical applications, as an alternative to autogenous bone grafts in the axial and appendicular skeleton. However, despite significant evidence of their potential benefit to bone repair there is, to date, a dearth of convincing clinical trials (Gautschi et al., 2007). On this regard, the main limitation of using recombinant proteins for inducing bone formation in clinical applications is the need for delivery systems that provide a sustained, biologically appropriate concentration of the osteogenic factor at the site of the defect (Lattanzi et al., 2008; Parrilla et al., 2010).

2.2.1 BMP receptors and intracellular signal transduction

BMP actions are mediated through the interaction with different sets of transmembrane serine/threonine kinase receptor complexes, grouped in two types, BMPRI and BMPRII (Massague, 1998; Zwijsen et al., 2003). BMP family members bind to their receptors with different affinities and in different combinations, determining the specificity of the downstream intracellular signals (F. Liu et al., 1995). BMPRI receptors include BMPR-IA (ALK-3), BMPR-IB (ALK-6), and ActR-IA (ALK-2) (Wan & Cao, 2005). BMPRII, activin type

IIA receptor (ActRIIA), and activin type IIB receptors (ActRIIB) are type II receptors, which bind exclusively BMP ligands, including BMP2, BMP4 and BMP7 (Wan & Cao, 2005). Generally, the type-I receptors are high-affinity binding receptors, whereas the type II receptors bind with lower affinity exclusively ligands belonging to the BMP family (X. Wu et al., 2007). BMPR-IB is the only receptor expressed within all types of cartilage and is required for correct chondrogenesis and osteogenic differentiation. ALK2 is expressed in isolated chick osteoblasts and chondrocytes, and overexpression of constitutively active ALK2 enhances chondrocyte maturation, suggesting that it is essential for normal endochondral ossification (X. Wu et al., 2007). Both type I and type II receptors are expressed on the cell surface; upon BMP2 binding, the type-II receptor transphosphorylates the type-I receptor. On its turn, the activated type I receptor phosphorylates of selected members of the Smad family of signal transduction proteins, namely Smad1, 5, and 8 (Kawabata et al., 1998; Nohe et al., 2002). The consequent activation of the Smad signaling cascade implies the formation of heterodimeric complexes with the common partner Smad (Co-Smad, Smad4), which translocate to the nucleus and recruit distinct transcription factors to regulate transcription, as illustrated in the following paragraphs (Wan and Cao, 2005; X.Wu et al., 2007). The cascade is sintetically depicted in Figure 1. As an alternative mechanism, BMP2 can also bind to preformed heteromeric receptor complexes and activate a Smad-independent transduction cascade, which results in the induction of alkaline phosphatase activity via p38-mitogen-activated protein kinase (MAPK; Kozawa et al., 2002; Guicheux et al., 2003; Nohe et al., 2002). BMP3 (osteogenin) appears to antagonize the osteogenic effects of BMP2 in stromal cells, likely acting via an activin-mediated pathway (Bahamonde et al., 2001).

2.2.2 BMP dowstream targets in bone biology

BMP2 is usually considered a paradigmatic model for studying bone formation mechanisms, since the original demonstration of its efficacy in inducing ectopic bone formation in muscles (E. A. Wang et al., 1990). *In vitro*, a wide number of studies demonstrated that BMP2 is able to induce the osteogenic differentiation of mesenchymal cells and transdifferentiation of myoblast into osteoblasts (reviewed by Ryoo et al., 2006). The BMP2 signaling involved in the osteoblast differentiation program, proceed downstream of the Smad cascade with the recruitment of osteo-specific transcription factors. The best characterized as the master osteogenic transcription factor induced by Bmp2 is the Runt-related transcription factor 2 (Runx2), because mice lacking Runx2 show complete arrest in osteoblast maturation and consequent absence of bone (Komori et al., 1997). Runx2 induces the expression of bone marker genes (including alkaline phosphatase, ALP, osteocalcin, osteopontin, bone sialoprotein and bone-specific collagens) through binding the osteoblast-specific cis-acting element-2 (OSE2), which is found in the promoter region of osteoblast-specific genes (Ziros et al., 2002). Runx2 is believed to function during the initial steps of osteogenic differentiation, from cell commitment to the chondro-osteogenic switch in endochondral ossification (Ryoo et al., 2006). The zinc finger-containing transcription factor Osterix (Osx) represents another piece in the mosaic work of Bmp2 action. Osx is expressed in developing bones and seems to act in the terminal differentiation of osteoblasts. As for Runx2, Osx-deficient mice display total absence of bone (Nakashima et al., 2002). Recent studies indicate that Runx2 and Osx mRNAs are not directly up-regulated by Bmp2, suggesting the existence of crucial intermediators, possibly represented by selected members of the Distal-less homeobox family (Dlx; further described in paragraph

2.10). Dlx5 is a homeodomain-containing transcription factor that is expressed in later stages during osteoblast differentiation and induces the expression of osteocalcin and the formation of a mineralized matrix (Ryoo et al., 2006). Dlx5 is believed to play an evolutionarily conserved role in skeletogenesis, as Dlx5-deficient mice display severe craniofacial abnormalities and delayed cranial ossification (Acampora et al., 1999). Dlx5 transcription is induced by Bmp2 signaling and could represent an upstream regulator of both Runx2 and Osx (Ryoo et al., 2006).

2.2.3 BMP antagnosists, inhibitors and further interactions

BMP signaling is modulated at different levels: extracellular BMP antagonists compete for receptor binding on the cell surface; inhibitory Smads and interacting molecules can interfere with the correct function of the intracellular Smad cascade; furthermore, alternative signals from co-existing transduction pathways converge on the same downstream targets to cooperate or antagonize BMP function on gene expression and protein processing.

BMP antagonists have been recently classified into three subfamilies based on the size of a cysteine-rich domain, known as cystine-knot, that characterizes many TGFβ superfamily members: the "Differential screening-selected gene aberrative in neuroblastoma" (DAN) family; the twisted gastrulation; and chordin and noggin. The DAN family is further subdivided in into four subgroups based on a conserved arrangement of additional cysteine residues outside of the cystine-knots: group 1 includes PRDC (Protein Related to Dan and Cerberus) and gremlin; group 2, coco and Cer1, homologue of Xenopus Cerberus; group 3 comprises the ; finally, group 4, sclerostin and USAG-1. All these molecules are involved in embryo development at various levels, representing also crucial node of intersection between Wnt- and BMP-signaling (Yanagita, 2005).

With regard to bone formation, the best studied antagonists of BMP signaling are noggin and chordin, which are structurally and fuctionally related, and regulate BMPs availability in the extracellular compartment (Rosen, 2006).

2.2.3.1 Noggin

Noggin (Nog) is a glycosylated chemokine protein, which is able to form a neutralizing complex that prevents BMPs from binding to BMPRs (Groppe et al., 2002; Krause et al., 2011). Nog action intervene as early as during gastrulation, where it antagonizes BMP-2, -4 and -7 and generates a dorsal-ventral BMP gradient which is crucial for the germ layer formation. Nog effects are pleiotropic during embryo development, although they are mainly explicated toward the formation of ectoderm and mesoderm derivatives (Krause et al. ,2011). In fact, Nog expression is essential for proper skeletal development, as excess BMP activity in Nog-null mice results in excess cartilage and failure to initiate joint formation, along with additional severe developmental abnormalities leading to premature embryo lethality (Brunet et al., 1998; McMahon et al., 1998; Tylzanowski et al., 2006). Conversely, ectopic expression of Nog in developing embryos results in suppression of lateral somite differentiation and complete inhibition of chondrogenesis in limbs (Capdevila & Johnson, 1998). Transgenic mice overexpressing noggin in mature osteoblasts show a dramatic decrease in bone mineral density and bone formation rate due to impaired osteoblast recruitment and function (X.B. Wu et al.., 2003). Most known Nog functions are based on its antagonism against BMP4 signalling, during both endochondral bone formation and teeth formation and eruption (Groppe et al., 2002; Tucker et al., 1998). Nog expression is regulated through a feedback system, as diverse BMPs (namely BMP2, -4, -5, -6 and -7) induce Nog expression in osteoblasts, while Indian hedgehog (Ihh) induce Nog expression in chondroytes (Krause et al., 2011). Finally, Nog expression is down-regulated by fibroblast growth factor-2 and -9 (FGF-2 and FGF-9) in the mesenchyme during cranial suture fusion in mice. Hence, it is speculated that the biological effects of gain-of-function mutations of the FGF receptor genes, typically associated to abnormal skeletal penotypes with cranial and limb malformations (see paragraph 2.6.2), are partially due to inappropriate inhibition of noggin expression (Warren et al., 2003).

2.2.3.2 Chordin

Similarly to noggin, chordin (CHRD) contains the cysteine-knot structure in its biochemical structure and is able to bind BMPs and sequester them in latent non-functional complexes. The formation of the Chrd-BMP complex completely prevents binding of Bmp2 to both BMPR1A and BMPR2 receptors, leading to dorsalization of early vertebrate embryo (Scott et al., 1999). Chrd binds predominantly to BMP2 and BMP4, although it has been demonstrated that BMP1 overexpression counteract the dorsalizing effects of chordin, suggesting that also BMP1 should be among the major chordin antagonists in early mammalian embryogenesis and in pre- and postnatal skeletogenesis (Scott et al., 1999). Furthermore, in mouse, Chrd binds also to Bmp7 with similar affinity (Zhang et al., 2007). Chordin is supposed to play a role during the very early embryo patterning, as it is expressed in the anterior primitive streak, in the node and subsequent axial meso-endoderm. Similarly to Nog, Chrd deficiency is early lethal in mice and is associated to a ventralized gastrulation phenotype. Stillborn animals have normal early development and neural induction but display later defects in inner and outer ear development and abnormalities in pharyngeal and cardiovascular organization (Bachiller et al., 2000). The expression and function of Chrd and Nog in the midgastrula strictly overlap. It seems that they can compensate for each other during early mouse development, as suggested by studying the phenotypic effects of combined Chrd/Nog mutations in mice. When both gene products are removed, antero-posterior, dorso-ventral, and left-right patterning are all affected in mice, with severe disruption of mesoderm development (Bachiller et al., 2000).

2.2.3.3 Sclerostin and USAG-1

Sclerostin (Sost), recently classified among BMP antagonists, was originally identified as the gene responsible for the autosomal recessive progressive sclerosing bone dysplasia, known as sclerosteosis (MIM#269500; Brunkow et al., 2001). In scleosteosis, loss of SOST prolongs the active bone-forming phase of osteoblasts, resulting in the increased bone mass. Sost is abundantly expressed in long bones and cartilages and binds to BMP-6 and -7 with highest affinity (Kusu et al., 2003; Winkler et al., 2003). Sost is expressed exclusively by osteocytes, and inhibits the differentiation and mineralization of murine preosteoblastic cells (van Bezooijen et al., 2004).

Transgenic mice overexpressing Sost exhibited low bone mass and decreased bone strength due to reduced osteoblast activity and bone formation (Winkler et al., 2003). The mechanism of action of Sost should be based on the inhibiton of BMP-induced Smad phosphorylation and alkaline phoaphatase (ALP) activity, though there are still controversies regarding this issue (Yanagita, 2005). It also acts as an inhibitor of the Wnt-signalling pathway, by binding and blocking the Wnt receptor LRP-5 (see paragraph 2.3.2).

Also another rare skeletal disease characterized by high bone mass, osteopetrosis or van Buchem's disease, already associated to LRP5 gene mutations, has been linked to inactivating mutations in the SOST gene (see Table 1 and 2). This finding highlighted the role of sclerostin in the homoeostasis of bone mass, and provided the rationale to target sclerostin with monoclonal antibodies to enhance bone formation. In a rat model of post-menopausal osteoporosis due to ovariectomy, treatment with a sclerostin antibody increased bone mass at all skeletal sites and completely prevented bone loss associated with oestrogen deficiency.
Another cysteine-knot secretory protein recently classified among the BMP antagonists is the uterine sensitization-associated gene-1 (USAG-1), originally found in rat endometrium upon sensitization, hence its name, and found expressed in the human kidney (Yanagita, 2005). USAG-1 share 38% identity to SOST aminoacid sequence, so that, also based on their functional overlap, the two moelcules could be grouped in a distinct family of BMP antagonists. Recombinant USAG-1 protein binds and inhibits BMP-2, -4, -6, and -7 with high affinity, reducing ALP activity in mesenchymal cells and pre-osteoblasts.

2.2.3.4 LIM-mineralization proteins

Among the BMP-interacting molecules, it is worth to mention the recently discovered Lim mineralization protein (LMP), an intracellular LIM-domain protein acting as a potent positive regulator of the osteoblast differentiation program (Bernardini et al., 2010). LMP was originally identified and cloned from rat calvarial osteoblasts stimulated by glucocorticoids, and subsequently emerged as a novel attractive osteogenic molecule able to induce the activation of the BMP signaling pathway (Boden et al., 1998; Boden et al., 1998b; Viggeswarapu et al., 2001). In humans, three different splice variants are transcribed from the LMP-coding gene (PDZ and LIM doamin-7, PDLIM7): LMP1 is the longest transcript, encodes the full-length protein isoform comprising conserved PDZ and LIM domains plus a non-conserved region, and has demonstrated osteogenic properties; LMP2, misses over 100 nucleotides within the non-conserved region and does not induce bone formation; finally the LMP3 isoform is the result of a more complex post-transcriptional processing that produces a smaller peptide missing all LIM domains while retaining a shorter non-conserved sequence (H.S. Kim et al., 2003; Y. Liu et al., 2002; Viggeswarapu et al., 2001). Despite the truncation of nearly two third of the full-length isoform, LMP3 retains efficient osteogenic properties, demonstrated *in vitro* and in different animal models (Lattanzi et al., 2008; Parrilla et al., 2010; Pola et al., 2004). *In vitro,* both LMP1 and LMP3 induce osteogenic differentiation of mesenchymal progenitors, fibroblasts and pre-osteoblasts, through the transcriptional activation of BMP-family members (mainly BMP2, BMP4 and BMP7) and TGFβ1 protein (Bernardini et al., 2010 ; Minamide et al., 2003). LMP1 osteogenic properties are also based on interactions with the Smad ubiquitin regulatory factor 1 (Smurf1), thus preventing Smads ubiquitination and potentiating BMP signaling, along with the insulin-growth factor biniding protein-6 (IGFBP6), a potent indcutor of osteoblast differnetiation (Sangadala et al., 2006; Strohbach et al., 2008). In addition, it suppresses osteoclast activity acting through the mitogen-activated protein kinase (MAPK)-signaling, which implies more pleiotropic effects to be exerted by the peptide (H. Liu et al., 2010). The effectiveness of LMPs in inducing bone formation *in vivo* has been demonstrated, using different strategy to deliver the gene/peptide at the site where the bone healing was required (H.S. Kim et al., 2003; Lattanzi et al., 2008; Parrilla et al, 2010; Pola et al., 2004; Sangadala et al., 2009; Strohbach et al., 2008b; X. Wang et al., 2011; Yoon et al., 2004). So far, the expression of human LMPs has been detected in the iliac crest bone, in teeth and in calvarial tissues and cells (Bernardini et al., 2011; Bunger et al., 2003; Fang et al., 2010; X. Wang et al., 2008).

2.2.4 Skeletal phenotypes associated to BMPs

At least four molecules that are directly involved in the BMP-TGFβ pathway are mutated in human syndromes comprising skeletal malformations in their phenotypes, due to the actions carried out during throughout development in mesoderm induction, tooth development, limb formation, bone induction, and fracture repair. Table 1 summarizes the mendelian disorders allelic to BMP-related gene mutations categorized in the "online mendelian inheritance in man" (OMIM) database (www.omim.org). Main differences in human phenotypes associated to different genes are evident, reflecting the diversified gene functions during skeletal development and patterning. In particular, while heterozygous mutations in the BMP4 gene are associated to minor facial malformations, different point mutations in the human homolog of the murine Nog (NOG) can cause five different phenotypes, invariably carachterized by limb malformations, and other skeletal anomalies due to impaired endochondral ossification. This could possibly reflect more pleiotropic roles for NOG (see Table 1).

Gene[a]	Diseases	MIM[b]
BMP4	Syndromic microphtalmia	607932
	Orofacial cleft	600625
BMPRIB	brachydactyly, type A2	112600
	Acromesomelic chrondrodysplasia with genital anomalies	609441
NOG	brachydactyly, type B2	611377
	multiple synostosis syndrome	186500
	stapes ankylosis with broad thumb/toe	184460
	proximal symphalangism	185800
	tarsal-carpal coalition syndrome	186570
SOST	Sclerosteosis	269500

a. gene symbol is provided; b. Mendelian Inheritance in Man (MIM) ID code.

Table 1. Mendelian diseases associated to BMP family mutations

2.3 WNT signaling

Since the original discoveries of the role of Wnt signalling in bone formation and skeletogenesis (Hartmann & Tabin, 2001; Lako et al., 1998), there has been a stream of research aimed at elucidating the complex roles that Wnt proteins, endogenous Wnt inhibitors and interacting molecules play in the regulation of bone mass, revelaing that they play a vital role in adult tissue maintenance (Milat & Ng, 2009).

2.3.1 Wnt proteins

The "wingless-type mouse mammary tumor virus (MMTV) integration site" family (WNT) consists of structurally related genes which encode secreted signaling glycoproteins, which are extremely conserved in evolution. They are implicated in oncogenesis and in several developmental processes, including regulation of cell fate, early axis specification, organ development and patterning during embryogenesis (Hartmann & Tabin, 2000, 2001). Hence, aberrations in Wnt signalling lead to complex developmental diseases.

WNT family members are defined by sequence homology to the Drosophila wingless (wg) and the murine int-1 proto-oncogene, hence the family name. The first Wnt gene was cloned 30 years ago (Nusse & Varmus, 1982); to date, nineteen Wnt genes have been identified in the mouse and human genomes (http://www.stanford.edu/rnusse/wntwindow.htlm; Milat & Ng, 2009). Wnt proteins are traditionally categorized into two classes, canonical and non-canonical, based on their *in vivo* and *in vitro* activities that are exerted through distinct molecular signal transduction mechanisms. Canonical Wnts (including Wnt1, Wnt3A, Wnt8, Wnt10b) activate a cascade that results in the translocation of β-catenin (cadherin-associated protein, beta 1, CTNNB1) to the nucleus, where it associates to the lymphoid-enhancer binding factor/T-cell specific transcription factors (TCF/LEF) that finally induces the expression of target genes (Logan et al., 2004; Milat & Ng, 2009). The canonical pathway, the best studied, initiate when a canonical Wnt-ligand binds to one of the Frizzled (Fz) receptors. This event inactivates the glycogen synthase kinase 3 (GSK3), through the developmental transducer phosphoprotein Dishevelled (Dvl), and therefore prevents phosphorylation and consecutive proteosomal-degradation of β-catenin (Westendorf et al., 2004; Behrens et al., 1996).

Non-canonical Wnts (including Wnt4, Wnt5a and Wnt11) activate transcription through β-catenin-independent signaling pathways, involving alternative intracellular second messengers. At least three alternative non-canonical Wnt pathways could be described. One is based on the intracellular release of Ca2+ that activates calcium-sensitive enzymes, which on their turn activate specific transcription factors (A.E. Chen et al., 2005). This Wnt-cGMP/Ca2+-protein kinase C dependent pathway plays important roles during dorso-ventral patterning of the embryo, regulating cell migration, as well as heart development, and might play a role during tumor suppression (Piters et al., 2008). The planar cell polarity (PCP) signaling (Mlodzik, 2002) represent another non-canonical Wnt-pathway, required for embryonic morphogenesis, activated through Fz receptors binding and results in the coactivation of Rho and Rac, two small GTPases that are able to regulate cytoskeletal architecture (Piters et al., 2008). Finally, the Wnt-protein kinase A (PKA) pathway is based on the increase cAMP levels, which activates PKA and the transcription factor CREB and has been implicated in myogenesis in mice (Kuhl et al., 2000; Semenov et al., 2007).

Recent evidences suggested that the distinct signaling pathways are alternatively activated through the binding of distinct sets of receptors, regardless of the original classification of canonical versus non-canonical Wnts (van Amerongen et al., 2008).

2.3.2 Wnt receptors

The mechanism by which Wnt binding to its receptors triggers the downstream signalling has been extensively studied, although a conclusive and comprehensive view has not been achieved so far (Fuerer et al., 2008). The best known Wnt receptors belong to the Frizzled (Fzd) family, which includes ten G protein-coupled transmembrane receptors (FZD1-to-10; Wodarz & Nusse, 1998). Thereafter, various members of the density lipoprotein receptor (LRP) family (LRP5 and LRP6) have been shown to be essential co-receptor for Wnt signalling (Tamai et al., 2000; Wehrli et al., 2000). LRP phosphorylation by activated Wnt is critical and requires the cooperative roles of FZD, the cytoplasmic scaffolding proteins dishevelled (Dsh/Dvl) and axin, and GSK3, within the canonical pathway (Bilic et al.., 2007; Davidson et al., 2005).

2.3.3 Wnt targets

A large number of Wnt target genes have been identified to date, in over twenty studies based on genome-wide approaches (e.g. microarray-based gene expression profiling) in different cell lines and tissues (http://www.stanford.edu/~rnusse/pathways/targets.html). Distinct *in vitro* studies provided the evidence of "feedback targets" of Wnt, that are Wnt signalling components whose expression can be regulated by the signaling itself, indicating that feedback control is a key feature of Wnt signaling regulation. In particular, over 150 genes have been identified as direct transcriptional targets of the Wnt canonical pathways, as they contain Tcf/Lef binding sites, including basic regulators of cell proliferation/tumorigenesis (c-myc, cyclin D, c-jun, among others), growth factors (FGF9, FGF20, VEGF, BMP4), transcription factors (RunX2), and a wide number of genes implicated in cell adhesion and differentiation (see the gene-lists available at the web site above indicated).

2.3.4 Wnt in bone biology

An extensive review of the scientifc literature reveals that Wnt proteins play a leading role in bone development and homeostasis. In this respect, the canonical Wnt pathway has been most extensively studied for its role in skeletogenesis,

There is *in vitro* evidence that Wnt proteins are produced by calvaria, primary osteoblasts (Wnt1, Wnt4, Wnt14) and osteosarcoma cell lines. Wnt genes (e.g. Wnt7b) are up-regulated during osteogenic differentiation of bone marrow stromal cells (Kato et al., 2002; Gregory et al, 2005). Some Wnt proteins (Wnt10b, Wnt1,Wnt2 and Wnt3a) have an effect on bone physiology, as they regulate bone marker gene expression (osteocalcin, RunX2, Osterix, alkaline phosphatase), stimulate osteoblastogenesis and inhibit adipogenesis, mainly through the canonical pathway (Takada et al, 2009). Mice lacking either Wnt10b or Wnt5a display impaired bone structure organization and reduced bone mass due to hypoplasia (Bennet et al., 2005; Takada et al., 2007). Wnt5a seems to act through CaMKII rather than TCF/LEF, thus suggesting that both the canonical and non-canonical Wnt signalling pathways play a role in osteoblastogenesis (Milat & Ng, 2009). Mice lacking Lrp5 display a low bone mass secondary to reduced osteoblast proliferation (Kato et al., 2002). Similarly in humans, a loss-of-function mutation in LRP5 occurs in the osteoporosis-pseudoglioma syndrome (OPPG, MIM#259770; Table 2), an autosomal recessive syndrome characterized low bone mass, ocular defects, and predisposition to fractures (Gong et al., 2001). Conversely, the gain-of-function mutation in Lrp5 may not have an effect on bone density when expressed in mature osteoblasts and can be associated to increased bone mass, due to inhibition of Wnt sigaling (Yadav et al., 2008).

Moreover, LRP5 inhibits tryptophan hydroxylase (Tph1) expression, a rate-limiting enzyme in the gut-derived serotonin biosynthetic pathway, impairing serotonin synthesis. Serotonin on its turn regulates the bone mass (Warden et al., 2005), in fact, gut-specific deletion of LRP5 results in low bone mass, similarly to the phenotype observed in LRP5-null mice (Yadav et al., 2008). Reasonably, this could provide the first possible explanation of the complex gut–bone interactions in the regulation of bone mass (Milat & Ng, 2009). Conversely, osteoblast-specific deletions of LRP5 do not cause osteoblast defects. LRP5 may be involved in postatal regulation of osteoblast differentiation and it is possible that LRP6, rather than LRP5, is the critical co-receptor for Wnt signalling in bone. As a proof of evidence, LRP6 loss of function bone phenotype is much more severe than that associated to LRP5 loss. The LRP6−/− genotype is lethal in mice, while heterozygous mice display reduced bone mass (Pinson et al., 2000). In humans, a missense mutation in LRP6, with consequent impairment of Wnt signalling, has been associated to an autosomal dominant early coronary artery disease, to metabolic risk factors and to osteoporosis (Mani et al.., 2007).

β-catenin (CTNNB1) mutations appeared to affect bone resorption by regulating, in differentiated osteoblasts, the expression of osteoprotegerin (OPG), which controls osteoclast differentiation (Glass et al., 2005; see paragraph 2.8). Also, conditional deletion of Ctnnb1 in mouse embryo limb and head mesenchyme resulted in blockage of osteoblastic differentiation of mesenchymal precursors (Day et al., 2005; Hill et al.,2005). Ctnnb1 is indeed crucial in determining the correct osteoblastic fate of mesenchymal progenitors in the developing embryo (Hill et al., 2005).

Wnt signaling is also involved in the transcriptional modulation of the molecular events leading to cartilage differentiation. Ectopic canonical Wnt signaling leads to enhanced ossification and suppression of chondrocyte formation during skeletogenesis (Day et al., 2005). On the other hand, during both intramembranous and endochondral ossification, b-catenin inactivation induces ectopic chondrocyte formation in place of osteoblast differentiation. Moreover, Wnt signaling is essential for skeletal lineage differentiation, preventing transdifferentiation of osteoblasts into chondrocytes, and control stem cell self renewal, proliferation and fate lineage specification, by regulating the balance between FGF and BMP signaling (Hill et al., 2005).

2.3.5 Wnt-signaling inhibitors

Other ligands can bind the Fzd–LRP5/6 receptor complex, thus antagonizing Wnt signal transduction pathway. Dickkopfs (Dkk) proteins, compete for the LRP5/6 receptor and prevent canonical signalling. Dkk are involved in epithelial-mesenchymal transition during mesodermal tissue development and play an important role in bone biology. DKKs role in vertebrate development is due to their local inhibitory funtion on Wnt-regulated processes, such as antero-posterior axial patterning, limb development, somitogenesis and eye formation (Pinzone et al, 2009).

Dkk1 binds to LRP6 with high affinity and is expressed by osteocytes and osteosarcoma cells. When overexpressed, DKK1 induce osteopenia, while Dkk1 loss induces increased bone formation in mice (Milat & Ng 2009). In humans, an increase of DKK1 expression in leukocytes was associated to the presence of bone lesions in myeloma patients (Milat & Ng, 2009). The role in bone homestasis of other Wnt inhibitors, such as the secreted frizzled related protein-1 (sFRP1) and the Wnt inhibitory factor 1, (WIF-1) has been explored and demonstrated so far exclusively in animal and cellular models (Milat & Ng, 2009).

It is worth to mention that close relationships between the BMP- and the WNT-signaling occur at this level; Dkk1 and Nog cooperate in mammalian head induction (del Barco Barrantes et al., 2003); the expression of DKK1 is regulated by BMP-4 in limb development (Grotewold et al., 2002). Furthermore, the mutlifunctional antagonist called Cerberus, a potent inducer of head formation during vertebrate development, has distinct binding sites for Wnt proteins and BMPs (Piccolo et al., 1999). Finally, USAG-1 might also have dual activities, and play as a molecular link between Wnt and BMP signaling pathway (Yanagita et al., 2004).

2.3.6 Skeletal phenotypes associated to Wnt signalling members

Over 70 mendelian syndromes presenting with skeletal abnormalities in humans are associated to mutations in Wnt signaling-related genes. This large group include complex developmental disorders with multi-system implication due to severe imbalance of body patterning in embryo. Besides very rare and incompletely characterized syndromes, some of the most significant WNT-associated skeletal phenotypes are summarized in table 2. Overall, these diversified phenotypes are characterized alternatively by limb malformations and defective/eccessive ossification.

Refer to the OMIM database (www.omim.org) for complete clinical information about the listed phenotypes and for additional Wnt-related genetic disorders.

Gene[a]	Diseases	MIM[b]
LRP5	Hyperostosis, endosteal	144750
	Osteopetrosis, autosomal dominant 1	607634
	Osteoporosis-pseudoglioma syndrome	259770
	Osteosclerosis	144750
	van Buchem disease, type 2	607636
	Bone mineral density variability 1	601884
WNT5A	Robinow syndrome, autosomal dominant	180700
SOX9	Acampomelic campomelic dysplasia	114290
	Campomelic dysplasia	
	Campomelic dysplasia with autosomal sex reversal	
WNT10B	Split-hand/foot malformation 6	225300
WISP3	Arthropathy, progressive pseudorheumatoid, of childhood	208230
	Spondyloepiphyseal dysplasia tarda with progressive arthropathy	
PRKAR1A	Acrodysostosis with hormone resistance	101800
FRZB	Osteoarthritis susceptibility 1	165720
ROR2	Brachydactyly, type B1	113000
	Robinow syndrome	268310

a. gene symbol is provided; b. Mendelian Inheritance in Man (MIM) ID code.

Table 2. Main mendelian syndromes associated to mutations in genes related to the Wnt-signaling

2.4 Hedgehog homologs family

Drosophila hedgehog (Hh) and its vertebrate orthologs, Sonic hedgehog (Shh), Indian hedgehog (Ihh), and Desert hedgehog (Ihh) are secreted proteins involved in the establishment cell fates at several points during development. The vast majority of information on the Hh system derives from the studies performed in Drosophila. Hh production occurs through a well documented process of synthesis and post-translational processing leading to cholesterol-modification. This biochemical feature allows the Hh proteins to permeate the plasma membrane and form diffusible multimeric complexes. These represent represent the biologically active forms required for long-range signaling across different tissues in the developing embryo (Ehlen et al., 2006). Further transduction depends on the presence of the tramsmembrane protein dispatched-1 (Disp1), which is essential for driving long-range Hh signaling in flies and mice (Burke et al., 1999). Once they reach the target site of action, Hh molecules bind to the surface receptor Patched-1 (Ptch1) and induce the release and functional activation of the transmembrane protein smoothened (Smo). Smo activation on its turn induce downstream signaling, including the de-repression of the transcription factors belonging to the glioma-associated family of zinc finger oncogenes (Gli-1, -2 and -3; vertebrate orthologs of the Drososphila Cubitus interruptus), resulting in the activation of target gene expression (Cohen, 2003). Gli proteins are DNA-binding transcription factors which localize in the cytoplasm and play important roles during embryogenesis (Lum & Beachy, 2004). This is also substantiated by the implication of human GLI genes in complex developmental disorders (see paragraph 2.4.2 and table 3).
The signal transduction events downstream of Smo are best understood in Drosophila, while the complete sequence of molecular events involved in Hh signaling in vertebrate skeletogenesis is still unclear. A growing number of studies during the last decade have been trying to clarify this issue (Ehlen, 2006). New evidences are taking root in suggesting that vertebrate Hh signaling is related to the function of the primary cilium, a specialized cell surface projection intensively involved in intercellular signaling, which is essential for the correct coordination of organogenesis. In fact, some molecules involved in the Hh signalling cascade localize to the primary cilium (Corbit et al., 2005; Haycraft et al., 2005; Singla and Reiter, 2006). In addition, mutations in components of the intraflagellar transport machynery are able to indirectly disrupt Hh signaling and lead to a wide range of human disorders, comprising severe impairment of organ patterning in their phenotypes (van Reeuwijk et al., 2011).

2.4.1 Hh in bone biology

Hedgehog signaling coordinates a variety of embryo patterning processes through a series of inductive interactions (Ehlen et al., 2006). In particular, in vertebrates Shh and Ihh are essential regulators of skeletogenesis as they provide positional information and initiate or maintain cellular differentiation programs, regulating the formation of cartilage and bone. They basically regulate endochondral ossification, acting either as paracrine modulators on adjacent cells or over long distances, leading to the axial and appendicular skeleton patterning (Ehlen et al., 2006). Indian hedgehog (Ihh) can be regarded as the osteogenic HH, being a signaling molecule expressed predominantly in pre-hypertrophic chondrocytes where it plays a major role in endochondral bone formation. Ihh functions in the growth plate are mediated through the parathyroid hormone-related peptide (PTHrP) (Vortkanp et al., 1996). In the absence of Ihh, PTHrP mRNA is undetectable in fetal bones (Kronenberg, 2006).

The parathyroid hormone-related peptide (PTHrP) also named PTH-like hormone (PTHLH), is a key regulator of endochondral bone formation synthesized by perichondrial cells and chondrocytes in growing bones. This hormone was originally discovered as a circulating peptide increased in the hypercalcemia occurring during malignancies (Suva et al., 1987). As a circulating hormone the PTHrP has pleiotropic functions, while during endochondral bone formation it acts in a juxtacrine/paracrine manner, binding to the same receptor as paratohomone (PTH/PTHrP Rec or PTHR1); the signal is transduced in the intracellular compartment via the recruitment of multiple G proteins and subsequent activation of adenylate cyclise, which generates cAMP. cAMP-dependent PKA then promote a downstream cascade leading to the suppression of target genes, including RunX2. PKA also phosphorylates and activate SOX9. The PTHR1 is expressed by chondrocytes as they stop proliferating. PTHrP then induces proliferation and delays chondrocyte hypertrophy (Kronenberg, 2006). Mice missing either the PTHrP or its receptor genes undergo a truncated endochondral sequence leading to shorter or absent column of proliferating chondrocytes in fetal bones and usually die shortly after birth, due to severe impairment of rib cage development (Amizuka et al., 1994; Chung et al., 1998). Conversely mice overexpressing either genes show bones with increased number of proliferating chondrocytes giving rise to delayed endochondral sequence (Weir et al., 1996).

2.4.2 Skeletal phenotypes associated to HH family members

Due to their essential role in embryo development, mutations of the HH family genes imply severe alteration of vertebrate body patterning and affect the cell proliferative homeostasis leading to tumorigenesis. There are at least three defined phenotypes that are directly ascribable to HH gene mutations in humans. Noticeably, being essential for the endochondral ossification throughout the developing skeleton, human IHH mutations in homozygosis lead to malformations involving both appendicular and axile skeletal structures (see table 3). Main mendalian disorders of the whole HH signaling are listed in table 3.

Gene[a]	Diseases	MIM[b]
IHH	Acrocapitofemoral dysplasia	607778
	Brachydactyly, type A1	112500
SHH	Single median maxillary central incisor	147250
PTHLH	Brachydactyly, type E2	613382
GLI3	Greig cephalopolysyndactyly syndrome	175700
	Pallister-Hall syndrome	146510
	Polydactyly, postaxial, types A1 and B	174200
	Polydactyly, preaxial, type IV	174700

a. gene symbol is provided; b. Mendelian Inheritance in Man (MIM) ID code.

Table 3. Selected mendealian malformation syndromes of HH signaling molecules

2.5 The FGF/FGFR signaling

Fibroblast growth factors (FGFs) and corresponding receptors (FGFRs) are known to play important roles during bone development. FGF signaling is essential for maintaining bone homeostasis and during fracture healing. The FGF family currently comprises over 20 structurally related members that bind to tyrosine kinase transmembrane receptors. Upon binding FGFR on its extracellular ligand-binding domain, FGF causes the dimerization of receptor monomers, leading to autophosphorylation of tyrosine residues on the intracellular signal transduction domain (Su et al., 2008). Alternative downstream signal transduction pathways have been described that basically imply the activation of the mitogen-activated protein kinase (MAPK) signaling. (Eswarakumar et al., 2005).

2.5.1 FGFs/FGFRs in bone biology

FGF sigaling is crucial in both endochondral and intramembranous ossification. Different FGF ligands are expressed in the mesenchyme of the limb bud at the stage of condensation and later in chondrocytes and osteoblasts in the growth plate of developing long bones (Colvin et al., 1999; Lazarus et al., 2007; Yu et al., 2003). During the cyclic proliferation/hypertrophy stages of endochondral bone formation, more then ten different FGF molecules are expressed in a perfectly spatio-temporal coordinated fahion (Lazarus et al., 2007). Particularly, converging evidences indicate FGF2 as the earliest marker gene to be expressed in prechondrocyte condensation stages, while FGF1 and FGF3 appear later in differentiated chondrocytes (Lazarus et al., 2007; Yu et al., 2003).

Lessons from genetically modified mouse models and *in vitro* studies indicated that excessive Fgf2 inhibits chondrogenesis, resulting in decreased bone elongation, hypertrophic diffentiation and abnormal chondrocyte proliferation (Montero et al., 2000; Sobue et al., 2005). Conversely, mice lacking Fgf2 display reduced bone formation and abnormal bone structure (Montero et al., 2000). Overall, the correct dosage of Fgf2 is essential for the bone growth and homeostasis (Su et al., 2008). Similarly, other FGF ligands have a documented role in limb outgrowth and patterning, from the stage of condensation till osteoblastic differentiation, indicating some kind of redundancy among FGF signaling (de Lapeyriere et al., 1993; Fiore et al. , 1997; Finch et al., 1995; Guo et al., 1996; Haub et al., 1991; Hebert et al., 1994).

With regard to intramembranous ossification, all Fgfs, except Fgf-3 and -4, are expressed in coronal suture in the mouse embryo and in other mesenchymal sutures during craniofacial development (Su et al., 2008). The role of FGF/FGFR signaling in promoting intramembranous ossification is indeed strongly supported by the association of FGFR1-3 genes in human craniosynostosis syndromes (see table 4). Increased FGF signaling cause increased proliferation rates in suture-derived calvarial cells leading to premature suture closure (i.e. synostosis; H.J. Kim et al., 1998). FGF signaling also regulates calvarial cell differentiation. Therefore, FGF signaling exerts a dual effect on osteoblast biology, inducing proliferation of immature osteoblasts and apoptosis in differentiated osteoblasts (Mansukhani et al., 2000). The pro-differentiation effects should be the result of Runx2-induced expression of osteocalcin, enhanced by Fgf2 (H.J. Kim et al., 2003). FGF signaling actually cross-talks with the other osteogenic pathways, including Msx2, Twist, Bmp and other TGF-β superfamily members, during calvarial suture morphogenesis (Opperman, 2000; Rice at al, 2005).

2.5.2 Skeletal phenotypes associated to FGF signaling; The FGFR syndromes

Missense mutations in either FGFs or FGFRs human genes cause a variety of congenital skeletal disorders, including syndromic craniosynostosis (CRS) and hypo/achondroplasia, among others (extensively reviewed by Su et al., 2008). In particular, both CRS syndromes and chondrodysplasias, are associated to gain-of-function mutations in either of the FGFR-1, -2 and -3 genes, which imply the constitutive activation of the kinase receptor activity regardless of ligand binding on the extracellular domain. A list of the best characterized malformation syndromes associated to FGFR gene mutations (the autosomal dominant "FGFR syndromes") is provided in table 4, as paradigmatic examples of the effects of FGF signaling impairment in human diseases. The functional relevance of the most common FGFR gene mutations of syndromic craniosynostosis has been further examined using animal models and *in vitro* studies (Su et al., 2008).

Gene[a]	Diseases	MIM[b]
FGFR2	Antley-Bixler syndrome	207410
	Apert syndrome	101200
	Beare-Stevenson cutis gyrata syndrome	123790
	Crouzon syndrome	123500
	Gastric cancer, somatic	137215
	Jackson-Weiss syndrome	123150
	LADD syndrome	149730
	Pfeiffer syndrome	101600
	Saethre-Chotzen syndrome	101400
	Scaphocephaly with maxillary retrusion and mental retardation	609579
FGFR3	Achondroplasia	100800
	CATSHL syndrome	610474
	Crouzon syndrome with acanthosis nigricans	612247
	Hypochondroplasia	146000
	LADD syndrome	149730
	Muenke syndrome	602849
	Thanatophoric dysplasia, type I	187600
	Thanatophoric dysplasia, type II	187601
FGFR1	Jackson-Weiss syndrome	123150
	Osteoglophonic dysplasia	166250
	Pfeiffer syndrome	101600
	Trigonocephaly	190440

Table 4. The FGFRs syndromes: skeletal malformations associated to FGFRs: a. gene symbol is provided; b. Mendelian Inheritance in Man (MIM) ID code.

2.6 TWIST

The Twist homolog 1 (Drosophila), TWIST1, belongs to the basic helix-loop-helix (bHLH) class of transcriptional regulators that dimerize to form a bipartite DNA binding groove, which recognize a consensus DNA element and alter the chromatin structure (Pan et al., 2009). Twist1 represents a critical modulator of mesenchymal cell fate during skeletal development, inducing differentiation toward both the chondrogenic and the osteogenic lineages, while inhibiting myogenesis (Miraoui & Marie, 2010). In Drosophila, twist homozygous mutations are associated to a lethal phenotype, due to disruption of gastrulation and failure in mesodermal-derived organ development and leading to complete eversion of head; the embryo was twisted in the egg, hence the name given to the gene

(Simpson, 1983). Heterozygous mutations in the Twist1 gene usually determine loss-of-function due to haploinsufficiency (Zackai and Stolle, 1998). In fact, mice heterozygous for a Twist null mutation exhibited cranial and limb defects (Bourgeois et al.. 1998; El Ghouzzi et al.. 1997). Such findings, allowed to confirm TWIST1 as the candidate gene for the Saethre-Chotzen syndrome (MIM#101400, autosomal dominant), characterized by craniofacial and limb malformations and indicated a key role of TWIST in n the mesodermal development of the head and limbs (El Ghouzzi et al., 1997; Gripp et al., 2000; see following sections). Thereafter, Twist role in calvarial bone/suture patterning and development has been intensively investigated (Miraoui & Marie, 2010). In this context. Twist1 appears to act as an upstream transcriptional regulator of FGFRs (Shishido et al., 1993).

2.7 The RANK/RANKL/OPG system in bone biology

Bone resorption, required during endochondral bone formation and bone remodeling, is driven by functional activation of osteoclasts. It is now clear that the complete maturation of osteoclasts occurs only in presence of osteoblasts (Grano et al., 1990; Teti et al, 1991). The molecular basis of this fundamental interaction resides in the interplay between the receptor activator of nuclear factor kappa B (RANK), its ligand (RANKL) and the osteoprotegerin (OPG).

RANK is a homotrimeric transmembrane receptor, belonging to the tumor necrosis factor (TNF) receptor superfamily, expressed on the cell surface of osteoclast precursors and mature osteoclasts. RANKL, also called OPG-ligand or osteoclast differentiation factor (ODF), also belong to the TNF superfamily and is expressed in osteoblasts (Boyce and Xing, 2008). The interaction between RANK and RANKL induces a downstream signalling, that involves the nuclear factor kB (NFKB), with subsequent transcriptional activation of target genes leading to recruitment, differentiation, activation and survival of osteoclasts.

OPG, also known as tumor necrosis factor receptor superfamily member 11 (TNFRSF11) or osteoclastogenesis inhibitory factor (OCIF) is a soluble receptor of RANK, exrpressed in osteoblasts, stromal cells and other non-skeletal cells. OPG acts as a decoy receptor for RANKL, as it prevents RANK/RANKL interaction and inhibits osteoclastogenesis and bone resorption (Khosla, 2001). The RANKL/OPG ratio represents a major determinant in bone mass regulation, as inferred from the OPG-deficient mouse, which displays an osteoporotic phenotype with increased osteoclasts (Bucay et al., 1998). Conversely, OPG overexpression leads to osteopetrosis (Simonet et al., 1997).

OPG expression is regulated by the canonical Wnt pathway, which regulates osteoclasts by increasing the OPG/RANKL ratio (Suzuki et al., 2008). The OPG/RANKL ratio in osteoblasts is also regulated by bone remodeling hormones. Both parathormone (PTH) and vitamin D decrease the ratio by the transcriptional up-regualtion of RANKL. Conversely, estrogens increase OPG production in osteoblasts, hence increase bone formation and reduce resorption (Zallone, 2006). More recently a role in the control of bone remodeling has been emerging for leptins, serotonin and insulin, probably acting through the RANKL/OPG system (Elefteriou, 2005; Huang et al, 2009).

2.7.1 Skeletal phenotypes associated to OPG mutations

Besides the documented involvement of the RANK/RANKL/OPG system in the pathogenesis of acquired multifactorial bone remodeling disorders, such as osteoporosis and osteoarthritis, OPG is also emerged as a genetic disease-associated gene.

Homozygous or compound heterozygous mutations of TNFRSF11 have been found in juvenile Paget disease of bone (MIM#239000), characterized by systemic hyperhostosis, with typically increased skull bone thickness, hyperphosphatemia and progressive skeletal deformities.

2.8 Notch signaling

Evolutionarily conserved Notch signaling plays an important role in developmental processes and adult tissue homeostasis by regulating cell fate determination, proliferation, differentiation and apoptosis in a spatio-temporal coordinated manner. The Notch receptor and its ligands are transmembrane proteins whose signaling requires cell to cell contact between neighboring cells (Engin & Lee, 2010). Four Notch receptors (Notch1-4) are known in mammals, while Notch ligands fall into two classes: Delta and Jagged. Subsequent cleavage steps occur upon Notch receptor/ligand interaction to activate the Notch intracellular domain (Notch ICD) that is then released from the membrane, and translocated to the nucleus (Hayes et al, 2003). In the nucleus, Notch ICD binds specific transcription factors and recruits transcriptional co-activators to induce the expression of a basic helix-loop-helix (bHLH) family of genes (Engin & Lee, 2010).

Notch signaling is involved in skeletal patterning and somitogenesis, as related molecules are expressed in the presomitic mesoderm (PSM) of mouse embryos. Notch1 null mouse embryos exhibits significantly delayed and disorganized somitogenesis (Conlon et al., 1995; Turnpenny et al., 2007).

Converging evidences suggest that Notch pathway is active in the early stages of osteoblast differentiation, also by acting on Runx2-dependent osteogenic gene expression (McLarren et al., 2000; Tezuka et al., 2002). Nonetheless, this issue is currently debated. Notch could also regulate osteoclastogenesis, through the up-regulation of RANKL and OPG genes, suggesting that the functional cross-talk between osteoblasts and osteoclasts might be also mediated by Notch signaling (Engin & Lee, 2010). Finally, Notch signaling is believed to act also in chondrogenic differentiation, although its exact role and its temporal effects during chondro/osteoblastogenesis are still unclear.

Getting into the clinical field, mutations in Notch pathway genes are the etiology of two genetic disorders with severe skeletal impairment: Spondylocostal dysostosis type 1 (SCDO1, MIM#602768) and Alagille syndrome (AGS, MIM#118450), both characterized by vertebral column defects (Bulman et al., 2000; L. Li et al., 1997). This clinical evidence, confirm the best characterized function of NOTCH signaling as a regulator of somitogenesis.

2.9 Homeobox genes

The homeobox genes belonging to the muscle segment homeobox gene (Msx) family, Msx-1 and Msx-2, are implicated in the regulation of craniofacial skeletal morphogenesis (Aïoub et al., 2007; Berdal et al., 2009; Orestes-Cardoso et al., 2002). Msx genes are expressed in the cranial neural crest (CNC) cells where they regulate migration and proliferation and specify tissue lineage differentiation fates. They preferentially support skeletal tissue development and they contribute extensively to the formation of the craniofacial skeleton (Bendall & Abate-Shen, 2000). Msx1 and Msx2 genes are expressed in osteoclasts and drive the membranous ossification. In particular, Msx1 has been functionally associated with mandible development, while Msx2 as been implicated in tooth eruption and elongation (Aïoub et al., 2007; Orestes-Cardoso et al., 2002).

The MSX homeoproteins are co-expressed with the distal-less homeobox gene (DLX) family in CNC cells and in various developing tissues. MSX and DLX molecules structurally and functionally interact *in vitro* by forming heterodimers via their homeodomains and reciprocally inhibit each other's activities (Bendall & Abate-Shen, 2000). These homeoprotein families are jointly implicated in the control of craniofacial, axial, and appendicular skeletal morphogenesis (Alappat et al., 2003; Kraus and Lufkin, 2006; Lallemand et al.., 2005). In osteoblast differentiation, Msx activity counteracts the osteogenic-inducing property of Dlx during osteoblast differentiation. In mouse, Msx2 was found indeed to repress the expression of osteocalcin (OC), while Dlx genes were recruited to initiate OC transcription via RunX2 , leading to the final mineralization stage of osteoblast differentiation (Hassan et al., 2004). Thus, functional antagonism through heterodimer formation may provide a mechanism for regulating the transcriptional actions of Msx and Dlx *in vivo*. They were also shown to regulate one another's expression , and to share target genes such as amelogenin (Alappat et al., 2003; Kraus and Lufkin, 2006). On the other hand, it has also been suggested that Msx and Dlx genes act independently in regulating the development of craniofacial skeleton (Levi et al., 2006).

2.9.1 Skeletal disorders associated to MSX2

The human homolog of Msx-2 (MSX2, MIM*123101), originally cloned in 1993 (X. Li et al., 1993), has been associated to three distinct phenotypes, inherited as autosomal dominant tracts and sharing distinctive clinical features, such as craniofacial deformities of variable degrees, no limb involvement, and neurological symptoms (mainly represented by headache and seizures) among others (see www.ncbi.nlm.nih.gov/omim for detailed descriptions). A proline-to-hystidine substitution in the homeodomain of MSX2 was found in the Boston-type Craniosynostosis syndrome (type 2 Craniosynostosis, MIM#604757), a skeletal developmental disorder characterized by skull malformations (from mild asymmetry to trilobular skull with craniosynostosis, the so-called cloverleaf skull) and neurological symptoms usually without mental retardation (Muller et al., 1993; Warman et al., 1993). Deletion of the entire gene or mutations affecting the DNA-binding affinity of MSX2 where found in kindreds affected by the parietal foramina type 1 syndrome (PFM1; MIM#168500), featured by symmetric calvarial defects in the parietal bone, variably associated with additional craniofacial malformations (including cleft lip/palate, scalp defects and cranium bifidum), headache and seizures. Finally, parietal foramina with cleidocranial dysplasia (PFMCCD, MIM#168550) has been recently classified as a distinct MSX2-related mendelian disorder, in which the PFM phenotype is associated with clavicular hypoplasia and mild craniofacial dysmorphisms . In this latter case, a frameshift mutation in the homeodomain leading to premature termination of MSX2 translation was found (Garcia-Minaur et al., 2003). The association of these three allelic genetic diseases, strengthened the idea of MSX2 involvement in the control of membranous ossification.

2.10 MicroRNAs

The fine regulation of gene function necessary for the correct orchestration of osteogenesis and skeletal development may occur at several levels. One mechanism possibly acting in this process is represented by the post-transcriptional modulation operated by micro ribonucleic acids (microRNA or miRNA). miRNAs are a growing group of small (~22 ribonucleotides), single-stranded, noncoding RNAs that generally attenuate gene function. They regulate the translation of specific messenger RNA (mRNA) by base pairing with target complementary sequences (Carthew & Sontheimer, 2009). miRNA were first discovered in the nematode *Caenorhabditis elegans* and then found in diverse species, showing high degrees of evolutionary conservation. MicroRNAs are involved in many developmental signaling pathways and in housekeeping regulation of organ physiology (Schramke & Allshire, 2003). Over 1400 human miRNAs are deposited in the widest miRNA database (Griffiths-Jones et al, 2004, 2006, 2008; Kozomara et al., 2011; http://www.mirbase.org/). With regard to the regulation of bone formation, a growing number of miRNAs are found to be expressed in the developing skeletal system of metazoan, where are reasonably involved in regulating skeletal tissue homeostasis and development (He et al, 2009). Besides the emerging role of miRNAs during embryo skeletogenesis, miRNA-dependent modulation of gene function can alter skeletal phenotypes across individuals and also within same individual over time. This interpretation derives from recent studies focusing on miRNA biology in the pathogenesis of osteoporosis. Different miRNAs are upregulated in sencescent mesenchymal cells, leading to reduced cell plasticity and multilineage potential. Being able to modify the cell differentiation fate, miRNAs should interfere with the main developmental signaling pathways. Particularly, recent evidences suggest that miRNAs might have a regulatory function in osteoblast differentiation (Z. Li et al, 2008). BMP signaling pathway can be modulated at various level by miRNA; relevant results that recently emerged on this issue are shortly cited as examples. Mir125b inhibits osteoblast differentiation by reducing the cell proliferation rate; miR26a has been shown to inhibit the osteogenic differentiation of adipose tissue-derived stromal cells through intereference on Smad1 translation ; on their turn, Smads participate in miRNA biogenesis (Mizuno et al, 2008); miR-2861 enhances BMP2-induced osteoblastogenesis by repressing the histone deacetylase 5 gene, which induce Runx2 degradation (H. Li et al, 2009). Another miRNA, namely miR-138, regulates the osteogenic differentiation of human mesenchymal stem cells *in vivo* (Eskildsen et al, 2011). In addition, during BMP2-induced osteogenic differentiation of mesenchymal cells, the expression of miRNAs that target osteogenic genes is decreased (Z. Li et al, 2008).

Hence, the pathogenic increase or decrease of miRNAs targeting osteogenic genes, along with the action of BMPs on miRNA biogenesis, may influence bone develoment, concurring in the pathogenesis of bone-defective or hyper-ossification disorders.

Interestingly, several miRNA-coding genes are located within HOX gene clusters on evolutionary conserved chromosomal loci, and share their expression pattern. How this genomic situation could imply a HOX-miRNA functional interaction is still unclear, although Hox genes figure among miRNA targets (Yekta et al, 2008).

Finally, distinct studies have demonstrated that sequence variations occurring in miRNA genes can be associated to human diseases or disease-predisposition (Calin et al, 2005; Duan et al, 2007; Jazdzewsky et al, 2008). A homozygous mutation in miR-2861 results in reduced osteoblast activity leading to osteoporosis (H. Li et al, 2009). The evolution of craniofacial variation among species, the development of human craniofacial disease, and the physiological changes leading to osteopenia/osteoporosis that increases with aging, could result from evolutionary variation in miRNA expression patterns and/or structural modifications in miRNA binding sites in mRNAs, thus depicting a brand new era in the genetics of human diseases (He et al, 2009).

3. Conclusion

Overall, the molecular scenario that has been systematically described in this chapter could allow understanding the complexity of bone tissue homeostasis. Far from being considered a "resting" differentiated tissue, bone appears to be extremely plastic, as the control of its homeostasis is driven by thousand of genes interacting in complex developmental networks, along with post-translational and epigenetic mechanisms that can modify the genome performance.

The number of actors playing in this scene is much wider than that described here, thus the screenplay of osteogenesis is still too complex to allow depicting an exhaustive overview. This complexity implies an extremely high number of human diseases affecting bone development, formation and integrity, that possibly can grow over as the genetic body of knowledge further develops.

4. References

Acampora, D., Merlo, G.R., Paleari, L., Zerega, B., Postiglione, M.P., Mantero, S., Bober, E., Barbieri, O., Simeone, A., Levi, G. (1999). Craniofacial, vestibular and bone defects in mice lacking the Distal-less-related gene Dlx5. Development, Vol. 126, pp. 3795–3809

Aïoub, M., Lézot, F., Molla, M., Castaneda, B., Robert, B., Goubin, G., Néfussi, J.R., Berdal, A. (2007). Msx2 -/- transgenic mice develop compound amelogenesis imperfecta, dentinogenesis imperfecta and periodental osteopetrosis. Bone, Vol. 41, No. 5, pp.: 851-9.

Alappat, S., Zhang, Z.Y., Chen, Y.P. (2003) Msx homeobox gene family and craniofacial development. Cell Res, Vol. 13, No. 6, pp. 429-42.

Amizuka, N., Warshawsky, H., Henderson, J.E., Goltzman, D., Karaplis, A.C. (1994). Parathyroid hormone-related peptide-depleted mice show abnormal epiphyseal cartilage development and altered endochondral bone formation. J Cell Biol, Vol. 126, No. 6, pp. 1611-23.

Bachiller, D., Klingensmith, J., Kemp, C., Belo, J.A., Anderson, R.M., May, S.R., et al. (2000). The organizer factors chordin and noggin are required for mouse Forebrain Development. Nature, Vol. 403, No. 6770, pp. 658–61.

Bahamonde, M.E. & Lyons, K.M. (2001). BMP3: to be or not to be a BMP. J. Bone Joint Surg, Vol. 83-A, Suppl. 1, pp. S56–S62

Balint, E., Lapointe, D., Drissi, H., van der, M.C., Young, D.W., Van Wijnen, A.J., Stein, J.L., Stein, G.S., Lian, J.B. (2003) Phenotype discovery by gene expression profiling: mapping of biological processes linked to BMP-2-mediated osteoblast differentiation. J. Cell Biochem, Vol. 89, pp. 401–426.

Behrens, J., von Kries, J.P., Kuhl, M., Bruhn, L., Wedlich, D., Grosschedl, R., Birchmeier, W. (1996) Functional interaction of beta-catenin with the transcription factor LEF-1. Nature, Vol. 382, pp. 638–642.

Bendall, A.J. & Abate-Shen, C. (2000). Roles for Msx and Dlx homeoproteins in vertebrate development. Gene, Vol. 247, No. 1-2, pp. 17-31.

Bennett, C.N., Longo, K.A., Wright, W.S., Suva, L.J., Lane, T.F., Hankenson, K.D., & MacDougald, O.A. (2005). Regulation of osteoblastogenesis and bone mass by Wnt10b. Proc Natl Acad Sci U S A, Vol. 102, No. 9, pp. 3324-9.

Berdal, A., Molla, M., Hotton, D., Aïoub, M., Lézot, F., Néfussi, J.R. & Goubin, G. (2009). Differential impact of MSX1 and MSX2 homeogenes on mouse maxillofacial skeleton. Cells Tissues Organs, Vol 189, No. 1-4, pp. 126-32.

Bernardini, C., Saulnier, N., Parrilla, C., Pola, E., Gambotto, A., Michetti, F., Robbins, P.D., & Lattanzi, W. (2010). Early transcriptional events during osteogenic differentiation of human bone marrow stromal cells induced by Lim mineralization protein 3. Gene Expr, Vol. 15, No. 1, pp. 27-42.

Bernardini, C., Barba, M., Novegno, F., Massimi, L., Tamburrini, G., Michetti, F., Di Rocco, C. & Lattanzi, W. (2011) Molecular Profiling of Human Sporadic Craniosynostosis. Abstracts of the European Human Genetics Conference, Eur J Hum Genet. Vol. 19, Suppl. 2, pp. P.11.040

Bilic, J., Huang, Y.L., Davidson, G., Zimmermann, T., Cruciat, C.M., Bienz, M., & Niehrs, C. (2007) Wnt induces LRP6 signalosomes and promotes dishevelled-dependent LRP6 phosphorylation. Science,; Vol. 316, No. 5831, pp. 1619-22.

Boden, S.D., Liu, Y., Hair, G.A., Helms, J.A., Hu, D., Racine, M., Nanes, M.S., & Titus, L. (1998) LMP-1, a LIM-domain protein, mediates BMP-6 effects on bone formation. Endocrinology, Vol. 139, No, 12, pp. 5125-34.

Boden, S.D., Titus, L., Hair, G., Liu, Y., Viggeswarapu, M., Nanes, M.S., & Baranowski, C. (1998b). Lumbar spine fusion by local gene therapy with a cDNA encoding a novel osteoinductive protein (LMP-1). Spine, Vol. 23, No. 23, pp. 2486-92.

Boden, S.D. (2005). The ABCs of BMPs. Orthop Nurs, Vol. 24, No. 1, pp. 49-52.

Bourgeois, P., Stoetzel, C., Bolcato-Bellemin, A.L., Mattei, M.G., & Perrin-Schmitt, F. (1996). The human H-twist gene is located at 7p21 and encodes a B-HLH protein that is 96% similar to its murine M-twist counterpart. Mamm Genome, Vol. 7, No. 12, pp. 915-7.

Boyce, B.F., & Xing, L. (2008). Functions of RANKL/RANK/OPG in bone modeling and remodeling. Arch Biochem Biophys, Vol. 473, No. 2, pp. 139-46.

Brunet, L. J., McMahon, J. A., McMahon, A. P., & Harland, R.M. (1998). Noggin, cartilage morphogenesis, and joint formation in the mammalian skeleton. Science, Vol. 280, pp. 1455-1457.

Brunkow, M.E., Gardner, J.C., Van Ness, J., Paeper, B.W., Kovacevich, B.R., Proll, S., et al. (2001) Bone dysplasia sclerosteosis results from loss of the SOST gene product, a novel cystine-knot-containing protein. Am J Hum Genet , Vol. 68, No. 3, pp. 577–89.

Bucay, N., Sarosi, I., Dunstan, C.R., Morony, S., Tarpley, J., Capparelli, C., Scully, S.,Tan, H.L., Xu, W., Lacey, D.L., Boyle, W.J., & Simonet, W.S. (1998) osteoprotegerin-deficient mice develop early onset osteoporosis and arterial calcification. Genes Dev, vol.12, No. 9, pp. 1260-8.

Bulman, M.P., Kusumi, K., Frayling, T.M., McKeown, C., Garrett, C., Lander, E.S., Krumlauf, R., Hattersley, A.T., Ellard, S., & Turnpenny PD. (2000). Mutations in the human delta homologue, DLL3, cause axial skeletal defects in spondylocostal dysostosis. Nat Genet, Vol. 24, pp. 438–441.

Bünger, M.H., Langdahl, B.L., Andersen, T., Husted, L., Lind, M., Eriksen, E.F., & Bünger, C.E. (2003). Semiquantitative mRNA measurements of osteoinductive growth factors in human iliac-crest bone: expression of LMP splice variants in human bone. Calcif Tissue Int, Vol. 73, No. 5, pp. 446-54.

Burke, R., Nellen, D., Bellotto, M., Hafen, E., Senti, K.A., Dickson, & B.J., Basler, K. (1999). Dispatched, a novel sterol-sensing domain protein dedicated to the release of cholesterol-modified hedgehog from signaling cells. Cell, Vol. 99, No. 7, pp. 803-15.

Calin, G.A., Ferracin, M., Cimmino, A., Di Leva, G., Shimizu, M., Wojcik, S.E., Iorio, M.V., Visone, R., Sever, N.I., Fabbri, M., Iuliano, R., Palumbo, T., Pichiorri, F., Roldo, C., Garzon, R., Sevignani, C., Rassenti, L., Alder, H., Volinia, S., Liu, C.G., Kipps, T.J., Negrini, M., & Croce, C.M. (2005). A MicroRNA signature associated with prognosis and progression in chronic lymphocytic leukemia. N Engl J Med, Vol. 353, No. 17, pp. 1793-801.

Canalis, E., Economides, A.N., & Gazzerro, E. (2003). Bone morphogenetic proteins, their antagonists, and the skeleton. Endocr. Rev, Vol. 24 , pp. 218–235.

Capdevila, J., & Johnson, R. L. (1998) Endogenous and ectopic expression of noggin suggests a conserved mechanism for regulation of BMP function during limb and somite patterning. Dev. Biol, Vol. 197, pp. 205–217.

Carthew, R.W. & Sontheimer, E.J. (2009). Origins and Mechanisms of miRNAs and siRNAs. Cell, Vol. 136, No, 4, pp. 642-55.

Chen, A.E., Ginty, D.B., & Fan, C-M. (2005). Protein kinase a signalling via CREB controls myogenesis induced by Wnt proteins. Nature, Vol. 433:317–22.

Chen, D., Zhao, M., & Mundy, G.R. (2004). Bone morphogenetic proteins. Growth Factors, Vol. 22, No. 4, pp. 233-41.

Chen, H., Shi, S., Acosta, L. et al. (2004). BMP10 is essential for maintaining cardiac growth during murine cardiogenesis. Development. Vol. 131, pp. 2219–2231.

Cheng, H., Jiang, W., Phillips, F. M., Haydon, R. C., Peng, Y., Zhou, L., et al. (2003). Osteogenic activity of the fourteen types of human bone morphogenetic proteins (BMPs). J. Bone Joint Surg American, Vol. 85-A, pp. 1544-1552.

Chung, U.I., Lanske, B., Lee, K., Li, E., & Kronenberg, H. (1998).The parathyroid hormone/parathyroid hormone-related peptide receptor coordinates endochondral bone development by directly controlling chondrocyte differentiation. Proc Natl Acad Sci USA, Vol. 95, No. 22, pp. 13030-5.

Cohen, M.M. Jr. (2003) The hedgehog signaling network. Am J Med Genet A, Vol. 123, pp. 5-28.

Cohen, M.M. Jr. (2006). The new bone biology: pathologic, molecular, and clinical correlates. Am J Med Genet A, Vol. 140, No. 23, pp. 2646-706.

Colvin, J. S., Feldman, B., Nadeau, J. H., Goldfarb, M. & Ornitz, D. M. (1999) Genomic organization and embryonic expression of the mouse fibroblast growth factor 9 gene. Dev Dyn, Vol. 216, pp. 72-88.

Conlon, R.A., Reaume, A.G., & Rossant, J. (1995). Notch1 is required for the coordinate segmentation of somites. Development, Vol. 121, pp. 1533–1545.

Corbit, K.C., Aanstad, P., Singla, V., Norman, A.R., Stainier, D.Y., & Reiter, JF. (2005). Vertebrate smoothened functions at the primary cilium. Nature, Vol. 437, pp. 1018-21.

Davidson, G., Wu, W., Shen, J., Bilic, J., Fenger, U., Stannek, P., Glinka, A., & Niehrs, C. (2005). Casein kinase 1 gamma couples Wnt receptor activation to cytoplasmic signal transduction. Nature, Vol. 438, No. 7069, pp. 867-72.

Day, T.F., Guo, X., Garrett-Beal, L., & Yang, Y. (2005) Wnt/beta-catenin signaling in mesenchymal progenitors controls osteoblast and chondrocyte differentiation during vertebrate skeletogenesis. Dev Cell, Vol. 8, No. 5, pp. 739-50.

del Barco Barrantes, I., Davidson, G., Grone, H.J.,Westphal, H., & Niehrs, C. (2003). Dkk1 and noggin cooperate in mammalian head induction. Genes Dev, Vol. 17, No. 18, pp. 2239–44.

deLapeyriere, O., Ollendorff, V., Planche, J., Ott, M. O., Pizette, S., Coulier, F., & Birnbaum, D. (1993). Expression of the Fgf6 gene is restricted to developing skeletal muscle in the mouse embryo. Development, Vol. 118, pp. 601-611.

Duan, R., Pak, C., & Jin, P. (2007). Single nucleotide polymorphism associated with mature miR-125a alters the processing of pri-miRNA. Hum Mol Genet, Vol. 16, No. 9, pp. 1124-31.

Dudley, A.T., Lyons, K.M. & Robertson. E.J. (1995). A requirement for bone morphogenetic protein-7 during development of the mammalian kidney and eye. Genes Dev, Vol.9, pp. 2795–2807.

Ehlen, H.W., Buelens, L.A., & Vortkamp, A. (2006). Hedgehog signaling in skeletal development. Birth Defects Res C Embryo Today, Vol. 78, No. 3, pp. 267-79.

el Ghouzzi, V., Le Merrer, M., Perrin-Schmitt, F., Lajeunie, E., Benit, P., Renier, D., Bourgeois, P., Bolcato-Bellemin, A.L., Munnich, A., & Bonaventure, J. (1997). Mutations of the TWIST gene in the Saethre-Chotzen syndrome. Nat Genet. Vol. 15, No. 1, pp. 42-6.

Elefteriou, F., Ahn, J.D., Takeda, S., Starbuck, M., Yang, X., Liu, X., Kondo, H., Richards, W.G., Bannon, T.W., Noda, M.,, Clement, K., Vaisse, C., & Karsenty, G. (2005). Leptin regulation of bone resorption by the sympathetic nervous system and CART. Nature, Vol. 434, No. 7032, pp. 514-20.

Engin, F. & Lee, B. (2010). NOTCHing the bone: Insights into multi-functionality. Bone. 2010 February ; 46(2): 274–280

Eskildsen T, Taipaleenmäki H, Stenvang J, Abdallah BM, Ditzel N, Nossent AY, Bak M, Kauppinen S, Kassem M. (2011). MicroRNA-138 regulates osteogenic differentiation of human stromal (mesenchymal) stem cells *in vivo*. Proc Natl Acad Sci U S A, Vol. 108, No. 15, pp. 6139-44.

Eswarakumar, V. P., Lax, I. & Schlessinger, J. (2005). Cellular signaling by fibroblast growth factor receptors. Cytokine Growth Factor Rev, Vol. 16, pp. 139-149.

Evans, C. (2011). Gene therapy for the regeneration of bone. Injury, Vol. 42, No. 6, pp. 599-604.

Fang, P., Wang, X., Zhang, L., Yuan, G., Chen, Z., & Zhang, Q. (2010). Immunohistochemical localization of LIM mineralization protein 1 during mouse molar development. J Mol Histol, Vol. 41, No. 4-5, pp. 199-203.

Finch, P. W., Cunha, G. R., Rubin, J. S., Wong, J. & Ron, D. (1995). Pattern of keratinocyte growth factor and keratinocyte growth factor receptor expression during mouse fetal development suggests a role in mediating morphogenetic mesenchymal-epithelial interactions. Dev Dyn, Vol. 203, pp. 223-240.

Fiore, F., Planche, J., Gibier, P., Sebille, A., deLapeyriere O., & Birnbaum, D. (1997). Apparent normal phenotype of Fgf6-/- mice. Int J Dev Biol, Vol. 41, pp. 639-642.

Fuerer, C., Nusse, R., & Ten Berge, D. (2008). Wnt signalling in development and disease. Max Delbruck Center forMolecular Medicine meeting on Wnt signaling in development and disease. EMBO Rep, Vol. 9, pp. 134–138.

Garcia-Minaur, S., Mavrogiannis, L. A., Rannan-Eliya, S. V., Hendry, M. A., Liston, W. A., Porteous, M. E. M., & Wilkie, A. O. M. (2003). Parietal foramina with cleidocranial dysplasia is caused by mutation in MSX2. Europ J Hum Gene,. Vol. 11, pp. 892-895.

Gautschi, O.P., Frey, S.P., & Zellweger, R. (2007). Bone morphogenetic proteins in clinical applications. ANZ J Surg.Vol. 77, No. 8, pp. 626-31.

Gimble, J.M., Morgan, C., Kelly, K., et al. (1995). Bone morphogenetic proteins inhibit adipocyte differentiation by bone marrowstromal cells. J. Cell. Biochem. Vol. 58, pp. 393–402.

Glass, D.A. 2nd, Bialek, P., Ahn, J.D., Starbuck, M., Patel, M.S., Clevers, H., Taketo, M.M., Long, F., McMahon, A.P., Lang, R.A., & Karsenty, G. (2005). Canonical Wnt signaling in differentiated osteoblasts controls osteoclast differentiation. Dev Cell, Vol. 8, No. 5, pp. 751-64.

Gong, Y., Slee, R.B., Fukai, N., Rawadi, G., Roman-Roman, S., Reginato, A.M., Wang, H., Cundy, T., Glorieux, F.H., Lev, D., Zacharin, M., Oexle, K., Marcelino, J., Suwairi, W., Heeger, S., Sabatakos, G., Apte, S., Adkins, W.N., Allgrove, J., Arslan-Kirchner, M., Batch, J.A., Beighton, P., Black, G.C., Boles, R.G., Boon, L.M., Borrone, C., Brunner, H.G., Carle, G.F., Dallapiccola, B., De Paepe, A., Floege, B., Halfhide, M.L., Hall, B., Hennekam, R.C., Hirose, T., Jans, A., Jüppner, H., Kim, C.A., Keppler-Noreuil, K., Kohlschuetter, A., LaCombe, D., Lambert, M., Lemyre, E., Letteboer, T., Peltonen, L., Ramesar, R.S., Romanengo, M., Somer, H., Steichen-Gersdorf, E., Steinmann, B., Sullivan, B., Superti-Furga, A., Swoboda, W., van den Boogaard, M.J., Van Hul, W., Vikkula, M., Votruba, M., Zabel, B., Garcia, T., Baron, R., Olsen, B.R., & Warman, M.L. (2001). Osteoporosis-Pseudoglioma Syndrome Collaborative Group. LDL receptor-related protein 5 (LRP5) affects bone accrual and eye development. Cell, Vol. 107, No. 4, pp. 513-23.

Grano, M., Colucci, S., Cantatore, F.P., Teti, A. & Zambonin Zallone A. (1990) Osteoclast bone resorption is enhanced in the presence of osteoblasts. Boll Soc Ital Biol Sper, Vol 66, No 11, pp.1051-7.

Gregory, C.A., Gunn, W.G., Reyes, E., Smolarz, A.J., Munoz, J., Spees, J.L., Prockop, D.J. (2005) How Wnt signaling affects bone repair by mesenchymal stem cells from the bone marrow. Ann N Y Acad Sci. Vol 1049, pp 97-106.

Griffiths-Jones, S., Grocock, R.J., van Dongen, S., Bateman, A., Enright, A.J. (2006) miRBase: microRNA sequences, targets and gene nomenclature NAR, Vol 34(Database Issue), pp D140-D144

Griffiths-Jones S., Saini, H.K., van Dongen, S., Enright, A.J. (2008) miRBase: tools for microRNA genomics. NAR, Vol 36(Database Issue), ppD154-D158

Griffiths-Jones, S. (2004) The microRNA Registry NAR, Vol 32(Database Issue), pp D109-D111

Gripp, K.W., Zackai, E.H., Stolle, C.A. (2000) Mutations in the human TWIST gene. Hum Mutat.;15(2):150-5.

Groppe, J., Greenwald, J., Wiater, E., Rodriguez-Leon, J., Economides, A. N., Kwiatkowski, W., Affolter, M., Vale, W. W., Belmonte, J. C., and Choe, S. (2002) Structural basis of

BMP signalling inhibition by the cystine knot protein Noggin. Nature, Vol 420, pp 636–642

Grotewold, L., Ruther, U. (2002) The Wnt antagonist Dickkopf-1 is regulated by Bmp signaling and c-Jun and modulates programmed cell death. EMBO J, Vol 21, No 5, pp 966–75.

Guicheux, J., Lemonnier, J., Ghayor, C., Suzuki, A., Palmer, G., Caverzasio, J. (2003) Activation of p38 mitogen-activated protein kinase and c-Jun-NH2-terminal kinase by BMP-2 and their implication in the stimulation of osteoblastic cell differentiation. J Bone Miner Res. Vol 18, No 11, pp 2060-8.

Guo, L., Degenstein, L. & Fuchs, E. (1996) Keratinocyte growth factor is required for hair development but not for wound healing. Genes Dev, Vol 10, pp 165-175

Hall, B.K. & Miyake, T. (1995). Divide, accumulate, differentiate: cell condensation in skeletal development revisited. Int. J. Dev. Biol., Vol 39, pp 881–893

Hartmann, C., Tabin, C.J. (2000) Dual roles of Wnt signaling during chondrogenesis in the chicken limb. Development. Vol 127, No 14, pp 3141-59

Hartmann, C., Tabin, C.J. (2001) Wnt-14 plays a pivotal role in inducing synovial joint formation in the developing appendicular skeleton. Cell. Vol 104, No 3, pp 341-51

Hassan, M.Q., Javed, A., Morasso, M. I., Karlin, J., Montecino, M., van Wijnen, A. J., Stein, G. S., Stein, J. L., Lian, J. B. (2004). Dlx3 transcriptional regulation of osteoblast differentiation: temporal recruitment of Msx2, Dlx3, and Dlx5 homeodomain proteins to chromatin of the osteocalcin gene. Molec. Cell. Biol. Vol 24, pp 9248-9261,

Haub, O. & Goldfarb, M (1991). Expression of the fibroblast growth factor-5 gene in the mouse embryo. Development Vol 112, pp 397-406

Haycraft, C.J., Banizs, B., Aydin-Son, Y., Zhang, Q., Michaud, E.J., Yoder, B.K. (2005) Gli2 and Gli3 localize to cilia and require the intraflagellar transport protein polaris for processing and function. PLoS Genet. Vol 1, No 4, pp e53.

Hayes, A.J., Dowthwaite, G.P., Webster, S.V., Archer, C.W. (2003) The distribution of Notch receptors and their ligands during articular cartilage development. J Anat Vol 202, pp 495–502.

He, X., Eberhart, J.K., Postlethwait, J.H. (2009) MicroRNAs and micromanaging the skeleton in disease, development and evolution. J Cell Mol Med. Vol 13, No 4. pp 606-18.

Hebert, J.M., Rosenquist, T., Gotz, J. & Martin, G.R. (1994) FGF5 as a regulator of the hair growth cycle: evidence from targeted and spontaneous mutations. Cell. Vol 78, pp 1017-1025

Hill, T.P., Später, D., Taketo, M.M., Birchmeier, W., Hartmann, C. (2005) Canonical Wnt/beta-catenin signaling prevents osteoblasts from differentiating into chondrocytes. Dev Cell. Vol 8, No 5, pp 727-38

Howship, J. (1815) Experiments and Observations in order to ascertain the means employed by the animal economy in the formation of bone. Med Chir Trans. Vol 6, pp 263-676.5.

Huang, H.H., Brennan, T.C., Muir, M.M., Mason, R.S. (2009) Functional alpha1- and beta2-adrenergic receptors in human osteoblasts. J Cell Physiol. Vol 220, No 1, pp 267-75.

Jazdzewski, K., Murray, E.L., Franssila, K., Jarzab, B., Schoenberg, D.R., de la Chapelle, A. (2008) Common SNP in pre-miR-146a decreases mature miR expression and predisposes to papillary thyroid carcinoma. Proc Natl Acad Sci U S A. Vol 20, No105, pp 7269-74.

Jena, N., Martin-Seisdedos, C., Mccue, P. & Croce, C.M. (1997). BMP7 null mutation in mice: developmental defects in skeleton, kidney, and eye. Exp. Cell Res. Vol 230:, pp 28–37.

Kanaan, R.A., Kanaan, L.A. Transforming growth factor beta1, bone connection. Med Sci Monit. 2006 Aug;12(8):RA164-9.

Katagiri, T, Yamaguchi, A,. Komaki, M., Abe, E., Takahashi, N., Ikeda, T., Rosen, V., Wozney, J.M., Fujisawa-Sehara, A., Suda, T. (1994) Bone morphogenetic protein-2 converts the differentiation pathway of C2C12 myoblasts into the osteoblast lineage. J Cell Biol. Vol 127, No 6 Pt 1, pp 1755-66.

Kato, M., Patel, M.S., Levasseur, R., Lobov, I., Chang, B.H., Glass, D.A. 2nd, Hartmann, C., Li, L., Hwang, T.H., Brayton, C.F., Lang, R.A., Karsenty, G., Chan, L. (2002) Cbfa1-independent decrease in osteoblast proliferation, osteopenia, and persistent embryonic eye vascularization in mice deficient in Lrp5, a Wnt coreceptor. J Cell Biol. Vol 157, No 2, pp 303-14.

Kawabata, M., Imamura, T., Miyazono, K. (1998). Signal transduction by bone morphogenetic proteins. Cytokine Growth Factor Rev. Vol 9, pp 49–61

Khosla, S. Minireview: the OPG/RANKL/RANK system. (2001) Endocrinology. Vol 142, No12, pp 5050-5.

Kim, H.J., Rice, D.P., Kettunen ,P.J. & Thesleff, I. (1998) FGF-, BMP- and Shh-mediated signalling pathways in the regulation of cranial suture morphogenesis and calvarial bone development. Development, Vol 125, pp 1241-1251

Kim, H.J., Kim, J.H., Bae, S.C., Choi, J.Y., Kim, H.J. & Ryoo, H.M. (2003) The protein kinase C pathway plays a central role in the fibroblast growth factor-stimulated expression and transactivation activity of Runx2. J Biol Chem. Vol 278, pp 319-326

Kim, H.S., Viggeswarapu, M., Boden, S.D., Liu, Y., Hair, G.A., Louis-Ugbo, J., Murakami, H., Minamide, A., Suh, D.Y., Titus, L. (2003) Overcoming the immune response to permit *ex vivo* gene therapy for spine fusion with human type 5 adenoviral delivery of the LIM mineralization protein-1 cDNA. Spine (Phila Pa 1976). Vol 1, No 28(3), pp 219-26.

Komori, T., et al., (1997). Targeted disruption of Cbfa1 results in a complete lack of bone formation owing to maturational arrest of osteoblasts. Cell. Vol 89, pp 755–764.

Kozawa, O., Hatakeyama, D., Uematsu, T. (2002) Divergent regulation by p44/p42 MAP kinase and p38 MAP kinase of bone morphogenetic protein-4-stimulated osteocalcin synthesis in osteoblasts. J Cell Biochem. Vol 84, No 3, pp 583-9.

Kozomara, A., Griffiths-Jones, S. (2011) miRBase: integrating microRNA annotation and deep-sequencing data. NAR Vol 39(Database Issue), pp D152-D157

Kraus, P., Lufkin, T. (2006) Dlx homeobox gene control of mammalian limb and craniofacial development. Am J Med Genet A. Vol 1, No 140(13), pp 1366-74.

Krause, C., Guzman, A., Knaus, P. (2011) Noggin. Int J Biochem Cell Biol. Vol 43, No 4, pp 478-81.

Kuhl, M., Sheldahl, L.C., Park, M., Miller, J.R., Moon, R.T. (2000) The Wnt/Ca+2 pathway: a new vertebrate Wnt signaling pathway takes shape. Trends Genet. Vol 16, pp 279–83

Kusu, N., Laurikkala, J., Imanishi, M., Usui, H., Konishi, M., Miyake, A., et al. (2003) Sclerostin is a novel secreted osteoclast-derived bone morphogenetic protein antagonist with unique ligand specificity. J Biol Chem. Vol 278, No 26, pp 24113-7.

Lako, M., Strachan, T., Bullen, P., Wilson, D.I., Robson, S.C., Lindsay, S. (1998) Isolation, characterisation and embryonic expression of WNT11, a gene which maps to 11q13.5 and has possible roles in the development of skeleton, kidney and lung. Gene. Vol 219, No 1-2, pp 101-10.

Lallemand, Y., Nicola, M.A., Ramos, C., Bach, A., Cloment, C.S., Robert, B. (2005) Analysis of Msx1; Msx2 double mutants reveals multiple roles for Msx genes in limb development. Development. Vol 132, No 13, pp 3003-14.

Lattanzi, W., Parrilla, C., Fetoni, A., Logroscino, G., Straface, G., Pecorini, G., Stigliano, E., Tampieri, A., Bedini, R., Pecci, R., Michetti, F., Gambotto, A., Robbins, P.D., Pola, E. (2008) *Ex vivo*-transduced autologous skin fibroblasts expressing human Lim mineralization protein-3 efficiently form new bone in animal models. Gene Ther. Vol 15, No 19, pp 1330-43.

Lattanzi, W., Pola, E., Pecorini, G., Logroscino, C.A., Robbins, P.D. (2005) Gene therapy for *in vivo* bone formation: recent advances. Eur Rev Med Pharmacol Sci. Vol 9, No 3, pp 167-74

Lazarus, J.E., Hegde, A., Andrade, A.C, Nilsson, O. & Baron, J. (2007) Fibroblast growth factor expression in the postnatal growth plate. Bone Vol 40, pp 577-586

Levi, G., Mantero, S., Barbieri, O., Cantatore, D., Paleari, L., Beverdam, A., Genova, F., Robert, B., Merlo, G.R. (2006) Msx1 and Dlx5 act independently in development of craniofacial skeleton, but converge on the regulation of Bmp signaling in palate formation. Mech Dev. Vol 123, No 1, pp3-16.

Li, H., Xie, H., Liu, W., Hu, R., Huang, B., Tan, Y.F., Xu, K., Sheng, Z.F., Zhou, H.D., Wu, X.P. & Luo, X.H. (2009) A novel microRNA targeting HDAC5 regulates osteoblast differentiation in mice and contributes to primary osteoporosis in humans. J Clin Invest. Vol 119, No 12, pp 3666-77.

Li, L., Krantz, I.D., Deng, Y., Genin, A., Banta, A.B., Collins, C.C., Qi, M., Trask, B.J., Kuo, W.L., Cochran, J., Costa, T., Pierpont, M.E., Rand, E.B., Piccoli, D.A., Hood, L., Spinner, N.B. (1997) Alagille syndrome is caused by mutations in human Jagged1, which encodes a ligand for Notch1. Nat Genet. Vol 16, pp 243-251.

Li, Z., Hassan, M.Q., Volinia, S., van Wijnen, A.J., Stein, J.L., Croce, C.M., Lian, J.B., Stein, G.S. (2008) A microRNA signature for a BMP2-induced osteoblast lineage commitment program. Proc Natl Acad Sci U S A. Vol 105, No 37, pp 13906-11.

Li, X., Ma, L., Snead, M., Haworth, I., Sparkes, R., Jackson, C., Warman, M., Mulliken, J., Maxson, R., Muller, U., Jabs, E. (1993) A mutation in the homeodomain of the MSX2 gene in a family affected with craniosynostosis, Boston type. (Abstract) Am. J. Hum. Genet. 53 (suppl.): A213 only,.

Liu, H., Bargouti, M., Zughaier, S., Zheng, Z., Liu, Y., Sangadala, S., Boden, S.D., Titus, L. (2010) Osteoinductive LIM mineralization protein-1 suppresses activation of NF-kappaB and selectively regulates MAPK pathways in pre-osteoclasts. Bone. Vol 46, No 5, pp 1328-35.

Liu, Y., Hair, G.A., Boden, S.D., Viggeswarapu, M., Titus, L. (2002) Overexpressed LIM mineralization proteins do not require LIM domains to induce bone. J Bone Miner Res Vol 17, No 3, pp 406-14.

Liu, F., F. Ventura, J. Doody & J. Massague. (1995). Human type II receptor for bone morphogenic proteins (BMPs): extension of the two-kinase receptor model to the BMPs. Mol. Cell Biol. Vol 15, pp 3479–3486

Logan, C.Y., Nusse, R. (2004) The Wnt signaling pathway in development and disease. Annu Rev Cell Dev Biol, Vol 20, pp 781–810

Lum, L. and Beachy, P.A. (2004). The hedgehog response network: sensors, switches, and routers. Science Vol. 304, No. 5678, pp. 1755-9.

Luo, G., C. Hofmann, A.L. Bronckers, et al. (1995). BMP-7 is an inducer of nephrogenesis, and is also required for eye development and skeletal patterning. Genes Dev. Vol 9, pp 2808–2820.

Mani, A., Radhakrishnan, J., Wang, H., Mani, A., Mani, M.A., Nelson-Williams, C., Carew, K.S., Mane, S., Najmabadi, H., Wu, D., Lifton, R.P. (2007) LRP6 mutation in a family with early coronary disease and metabolic risk factors. Science. Vol 315, No 5816 pp 1278-82.

Mansukhani, A., P. Bellosta, M. Sahni & C. Basilico. (2000) Signaling by fibroblast growth factors (FGF) and fibroblast growth factor receptor 2 (FGFR2)-activating mutations blocks mineralization and induces apoptosis in osteoblasts. J Cell Biol Vol 149, pp 1297-1308

Massagué, J. (1998). TGF-beta signal transduction. Annu. Rev. Biochem, Vol. 67, pp. 753–791.

McLarren, K.W., Lo, R., Grbavec, D., Thirunavukkarasu, K., Karsenty, G., Stifani, S. (2000) The mammalian basic helix loop helix protein HES-1 binds to and modulates the transactivating function of the runt-related factor Cbfa1. J Biol Chem, Vol 275, pp 530–538.

McMahon, J.A., Takada, S., Zimmerman, L.B., Fan, C.M., Harland, R.M., McMahon, A.P. (1998) Nogginmediated antagonism of BMP signaling is required for growth and patterning of the neural tube and somite. Genes Dev, Vol 12, pp 1438–52

Mcpherron, A.C., A.M. Lawler & S.J. Lee. (1999). Regulation of anterior/posterior patterning of the axial skeleton by growth/differentiation factor 11. Nat. Genet. Vol 22, pp 260–264.

Milat, F., Ng, K.W. (2009) Is Wnt signalling the final common pathway leading to bone formation? Mol Cell Endocrinol. Vol 310, No(1-2), pp 52-62.

Minamide, A., Boden, S.D., Viggeswarapu, M., Hair, G.A., Oliver, C., Titus, L. (2003) Mechanism of bone formation with gene transfer of the cDNA encoding for the intracellular protein LMP-1. J Bone Joint Surg Am. Vol 85-A(6), pp 1030-9.

Miraoui, H., Marie, P.J. (2010) Pivotal role of Twist in skeletal biology and pathology. Gene Vol 468, No (1-2), pp 1-7

Miyazono, K., Maeda, S., Imamura, T. (2005) BMP receptor signaling: transcriptional targets, regulation of signals, and signaling cross-talk. Cytokine Growth Factor Rev. Vol 16, No 3, pp 251-63

Miyazono, K. (2000) Positive and negative regulation of TGF-beta signaling. J Cell Sci. Vol 113 (Pt 7), pp 1101-9.

Mizuno,Y., Yagi, K., Tokuzawa, Y., Kanesaki-Yatsuka, Y., Suda, T., Katagiri, T., Fukuda, T., Maruyama, M., Okuda, A., Amemiya, T., Kondoh, Y., Tashiro, H., Okazaki, Y. (2008) miR-125b inhibits osteoblastic differentiation by down-regulation of cell proliferation. Biochem Biophys Res Commun. Vol 368, No 2, pp 267-72.

Mlodzik, M. (2002) Planar cell polarization: do the same mechanisms regulate drosophila tissue polarity and vertebrate gastrulation? Trends Genet Vol 18, pp 564–71

Montero, A., Okada, Y., Tomita, M., Ito, M., Tsurukami, H., Nakamura, T., Doetschman, T., Coffin, J.D. & Hurley, M.M (2000) Disruption of the fibroblast growthfactor-2 gene results in decreased bone mass and bone formation. J Clin Invest Vol 105, pp 1085-1093

Muller, U., Warman, M.L., Mulliken, J.B., Weber, J.L. (1993) Assignment of a gene locus involved in craniosynostosis to chromosome 5qter. Hum. Molec. Genet. Vol 2, pp 119-122.

Nakashima, K., et al., (2002). The novel zinc finger-containing transcription factor osterix is required for osteoblast differentiation and bone formation. Cell Vol 108, pp 17–29.

Nohe, A., Hassel, S., Ehrlich, M., et al. (2002). The mode of bone morphogenetic protein (BMP) receptor oligomerization determines different BMP-2 signaling pathways. J. Biol. Chem. Vol 277, pp 5330–5338

Nusse, R., Varmus, H.E. (1982) Many tumors induced by the mouse mammary tumor virus contain a provirus integrated in the same region of the host genome. Cell. Vol 31, No 1, pp 99-109

Okamoto, M., Murai, J., Yoshikawa, H., Tsumaki, N. (2006) Bone morphogenetic proteins in bone stimulate osteoclasts and osteoblasts during bone development. J Bone Miner Res. Vol 21, No 7, pp 1022-33.

Opperman, L.A.(2000) Cranial sutures as intramembranous bone growth sites. Dev Dyn Vol 219, pp 472-485

Orestes-Cardoso, S., Nefussi, J.R., Lezot, F., Oboeuf, M., Pereira, M., Mesbah, M., Robert, B., Berdal. A. (2002) Msx1 is a regulator of bone formation during development and postnatal growth: *in vivo* investigations in a transgenic mouse model. Connect Tissue Res. Vol 43, No (2-3), pp 153-60.

Ozkaynak, E., Rueger, D.C., Drier, E.A., Corbett, C., Ridge, R.J., Sampath, T.K., Oppermann, H. (1990) OP-1 cDNA encodes an osteogenic protein in the TGF-beta family. EMBO J. Vol 9, No 7, pp 2085-93.

Pan, D., Fujimoto, M., Lopes, A., Wang, Y.-X. (2009) Twist-1 is a PPAR-delta-inducible, negative-feedback regulator of PGC-1-alpha in brown fat metabolism. Cell Vol 137, pp 73-86,.

Parrilla, C., Lattanzi, W., Fetoni, A., Bussu, F., Pola, E., Paludetti, G. (2010) *Ex vivo* gene therapy using autologous dermal fibroblasts expressing hLMP3 for rat mandibular bone regeneration. Head Neck. Vol 32, No 3, pp 310-8.

Pham, L., Beyer, K., Jensen, E.D., Rodriguez, J.S., Davydova, J., Yamamoto, M., Petryk, A., Gopalakrishnan, R., Mansky, K.C. (2011) Bone morphogenetic protein 2 signaling in osteoclasts is negatively regulated by the BMP antagonist, twisted gastrulation. J Cell Biochem. Vol 112, No 3, pp 793-803.

Piccolo, S., Agius, E., Leyns, L., Bhattacharyya, S., Grunz, H., Bouwmeester, T., De Robertis, E.M. (1999) The head inducer Cerberus is a multifunctional antagonist of Nodal, BMP and Wnt signals. Nature. Vol 397, No 6721, pp 707-10.

Pinson, K.I., Brennan, J., Monkley, S., Avery, B.J., Skarnes, W.C. (2000) An LDL-receptor-related protein mediates Wnt signalling in mice. Nature. Vol 40, No 6803, pp 535-8.

Pinzone, J.J., Hall, B.M., Thudi, N.K., Vonau, M., Qiang, Y.W., Rosol, T.J., Shaughnessy, J.D. Jr. (2009) The role of Dickkopf-1 in bone development, homeostasis, and disease. Blood. Vol 113, No 3, pp 517-25.

Piters, E., Boudin, E., Van Hul, W. (2008) Wnt signaling: a win for bone. Arch Biochem Biophys. Vol 473, No 2, pp 112-6.

Pola, E., Gao, W., Zhou, Y., Pola, R., Lattanzi, W., Sfeir, C., Gambotto, A., Robbins, P.D. (2004) Efficient bone formation by gene transfer of human LIM mineralization protein-3. Gene Ther. Vol 11, No 8, pp 683-93.

Rice, R., Rice, D.P. & Thesleff I. (2005) Foxc1 integrates Fgf and Bmp signalling independently of twist or noggin during calvarial bone development. Dev Dyn Vol 233, pp 847- 852.

Ripamonti, U., Ferretti, C., & Heliotis M. (2006). Soluble and insoluble signals and the induction of bone formation: molecular therapeutics recapitulating development. J Anat, Vol. 209, No. 4, pp. 447-68.

Rosen V. (2006) BMP and BMP inhibitors in bone. Ann N Y Acad Sci. Vol 1068, pp 19-25.

Ryoo, H.M., Lee, M.H., Kim, Y.J. (2006) Critical molecular switches involved in BMP-2-induced osteogenic differentiation of mesenchymal cells. Gene. Vol 17, No 366(1), pp 51-7.

Sangadala, S., Boden, S.D., Viggeswarapu, M., Liu, Y., Titus, L. (2006) LIM mineralization protein-1 potentiates bone morphogenetic protein responsiveness via a novel interaction with Smurf1 resulting in decreased ubiquitination of Smads. J Biol Chem. Vol 281, No 25, pp 17212-9.

Sangadala, S., Okada, M., Liu, Y., Viggeswarapu, M., Titus, L., Boden, S.D. (2009) Engineering, cloning, and functional characterization of recombinant LIM mineralization protein-1 containing an N-terminal HIV-derived membrane transduction domain. Protein Expr Purif. Vol 65, No 2, pp 165-73.

Schramke, V. & Allshire, R. Hairpin (2003) RNAs and retrotransposon LTRs effect RNAi and chromatin-based gene silencing. Science. Vol 301, No 5636, pp 1069-74

Scott, I.C., Blitz, I.L., Pappano, W.N., Imamura, Y., Clark, T.G., Steiglitz, B.M., Thomas, C.L., Maas, S.A., Takahara, K., Cho, K. W.Y., Greenspan, D.S. (1999) Mammalian BMP-1/Tolloid-related metalloproteinases, including novel family member mammalian Tolloid-like 2, have differential enzymatic activities and distributions of expression relevant to patterning and skeletogenesis. Dev. Biol. Vol 213, pp 283-300.

Semenov, M.V., Habas, R., Macdonald, B.T., & He, X. (2007). SnapShot: Noncanonical Wnt Signaling Pathways. Cell, Vol. 131, No. 7, pp. 1378.

Shishido, E., Higashijima, S., Emori, Y., & Saigo, K. (1993). Two FGF-receptor homologues of Drosophila: one is expressed in mesodermal primordium in early embryos. Development, Vol. 117, pp. 751-761.

Simonet, W.S., Lacey, D.L., Dunstan, C.R., Kelley, M., Chang, M.S., Lüthy, R., Nguyen, H.Q., Wooden, S., Bennett, L., Boone, T., Shimamoto, G., DeRose, M., Elliott, R., Colombero, A., Tan, H.L., Trail, G., Sullivan, J., Davy, E., Bucay, N., Renshaw-Gegg, L., Hughes, T.M., Hill, D., Pattison, W., Campbell, P., Sander, S., Van, G., Tarpley, J., Derby, P., Lee, R., & Boyle, W.J. (1997). Osteoprotegerin: a novel secreted protein involved in the regulation of bone density. I, Vol. 89, No. 2, pp. 309-19.

Simpson, P. (1983). Maternal-Zygotic Gene Interactions during Formation of the Dorsoventral Pattern in Drosophila Embryos. Genetics, Vol. 105, No. 3, pp. 615-32.

Singla, V. & Reiter, J.F. (2006). The Primary Cilium as the Cell's Antenna: Signaling at a Sensory Organelle. Science, Vol. 313, No. 5787, pp. 629-33.

Sobue, T., Naganawa, T., Xiao, L., Okada, Y., Tanaka, Y., Ito, M., Okimoto, N., Nakamura, T., Coffin, J. D.& Hurley, M. (2005). Over-expression of fibroblast growth factor-2 causes defective bone mineralization and osteopenia in transgenic mice. J Cell Biochem, Vol. 95, pp. 83-94.

Solloway, M.J., Dudley, A.T., Bikoff, E.K., et al. (1998). Mice lacking Bmp6 function. Dev. Genet, Vol. 22, pp. 321–339. 15.

Strohbach, C., Kleinman, S., Linkhart, T., Amaar, Y., Chen, S.T., Mohan, S., & Strong, D. (2008). Potential involvement of the interaction between insulin-like growth factor binding protein (IGFBP)-6 and LIM mineralization protein (LMP)-1 in regulating osteoblast differentiation. J Cell Biochem, Vol. 104, No. 5, pp. 1890-905.

Strohbach, C.A., Rundle, C.H., Wergedal, J.E., Chen, S.T., Linkhart, T.A., Lau, K.H., Strong, & D.D. (2008b). LMP-1 retroviral gene therapy influences osteoblast differentiation and fracture repair: a preliminary study. Calcif Tissue Int, Vol. 83, No. 3, pp. 202-11.

Su, N., Du, X., & Chen, L. (2008). FGF signaling: its role in bone development and human skeleton diseases. Front Biosci. Vol. 13, pp. 2842-65.

Suva, L.J., Winslow, G.A., Wettenhall, R.E., Hammonds, R.G., Moseley, J.M., Diefenbach-Jagger, H., Rodda, C.P., Kemp, B.E., Rodriguez, H., Chen, E.Y., et al. (1987). A parathyroid hormone-related protein implicated in malignant hypercalcemia: cloning and expression. Science, Vol. 237, No. 4817, pp. 893-6.

Suzuki, A., Ozono, K., Kubota, T., Kondou, H., Tachikawa, K., & Michigami, T. (2008). PTH/cAMP/PKA signaling facilitates canonical Wnt signaling via inactivation of glycogen synthase kinase-3beta in osteoblastic Saos-2 cells. J Cell Biochem, Vol. 104, No. 1, pp. 304-17.

Takada, I., Kouzmenko, A.P., & Kato, S. (2009). Wnt and PPARgamma signaling in osteoblastogenesis and adipogenesis. Nat Rev Rheumatol, Vol. 5, No. 8, pp. 442-7.

Takada, I., Mihara, M., Suzawa, M., Ohtake, F., Kobayashi, S., Igarashi, M., Youn, M.Y., Takeyama, K., Nakamura, T., Mezaki, Y., Takezawa, S., Yogiashi, Y., Kitagawa, H., Yamada, G., Takada, S., Minami, Y., Shibuya, H., Matsumoto, K., & Kato, S. (2007). A histone lysine methyltransferase activated by non-canonical Wnt signalling suppresses PPAR-gamma transactivation. Nat Cell Biol, Vol. 9, No. 11, pp. 1273-85.

Tamai, K., Semenov, M., Kato, Y., Spokony, R., Liu, C., Katsuyama, Y., Hess, F., Saint-Jeannet, J.P., & He, X. (2000) LDL-receptor-related proteins in Wnt signal transduction. Nature, Vol. 407, No. 6803, pp. 530-5.

Teti, A., Grano, M., Colucci, S., Cantatore, F.P., Loperfido, M.C., & Zallone, A.Z. (1991). Osteoblast-osteoclast relationships in bone resorption: osteoblasts enhance osteoclast activity in a serum-free co-culture system. Biochem Biophys Res Commun, Vol. 179, No. 1, pp. 634-40.

Tezuka, K., Yasuda, M., Watanabe, N., Morimura, N., Kuroda, K., Miyatani, S., & Hozumi, N.. (2002). Stimulation of osteoblastic cell differentiation by Notch. J Bone Miner Res, Vol. 17, pp. 231–239.

Tucker, A. S., Matthews, K. L.,& Sharpe, P. T. (1998). Transformation of tooth type induced by inhibition of BMP signaling. Science, Vol. 282, pp. 1136-1138.

Turnpenny, P.D., Alman, B., Cornier, A.S., Giampietro, P.F., Offiah, A., Tassy, O., Pourquie, O., Kusumi, K., & Dunwoodie, S. (2007). Abnormal vertebral segmentation and the notch signaling pathway in man. Dev Dy,; Vol. 236, pp. 1456–1474.

Tylzanowski, P., Mebis, L., Luyten, F.P. (2006). The Noggin null mouse phenotype is strain dependent and haploinsufficiency leads to skeletal defects. Dev Dyn, Vol. 235, pp. 1599–607.

Urist, M.R. 1965. Bone: formation by autoinduction. Science, Vol. 150, pp. 893–899.

van Amerongen, R., Mikels, A., & Nusse, R. (2008). Alternative wnt signaling is initiated by distinct receptors. Sci Signal. Vol. 1, No. 35, pp. re9.

van Bezooijen, R.L., Roelen, B.A., Visser, A., van derWee-Pals, L., deWilt, E., Karperien, M., et al. (2004). Sclerostin is an osteocyte-expressed negative regulator of bone formation, but not a classical BMP antagonist. J Exp Med , Vol. 199, No. 6, pp. 805–14.

van Reeuwijk, J., Arts, H.H., & Roepman, R. (2011). Scrutinizing ciliopathies by unraveling ciliary interaction networks. Hum Mol Genet, Vol., No. 20(R2), pp. R149-57.

Viggeswarapu, M., Boden, S.D., Liu, Y., Hair, G.A., Louis-Ugbo, J., Murakami, H., Kim, H.S., Mayr, M.T., Hutton, W.C., & Titus, L. (2001). Adenoviral delivery of LIM mineralization protein-1 induces new-bone formation *in vitro* and *in vivo*. J Bone Joint Surg Am, Vol. 83, No. A(3), pp. 364-76.

Vortkamp, A., Lee, K., Lanske, B., Segre, G.V., Kronenberg, H.M., & Tabin, C.J. (1996). Regulation of rate of cartilage differentiation by Indian Hedgehog and PTH-related protein. Science, Vol. 273, pp. 613-22.

Wan, M., & Cao, X. (2005). BMP signaling in skeletal development. Biochem Biophys Res Commun. Vol. 328, No. 3, pp. 651-7.

Wang, X., Cui, F., Madhu, V., Dighe, A.S., Balian, G., & Cui, Q. (2011). Combined VEGF and LMP-1 delivery enhances osteoprogenitor cell differentiation and ectopic bone formation. Growth Factors. Vol. 29, Vol. 1, pp. 36-48.

Wang, X., Zhang, Q., Chen, Z., & Zhang, L. (2008). Immunohistochemical localization of LIM mineralization protein 1 in pulp-dentin complex of human teeth with normal and pathologic conditions. J Endod, Vol. 34, No. 2, pp. 143-7.

Wang, E.A., Wang, E.A., Rosen, V., D'Alessandro, J.S., Bauduy, M., Cordes, P., Harada, T., Israel, D.I., Hewick, R.M., Kerns, K.M., LaPan P, et al., (1990). Recombinant human bone morphogenetic protein induces bone formation. Proc. Natl. Acad. Sci. U. S. A, Vol. 87, pp. 2220–2224.

Warden, S.J., Robling, A.G., Sanders, M.S., Bliziotes, M.M., & Turner, C.H. (2005). Inhibition of the serotonin (5-hydroxytryptamine) transporter reduces bone accrual during growth. Endocrinology, Vol. 146, No. 2, pp. 685-93.

Warman, M.L., Mulliken, J.B., Hayward, P.G., & Muller, U. (1993). Newly recognized autosomal dominant disorder with craniosynostosis. Am. J. Med. Genet., Vol. 46, pp. 444-449.

Warren, S.M., Brunet, L.J., Harland, R.M., Economides, A.N., & Longaker, M.T. (2003). The BMP antagonist noggin regulates cranial suture fusion. Nature, Vol. 422, pp. 625–9.

Wehrli, M., Dougan, S.T., Caldwell, K., O'Keefe, L., Schwartz, S., Vaizel-Ohayon, D., Schejter, E., Tomlinson, A., & Di Nardo, (2000). S. arrow encodes an LDL-receptor-related protein essential for Wingless signalling. Nature, Vol. 407, No. 6803, pp. 527-30

Weir, E.C., Philbrick, W.M., Amling, M., Neff, L.A., Baron, R., & Broadus, A.E. (1996). Targeted overexpression of parathyroid hormone-related peptide in chondrocytes causes chondrodysplasia and delayed endochondral bone formation. Proc Natl Acad Sci U SA., Vol. 93, No. 19, pp. 10240-5.

Westendorf, J.J., Kahler,R.A., & Schroeder. T.M. (2004). Wnt signaling in osteoblasts and bone diseases. Gene, Vol. 341, pp. 19–39.

Winkler, D.G., Sutherland, M.K., Geoghegan, J.C., Yu, C., Hayes, T., Skonier, J.E., et al. (2003). Osteocyte control of bone formation via sclerostin, a novel BMP antagonist. EMBO J, Vol. 22, No. 23, pp. 6267–76.

Wodarz, A., & Nusse, R., (1998). Mechanisms of Wnt signaling in development. Annu. Rev. Cell Dev. Biol., Vol. 14, pp. 59–88.

Wu, X., Shi, W., & Cao, X. (2007). Multiplicity of BMP signaling in skeletal development. Ann N Y Acad Sci, Vol. 1116, pp. 29-49.

Wu, X.B., Li, Y., Schneider, A., Yu, W., Rajendren, G., Iqbal, J., et al. (2003). Impaired osteoblastic differentiation, reduced bone formation, and severe osteoporosis in noggin overexpressing mice. J Clin Invest, Vol. 112, No. 924–34.

Yadav, V.K., Ryu, J.H., Suda, N., Tanaka, K.F., Gingrich, J.A., Schütz, G., Glorieux, F.H., Chiang, C.Y., Zajac, J.D., Insogna, K.L., Mann, J.J., Hen, R., Ducy, P. & Karsenty, G. (2008). Lrp5 controls bone formation by inhibiting serotonin synthesis in the duodenum. Cell, vol. 135, No. 5, pp. 825-37.

Yamaguchi, A., Komori, T., & T. Suda, (2000). Regulation of osteoblast differentiation mediated by bone morphogenetic proteins, hedgehogs, and Cbfa1. Endocr. Rev, Vol. 21, pp. 393–411.

Yanagita, M., Oka, M.,Watabe, T., Iguchi, H., Niida, A., Takahashi, S., et al. (2004). USAG-1: a bone morphogenetic protein antagonist abundantly expressed in the kidney. Biochem Biophys Res Commun, Vol. 316, No. 2, pp. 490–500.

Yanagita, M. (2005). BMP antagonists: their roles in development and involvement in pathophysiology. Cytokine Growth Factor Rev, Vol. 16, No 3, pp. 309-17.

Yekta, S., Tabin, C.J., & Bartel, D.P. (2008). MicroRNAs in the Hox network: an apparent link to posterior prevalence. Nat Rev Genet., Vol. 9, No. 10, pp. 789-96.

Yoon, S.T., Park, J.S., Kim, K.S., Li, J., Attallah-Wasif, E.S., Hutton, W.C., & Boden, S.D. (2004). ISSLS prize winner: LMP-1 upregulates intervertebral disc cell production of proteoglycans and BMPs *in vitro* and *in vivo*. Spine (Phila Pa 1976), Vol. 29, No. 23, pp. 2603-11.

Yu, K.,Xu, J., Liu, Z., Sosic, D., Shao, J., Olson, E. N., Towler, D.A.& Ornitz, D.M.(2003). Conditional inactivation of FGF receptor 2 reveals an essential role for FGF signaling in the regulation of osteoblast function and bone growth. Development, Vol. 130, pp.3063-3074.

Zackai, E.H. & Stolle CA. (1998). A New Twist: Some Patients with Saethre-Chotzen Syndrome Have a Microdeletion Syndrome. Am. J. Hum. Genet, Vol. 63, pp. 1277–1281.

Zaidi, M., (2007). Skeletal remodeling in health and disease. Nat. Med., Vol. 13, pp. 791–801.

Zallone, A. (2006). Direct and indirect estrogen actions on osteoblasts and osteoclasts. Ann N Y Acad Sci, Vol. 1068, pp. 173-9.

Zhang, J.-L., Huang, Y., Qiu, L.-Y., Nickel, J., Sebald, W. (2007). von Willebrand factor type C domain-containing proteins regulate bone morphogenetic protein signaling through different recognition mechanisms. J. Biol. Chem, Vol. 282: 20002-20014.

Zhao, G.Q., Deng, K., Labosky, P.A., et al. (1996). The gene encoding bone morphogenetic protein 8B is required for the initiation and maintenance of spermatogenesis in the mouse. Genes Dev, Vol. 10, No. 1657–1669.

Ziros, P.G., Gil, A.-P R., Georgakopoulos, T., Habeos, I., Kletsas, D., Basdra, E. K., Papavassiliou, A.G. (2002). The bone-specific transcriptional regulator Cbfa1 is a target of mechanical signals in osteoblastic cells. J. Biol. Chem., Vol. 277, pp. 23934-23941,.

Zwijsen, A., Verschueren, K., & Huylebroeck, D. (2003). New intracellular components of bone morphogenetic protein/Smad signaling cascades. FEBS Lett, Vol. 546, pp. 133–139.

3

Detrimental Effects of Alcohol on Bone Growth

Russell T. Turner, Elizabeth Doran and Urszula T. Iwaniec
Oregon State University,
USA

1. Introduction

Heavy drinking during adolescence may have immediate as well as long-term detrimental consequences to bone health. The growing skeleton is especially prone to fracture and alcohol may exacerbate fracture risk. Furthermore, a disproportionate amount of peak bone mass is acquired during adolescence. Alcohol, by decreasing bone formation, may decrease peak bone mass, predisposing the skeleton to early onset osteoporosis. Although it is well known that heavy drinking can have detrimental skeletal effects in adults (Turner 2000), few studies have focused specifically on the skeletal consequences of underage drinking in human subjects, in part, due to the difficulty in performing alcohol intervention studies in underage drinkers. As a result, the significance of alcohol consumption during this interval of rapid bone accretion on skeletal health is largely unknown. Thus, relevant animal models are critical for identifying the effects and mechanisms of action of alcohol on bone metabolism during bone growth. This chapter will focus on the detrimental effects of alcohol on the maturing skeleton using the laboratory rat as a model. We will also present evidence that these effects are mediated, at least in part, by alcohol-induced alterations in energy homeostasis.

2. Underage drinking

2.1 Magnitude of problem

Underage alcohol consumption is a major public health concern, especially in industrialized nations. The 2009 National Survey on Drug Use and Health reported that 10.4 million Americans between the ages of 12 and 17 had consumed alcohol during the month preceding the survey. Nearly 7 million of these teens reported engaging in binge drinking (5+ drinks on the same occasion) and 2.1 million classified themselves as heavy drinkers (5+ drinks per occasion on more than 5 days within the last month) (Department of Health and Human Services 2010). Rates of alcohol use, including binge and heavy drinking, have declined slightly since 2002; however alcohol consumption still occurs regularly in over 27% of American teenagers (Department of Health and Human Services 2010). High rates of alcohol consumption in youth were also reported in a 2008 survey of Australian secondary school students (White & Smith 2009). The European School Survey Project on Alcohol and Other Drugs, a survey of adolescent students in 35 European countries, reports even higher rates of alcohol use for European adolescents. The 2007 survey reported that within the month preceding the survey, 61% of students drank, 43% drank heavily, and 18% had been intoxicated (Hibell et al. 2009). However, none of these surveys provide insight regarding the effects of underage drinking on bone growth or, if an injury were to occur, on bone repair following the injury.

Globally, risky alcohol use among adolescents is on the rise (World Health Organization 2011). Although most under-age drinkers do not become alcohol-dependent, they are at increased risk for a variety of injuries and disorders. Liver cirrhosis, epilepsy, various forms of cancer, cardiovascular disease, and diabetes are just a few of the disorders that have been causally linked to alcohol consumption (Department of Health and Human Services 2010). Furthermore, alcohol use increases the chances of both intentional and unintentional injuries to bone due to violence and accidents.

2.2 Bone growth and maturation during adolescence

The attainment of peak bone mass occurs sometime during the third decade of life (Recker et al. 1992; Lin et al. 2003) but adolescence is a key time period in determining peak bone mass. Bone accrued during the 2 years surrounding the pubertal growth spurt accounts for approximately 25% of peak bone mass (Kontulainen et al. 2007). Roughly 90% of bone mass is achieved by late adolescence (Henry et al. 2004; Whiting et al. 2004). Modifiable factors such as diet are important determinants of peak bone mass (Eisman 1999; Bergmann et al. 2010; Ohlsson et al. 2011) and these effects may be compounded during the pubertal growth spurt. The introduction of factors inhibiting bone accrual during adolescence could lower peak bone mass and lead to decreased bone strength. A low peak bone mass, combined with age-related bone loss, has been shown to increase the likelihood of early onset osteoporosis, and the associated risk of fracture (Cooper et al. 2006; Xu et al. 2011). Reducing fracture risk in elderly osteoporotic populations is important, but 75% of the 6.8 million fractures occurring annually in the United States are <u>not</u> caused by osteoporosis. In fact, the group that accounts for the highest overall fracture rate is adolescent males (Goulding 2007). Heavy alcohol consumption may contribute to the high rate of fractures in this group.

3. Effects of alcohol on bone metabolism in growing animals

3.1 Animal models for investigating the effects and underlying mechanisms of action of alcohol on the maturing skeleton

Due to size and cost considerations, rats and mice are generally the preferred animals for investigating the actions of alcohol on bone metabolism. The reader is directed to our review of the strengths and weaknesses of rodents as animal models for osteoporosis (Iwaniec & Turner 2008). In brief, rodents are similar to humans in that bone grows by a combination of endochondral ossification and periosteal bone formation. Similarly, following the pubertal growth spurt, endochondral ossification slows in magnitude and ultimately ceases (Martin et al. 2003), while periosteal bone formation continues at a slow rate throughout the remainder of life. Humans, rats and mice undergo age-related bone loss, but it is unclear whether the mechanisms for the bone loss are the same across species.

Once formed, bone in humans is continuously remodeled. By repairing fatigue damage to bone, bone remodeling serves to maintain bone quality. Bone remodeling in rats is largely limited to endocortical and cancellous bone surfaces. Mice have very high rates of cancellous bone turnover but it is uncertain whether the close temporal and spatial integration of bone formation and resorption that characterizes bone remodeling in humans and rats occurs in mice. Haversion remodeling, the process by which cortical bone is remodeled in humans, is generally absent in small animals such as rats and mice. In spite of differences from humans, rodents, especially rats, have proven extremely valuable as preclinical animal models for osteoporosis. Regarding alcohol, not only has the rat accurately modeled the skeletal effects of chronic alcohol abuse in adults, some of the changes in bone and mineral homeostasis originally reported in the rat were subsequently shown to occur in human alcoholics (Turner et al. 1987; Turner et al. 1988).

There is no single pattern of alcohol consumption by underage drinkers. Drinking patterns range from occasional to regular, to binge. Based on dose-response and time-course studies in rats, the effects of alcohol on bone metabolism depend upon peak blood alcohol concentration and duration of exposure (Turner et al. 1998; Turner et al. 2001). As a consequence, no single animal model can replicate all of the actions of alcohol.

To model chronic alcohol consumption, alcohol can be delivered to animals in drinking water, as a component of a liquid diet or as a component of total intragastric nutrition (Lieber et al. 1989; French 2001). Addition of alcohol to drinking water is the simplest method but has significant disadvantages. Because of aversion to alcohol, high concentrations decrease fluid intake which may result in dehydration (Lieber et al. 1989). In addition, it is difficult to equalize macro and micronutrient levels among treatment groups. In particular, the controls receive all of their energy and nutrients from a standard rodent chow diet. This contrasts with the alcohol fed animals who receive their energy from both alcohol and diet, and other nutrients from the chow diet only. Lieber and colleagues, recognizing the limitations of delivering alcohol in drinking water, developed a liquid diet in which alcohol replaced carbohydrates isocalorically (Lieber et al. 1989). We have found this diet to be very useful for investigating the effects of alcohol on bone metabolism.

Total intragastric nutrition, while invasive and very labor intensive, is an alternative method which allows even better control of total nutrition. This method provides the investigator with complete control of the duration of exposure to alcohol. Thus, total intragastric nutrition is especially beneficial for delivering very high amounts of alcohol to induce a specific pathological response. However, because of exquisite sensitivity of the rodent skeleton to the metabolic effects of alcohol consumption, it is rarely necessary to employ alcohol levels that are high enough to require intragastric delivery.

Binge drinking is typically modeled by oral gavage or by intraperitoneal injection. Alcohol can also be delivered by intermittent intragastric infusion. We have experience using the first two methods. Although intraperitoneal injection is a convenient method to deliver alcohol for short duration studies (Turner et al. 1998), we have found that intraperitoneal injection of alcohol over multiple days does not reproduce the response obtained following oral administration. Daily delivery of alcohol (~1.2 g/kg) by either gavage or intraperitoneal injection resulted in a peak blood alcohol level of ~0.1 %. This dose rate had no significant effects on body weight gain, uterine weight or bone parameters in animals where alcohol was delivered by gavage (unpublished data). In contrast, alcohol delivered by intraperitoneal injection injection resulted in decreased cortical bone mass and drastic reductions in bone formation and mRNA levels for bone matrix proteins (Turner et al. 1998). We conclude from this and similar experiments that multiple intraperitoneal injections have severe effects on the skeleton that do not model the normal physiological response to alcohol.

Consistent with our data, Sampson et al. reported no detrimental effects on bone in growing rats using a model for binge drinking in which alcohol was administered by gavage on two consecutive days a week (Sampson et al. 1999). Based on the observation that longer exposure to relatively low blood levels of alcohol has greater effects on bone metabolism than brief exposure to high blood levels of alcohol, we have focused on skeletal response of growing rats to chronic alcohol consumption.

3.2 Effects of alcohol on the skeleton in growing rats

Long duration studies in growing rats have shown that chronic alcohol consumption decreases peak bone mass. For example, administration of alcohol (38% caloric intake) to post-pubertal Long Evans hooded rats for 10 months resulted in a decrease in tibia length, an increase in the size of the marrow cavity and a decrease in cancellous bone mass (Turner et al. 1988). The latter is important because reduced cancellous bone mass plays a key role in the etiology of osteoporotic fractures. Studies designed to evaluate bone growth have shown that alcohol inhibits the rate of bone elongation as well as addition of bone onto periosteal and endocortical endocortical surfaces of rapidly growing male rats (Figure 1) (Turner et al. 1987). These reductions in bone growth contribute to a decrease in bone mass. Similar changes were observed by Sampson and colleagues in growing female Sprague Dawley rats fed alcohol (Sampson et al. 1996; Hogan et al. 1997; Sampson et al. 1997; Sampson & Spears 1999).

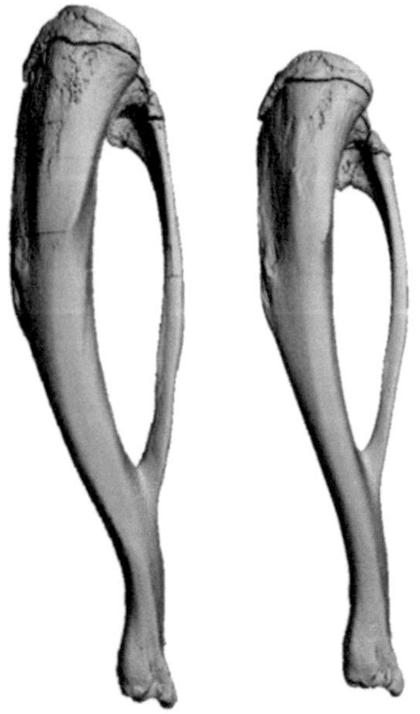

Fig. 1. Representative microcomputed tomography images of tibiae from rats fed control or alcohol diets. In this study, 4-week-old male rats were fed a liquid diet containing alcohol for 4 months. Except for isocaloric replacement of ethanol with maltose dextran, the controls were fed the same diet *ad libitum*. Chronic alcohol consumption (35% caloric intake) during post pubertal growth reduced peak bone mass as illustrated above for the tibia.

Bone formation is the product of osteoblast number and osteoblast activity. In growing rats, high levels of alcohol consumption were consistently found to decrease the extent of bone surface covered by active osteoblasts. The effect of alcohol on indices of osteoblast activity is less consistent, ranging from no effect to a moderate decrease. Alcohol results in a dose-associated decrease in osteoclast-lined bone surface (Turner et al. 2001). Thus, in addition to inhibiting bone formation, alcohol appears to inhibit bone resorption. Typical of low bone turnover forms of osteoporosis, bone loss in alcohol-fed rats is relatively slow (Hogan et al. 2001; Turner et al. 2001), a finding consistent with the slow rate of bone loss observed in adult chronic alcohol abusers (Odvina et al. 1995; Pumarino et al. 1996).

Chronic consumption of high levels of alcohol during growth reduces peak bone mass by inhibiting bone acquisition. However, there is conflicting evidence as to whether alcohol also impacts the extent of mineralization of bone matrix. Some, but not all, studies suggest that heavy drinking results in under-mineralization of bone matrix (Schnitzler & Solomon 1984; Turner et al. 1987; Diamond et al. 1989; Bikle et al. 1993; Schnitzler et al. 1994). To investigate this issue more fully, we determined the effects of alcohol consumption on bone formed following osteoinduction by demineralized bone matrix. In this model, ectopic bone is induced to form at extraskeletal sites in an animal by subcutaneous implantation of demineralized bone matrix. Used clinically in orthopedic practice to augment bone formation during fracture repair, osteoinduction is an ideal method to investigate the effect of alcohol on mineralization because experiments can be designed in which bone is not present until introduction of alcohol into the diet. In our studies, described elsewhere in detail (Trevisiol et al. 2007), subcutaneously implanted demineralized allogeneic bone matrix cylinders were used to model osteoinduction. Demineralized allogeneic bone matrix cylinders, prepared from femurs and tibiae of rats fed a normal diet, were implanted into sexually mature male rats adapted to alcohol (ethanol contributed 35% of caloric intake) or control liquid diets. Food intake in the control rats was restricted to match food intake of alcohol-fed animals. The implants were recovered 6 weeks later and analyzed by histology, microcomputed tomography and chemical analysis. Histological evaluation revealed a robust osteoinductive response, resulting in mature bone formation, in implants in rats fed the control diet. Alcohol consumption affected architecture of the implants but not volumetric density or mineral composition. Specifically, alcohol consumption resulted in significant decreases in demineralized allogeneic bone matrix-induced bone volume, bone volume/mg original cylinder weight, connectivity density, trabecular number and thickness, ash weight and % ash weight. There were, however, no changes in mineral (ash) density nor in the relative amounts of calcium, magnesium, iron, selenium and zinc (μg/mg ash), indicating that alcohol consumption reduced the amount of new bone formation but did not reduce mineral content of bone.

Osteoinduction is a key component in fracture repair. The decrease in osteinduction observed in the rats described above and in subsequent studies (Iwaniec et al. 2008) suggest that alcohol may impair fracture healing. Chronic exposure to dietary alcohol inhibits healing in a variety of models involving injury to bone (Chakkalakal et al. 2005; Wahl et al. 2005). However, it is not clear whether alcohol consumption has a clinically relevant effect on fracture healing in either humans or animal models. Addressing this important question should be a priority of future animal and human research.

4. Alcohol metabolism

It is not known whether the detrimental skeletal effects of alcohol on bone metabolism are due to the parent compound or a metabolite. The metabolism of ethanol occurs predominantly in the liver where ethanol is metabolized to acetaldehyde, a highly toxic metabolite, which in turn is rapidly metabolized to acetate. In addition to being released into circulation from the liver, it is conceivable that acetaldehyde is produced in skeletal tissue. Such a mechanism could lead to local levels of acetaldehyde that exceed circulating levels. However, based on the inability of cultured osteoblasts to reduce ethanol levels in culture media, it seems unlikely that osteoblasts produce acetaldehyde (Maran et al. 2001). This observation does not preclude the possibility that other cells within the local skeletal environment metabolize alcohol or that circulating levels of acetaldehyde are sufficient to have direct actions on bone cells. Further investigation is required to establish the contribution of acetaldehyde to the detrimental effects of alcohol on bone.

5. Does consuming alcohol have irreversible toxic effects on bone cells?

The question as to whether alcohol leads to irreversible toxic effects on the skeleton is important but has not been fully resolved. Alcohol consumption results in a dose-dependent decrease in bone formation that is paralleled by reductions in osteoblast-lined bone surface and osteoblast precursor pool in bone marrow (Dyer et al. 1998; Rosa et al. 2008). Reduced bone formation is preceded by lower mRNA levels for bone matrix proteins (Turner et al. 2001). These and similar data are often interpreted as evidence of toxicity. In support of toxicity, there is incomplete catch-up growth following cessation of alcohol feeding in growing rats (Sampson & Spears 1999). Similarly, bone mass does not return to normal when alcohol feeding is discontinued in skeletally mature rats (Sibonga et al. 2007). Taken together, these findings suggest that alcohol has irreversible toxic effects on the osteoblast. This conclusion appears to be supported by *in vitro* studies reporting that direct exposure to alcohol decreases proliferation of cultured osteoblasts and inhibits their synthesis of bone matrix proteins (Giuliani et al. 1999; Vignesh et al. 2006). However, the concentrations of alcohol necessary to achieve the detrimental effects in cell culture described above are generally very high, suggesting that mature osteoblasts are quite resistant to direct toxic effects of alcohol (Maran et al. 2001). In this regard, no direct toxicity was detected in dose-response studies performed on cultured human osteoblasts. Specifically, concentrations of ethanol that would be incompatible with human life had no effect on osteoblast number, proliferation or expression of genes for bone matrix proteins.

In contrast to the high concentrations of ethanol (50mM or greater) required to have direct inhibitory effects on osteoblasts in cell culture, much lower levels of alcohol reduce bone formation *in vivo*. This finding suggests that the inhibitory effects of alcohol on bone formation are primarily indirect (Turner et al. 2001). To further evaluate whether alcohol has irreversible indirect toxic effects on osteoblasts, we performed studies in which we administered parathyroid hormone to rats that had been fed alcohol (Turner et al. 2001). The bone anabolic effects of intermittent parathyroid hormone have been studied in humans and laboratory animals and currently, parathyroid hormone is the only bone anabolic therapy approved by the Federal Drug Administration for the treatment of postmenopausal osteoporosis. Parathyroid hormone is effective in increasing bone mass in most but not all subjects. Thus, lifestyle factors such as alcohol consumption, may inhibit the skeletal response to parathyroid hormone. However, studies to date in rats suggest that parathyroid hormone and alcohol have opposite but independent effects on bone formation. In other words, alcohol lowered the basal rate of bone formation compared to animals fed a normal diet and parathyroid hormone increased bone formation by the same magnitude in animals fed normal and alcohol diets (Turner et al. 2001; Sibonga et al. 2007; Iwaniec et al. 2008;

Howe et al. 2011). Additionally, administration of parathyroid hormone reversed bone loss in alcohol-fed rats (Sibonga et al. 2007). Taken together, these findings do not support an irreversible toxic effect of alcohol on bone cells. Indeed, they suggest that bone formation returns to normal following removal of alcohol from the diet, but a pharmacological intervention may be required to restore the bone that had been lost.

6. Mechanisms of action of alcohol on the growing skeleton

6.1 Alcohol is an endocrine disruptor

Bone metabolism is under tight endocrine control and it is well established that excessive alcohol consumption disrupts numerous endocrine functions. For example, alcohol consumption has been reported to alter the levels and skeletal responses to estrogen, vitamin D and parathyroid hormone (Dumitrescu & Shields 2005; Ronis et al. 2007; Sibonga et al. 2007). Each of these hormones play a key role in bone metabolism. As previously reviewed (Turner 2000; Turner & Sibonga 2001), disturbances in signaling by these hormones may contribute to the skeletal response to alcohol in adults. Less investigated, however, are the effects of alcohol on pituitary- (e.g., growth hormone) and adipocyte-derived (e.g, leptin) hormones. Disruption of signalling of hormones that function to integrate growth and energy metabolism by alcohol has not been intensively studied, but may be especially important to the effects of underage drinking on bone growth and maturation. As discussed below, alcohol alters local production and/or circulating levels of bone regulating hormones, proinflammatory cytokines (TNF-α) and adipokines related to energy intake and expenditure. In addition, there is evidence that alcohol results in end-organ resistance to two of the key mediators of energy homeostasis, growth hormone and leptin.

6.2 Impact of alcohol on energy metabolism

6.2.1 Energy metabolism

Bone growth during adolescence is tightly coupled to energy availability (Devlin et al. 2010). Regulation of energy metabolism involves the integration of signals from the digestive system, pancreas, liver, adipose tissue, hypothalamus and pituitary. The messengers that signal energy status and induce physiological adaptations consist of hormones, adipokines, cytokines, growth factors and neuronal networks. Alcohol consumption influences food intake and energy balance by altering the production and target organ response to these signals (Leibowitz 2005; Pravdova & Fickova 2006). As a consequence, we hypothesize that alcohol disrupts the tight coupling between energy availability and bone growth, maturation and turnover.

6.2.2 Effect of alcohol on energy intake

Alcohol has profound, dose-dependent effects on energy intake. Low concentrations of alcohol in the diet (0.5% and 3% caloric intake) were shown to enhance food consumption in rats (Turner et al. 2001; Turner & Iwaniec 2010). In contrast, higher alcohol concentrations generally suppress energy intake. Heavy alcohol consumption reduces bone formation in growing rats compared to pair-fed controls. However, pair-feeding underestimates the detrimental skeletal effects of alcohol consumption because self-selected caloric restriction in alcohol-fed rats also has detrimental effects on bone homeostasis (Maddalozzo et al. 2009).

6.2.3 Effect of alcohol on energy expenditure

Total energy expenditure reflects the sum of basal metabolic rate and energy consumed performing physical activity. The effect of alcohol consumption on total energy expenditure appears to be context dependent. In short-duration studies, pair-feeding control rats to animals fed a diet containing alcohol usually equalizes weight gain among treatment groups, but not necessarily body composition (see below). Also, in a 10-month-long study, slightly more energy was required to achieve the same weight gain in rats fed a diet containing ethanol (38% caloric intake) than the rats fed the control diet (Turner et al. 1988). In a 4-month-long study investigating the skeletal response to physical activity, treadmill-exercised rats fed a diet in which alcohol contributed 35% of caloric intake gained weight in parallel with exercised animals fed the control diet. Furthermore, exercise decreased weight gain compared to pair-fed non-exercising controls. Thus alcohol did not influence the increased energy requirements associated with a higher rate of physical activity. Overall, these findings suggest that alcohol does not have a major influence on overall energy expenditure.

There are, however, situations where alcohol consumption does influence energy metabolism. Specifically, changes in hormonal regulators of energy homeostasis may alter the relationship between alcohol consumption and energy expenditure. For example, estrogen acts physiologically to reduce energy intake and increases expenditure. In ovariectomized rats, estrogen deficiency results in increased weight gain which is due to a combination of hyperphagia and reduced energy expenditure. Similar to estrogen, alcohol increased energy expenditure in ovariectomized rats. As a consequence, pair-fed ovariectomized rats consuming a control diet gain more weight than animals fed the alcohol containing diet (Kidder & Turner 1998).

6.2.4 Body composition

Body composition was altered in sexually mature male rats fed alcohol (35% caloric intake) for 3 months. The alcohol-fed animals had less peripheral fat and a lower whole body bone mineral content compared to age-matched controls (Maddalozzo et al. 2009). In spite of an overall reduction in fat mass, bone marrow adiposity was increased in the rats fed alcohol (Maddalozzo et al. 2009). Similar to rodents, reduced peripheral fat and increased bone marrow adiposity is associated with chronic alcohol abuse in men (Liangpunsakul et al. 2010). In contrast, in a recent study investigating the role of estrogen in the skeletal response to alcohol we noted that heavy (35% caloric intake) alcohol consumption in slowly growing ovariectomized rats reduced overall body weight gain but increased white adipose tissue mass. Thus, there may be gender differences in the effects of alcohol on energy homeostasis.

The role of peripheral and bone marrow fat in regulation of bone metabolism appears complex and has generated a great deal of interest in recent years. As discussed below, alcohol-induced changes in peripheral and bone marrow fat depots may play an indirect but nevertheless important role in mediating the detrimental effects of alcohol consumption on the adolescent skeleton.

7. Alcohol disrupts the actions of key hormones that regulate energy metabolism

7.1 Leptin signaling is required for normal bone growth

As mentioned above, skeletal growth is tightly coupled to energy balance via complex and incompletely understood mechanisms. Leptin, the protein product of the *ob* gene, is produced by adipocytes and functions as a messenger in a feedback loop between adipose tissue and the hypothalamus. As such, leptin contributes to the regulation of energy intake and expenditure (Figure 2). Leptin also acts on other organs, including bone. Leptin-deficient *ob/ob* mice are morbidly obese and develop multiple pathologies associated with metabolic syndrome. Additionally, *ob/ob* mice have notable skeletal abnormalities. Initially, the *ob/ob* mouse was described as having high bone mass, but subsequent studies revealed a complex skeletal phenotype; compared to wild type (WT) mice, ob/ob mice have a low total and cortical bone but increased vertebral cancellous bone (Ducy et al. 2000; Bartell et al. 2011). The decrease in cortical bone in *ob/ob* mice is in part due to a decrease in bone length.

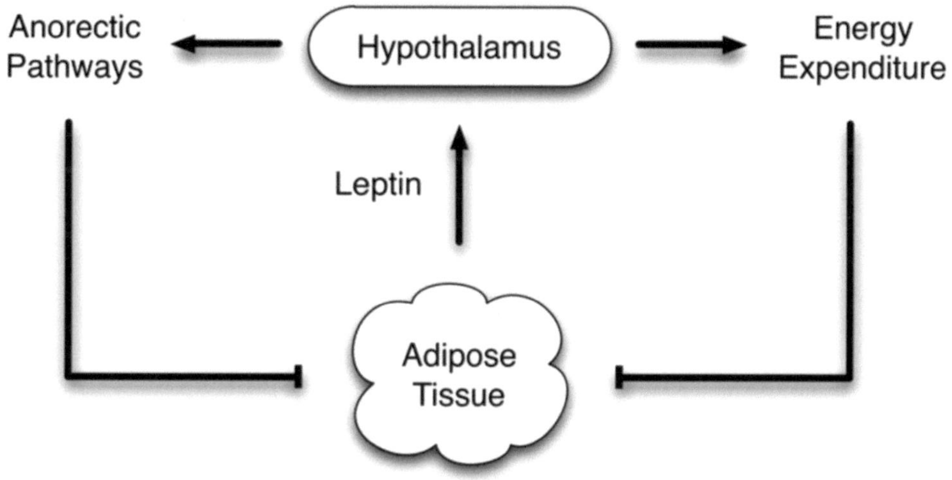

Fig. 2. Regulation of energy metabolism by leptin. Adipose tissue-derived leptin acts on the hypothalamus to increase energy expenditure and decrease appetite. These metabolic changes contribute to a negative feedback loop antagonizing further fat accumulation. Chronic alcohol consumption disrupts energy homeostasis by causing hypophagia, increased energy expenditure, and hypoleptinemia. Peripheral (serum) leptin functions physiologically to couple systemic growth (including bone growth) to energy availability. We hypothesize that chronic alcohol consumption during adolescence, by decreasing serum leptin levels, reduces bone growth which in turn contributes to the reduced peak bone mass observed in growing rats fed a diet containing alcohol.

To evaluate the effect of hypothalamic signaling as a mediator of the skeletal response to leptin, we performed a study in which growing *ob/ob* mice were injected in the hypothalamus with either adeno-associated virus-leptin (rAAV-lep) or a control vector coding for green fluorescent protein (rAAV-GFP). Treatment with rAAV-lep restored the *ob/ob* skeletal phenotype to WT by increasing femoral length and total bone volume, and decreasing femoral and vertebral cancellous bone volume. As a consequence, at 15 weeks post-rAAV-lep injection the *ob/ob* mice no longer differed from WT mice (Iwaniec et al. 2007). In recent unpublished studies we have shown that daily subcutaneous administration of leptin increases the longitudinal rate of bone growth in *ob/ob* mice as well as bone formation on cortical and cancellous bone surfaces. Taken together, these results suggest that leptin functions as an essential factor for normal bone growth and turnover.

7.2 Reduced leptin signaling as a mechanism for the detrimental effects of alcohol on bone growth

Alcohol alters serum leptin levels in humans and animals (Nicolas et al. 2001; Santolaria et al. 2003; Calissendorff et al. 2004; Otaka et al. 2007; Maddalozzo et al. 2009). Decreased leptin levels are often associated with chronic alcohol consumption in humans, even after accounting for alcohol-induced reductions in fat mass (Nicolas et al. 2001; Calissendorff et al. 2004; Otaka et al. 2007). However, the change in leptin levels depends upon the level and pattern of alcohol consumption. In our model of chronic adolescent drinking, there is a substantial decrease in serum leptin levels (Figure 3). Additionally, there are studies suggesting that alcohol impairs leptin signaling by inducing target organ resistance to the hormone (Gordeladze et al. 2002).

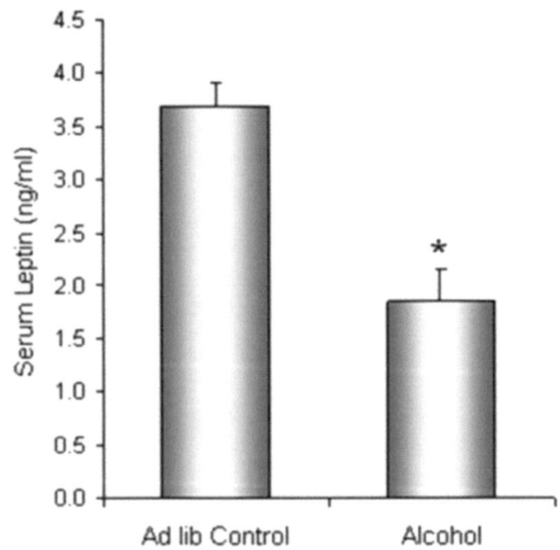

Fig. 3. Evidence for decreased leptin levels in serum of alcohol-fed rats compared to *ad labium*-fed (Ad lib) controls. Four-week-old male rats were fed alcohol containing (35%caloric intake) or control diets for 3 months. Data are mean ± SE, *P<0.05.

Leptin, in addition to having central actions mediated through the hypothalamus, has the potential to act directly on target organs, including bone (Burguera et al. 2001; Reseland et al. 2001; Gordeladze et al. 2002; Thomas 2004). The putative hypothalamic-mediated and direct pathways of leptin action on bone metabolism have been reviewed by Hamrick (Hamrick et al. 2004; Hamrick & Ferrari 2008). By transplanting bone marrow cells from leptin receptor-deficient *db/db* mice into WT mice, we have shown that the physiological actions of leptin on bone turnover are primarily due to peripheral leptin signaling (Unpublished data).

Leptin deficiency results in skeletal abnormalities that, in many ways, are similar to effects of chronic alcohol abuse. Specifically, leptin deficiency and alcohol consumption in growing rodents each result in decreases in longitudinal bone growth, radial bone growth, and cancellous bone turnover (Turner 2000; Iwaniec et al. 2007). Also, leptin deficiency and alcohol consumption in growing rodents each result in elevated bone marrow adiposity (Steppan et al. 2000; Hamrick et al. 2004; Hamrick et al. 2005; Hamrick & Ferrari 2008). Thus, one mechanism by which alcohol consumption may decrease bone acquisition during adolescence is by reducing leptin levels. Further studies are required to determine whether normalization of leptin levels in alcohol-fed growing rats corrects the detrimental effects of alcohol on bone growth, architecture and turnover.

8. Osteoblasts and adipocytes

As discussed, we have shown that alcohol consumption increases bone marrow adiposity and decreases both bone formation and peak bone mass in a rat model for chronic alcohol abuse (Maddalozzo et al. 2009). Adipocytes and osteoblasts are derived from bone marrow mesenchymal stromal cells (Vaananen 2005; Gimble et al. 2006) (Figure 4). An inverse association between bone mass and bone marrow adiposity is commonly observed (Pei & Tontonoz 2004; Morita et al. 2006) and, although yet to be firmly established, several lines of evidence suggest that there is a cause and effect relationship. A deficiency in PPARγ, a key mediator of adipocyte differentiation, reduced fat and enhanced osteogenesis (Akune et al. 2004), suggesting that suppression of adipogenesis leads to increased bone formation. Based primarily on cell culture studies, some investigators have concluded that increased adipocyte differentiation inevitably occurs at the expense of osteoblast differentiation. If correct, the increase in bone marrow fat in alcohol-fed rats may play a causative role in the decrease in bone formation. In support of this idea, alcohol increased PPARγ expression, increased adipocyte differentiation and decreased osteoblast differentiation in an immortalized mesenchymal stem cell line (Wezeman & Gong 2004). It should be mentioned, however, that a close inverse association between bone marrow fat and bone formation is not always apparent (Menagh et al. 2010; Turner & Iwaniec 2011). This has led us to suggest that changes in osteoblast differentiation are not inevitably coupled to changes in adipocyte differentiation. Instead, we have proposed that some regulatory factors have opposite effects on osteoblast and adipocyte differentiation but others have actions that are limited to one or the other cell lineage.

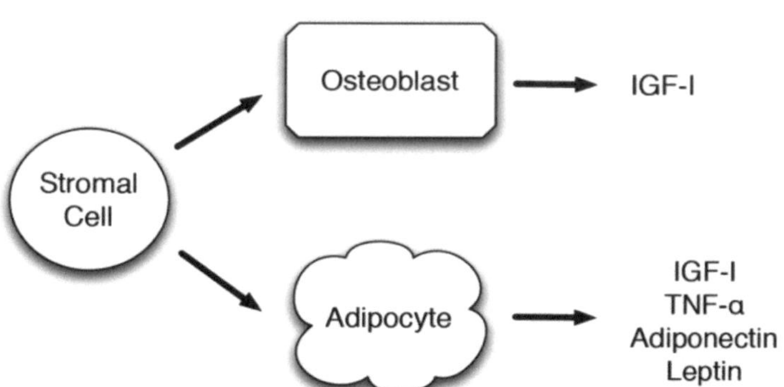

Fig. 4. Osteoblasts and adipocytes are derived from bone marrow stromal cells. They produce factors that act locally to influence bone growth and turnover. Whereas leptin and IGF-I enhance bone formation, adiponectin and TNF-α inhibit osteoblast differentiation.

There is an alternative, non-mutually exclusive mechanism by which peripheral and/or bone marrow fat can influence bone metabolism. More than 50 adipocyte-derived adipokines, growth factors, and proinflammatory cytokines have been identified. Several of these factors, including leptin, adiponectin, tumor necrosis factor-alpha (TNF-α) and insulin-like growth factor-I (IGF-I) are known to have direct effects on bone cells. Adipocytes produce IGF-I in response to growth hormone and are reported to be an important source of systemic IGF-I (Vikman et al. 1991). Although bone marrow adipocytes produce a spectrum of factors with differing effects on bone formation, most investigators believe that the factors which inhibit bone formation generally predominate. This belief is based on the observation that increased marrow fat is typically associated with osteopenia. If this interpretation is correct, chronic consumption of alcohol would tend to perpetuate a continued cycle where increased bone marrow fat would lead to additional fat accumulation and additional bone loss.

Genes Related to Lipid Synthesis and Storage	**Change**
Sortilin	+4.7 fold
Very-long-chain Acyl-CoA dehydrogenase	+4.5 fold
Glycerol-3-phosphate acyltransferase	+6.7 fold
Lipoprotein lipase	+7.9 fold
Non specific lipid transfer protein	+2.9 fold
Fatty acid synthase	+3.8 fold
Lysophospholipase	+5.6 fold
sn-glycerol-3-phosphate acyltransferase	+4.7 fold
Non-specific lipid transfer protein	+2.9 fold
Phosphatidate phospohydrolase type 2	+4.9 fold
Phospholipase C	+3.6 fold
Phosphocholine cytidyltransferase	+5.3 fold
Branched chain α-keto acid dehydrogenase E1	+14.4 fold
Genes Related to Lipolysis and β-Oxidation	
3-Oxoacyl-CoA thiolase	-3.2 fold
DcoH	-5.3 fold
Ryudocan (Syndecan-4)	-4.8 fold
D-β-hydroxybutyrate dehydrogenase	-3.2 fold
Genes Related to Adipocyte Differentiation, Function and/or IGF-I Signaling	
Glucocorticoid receptor	+2.5 fold
Glucocorticoid regulated kinase	+7.0 fold
11-β-hydroxysteroid dehydrogenase, type 2	+4.2 fold
Stat5b	-2.6 fold
Alpha-1β adrenergic receptor	+3.6 fold
GPAT	+4.7 fold
PI3K	-3.0 fold
IP3	+3.2 fold
Natriuretic factor precursor	+6.1 fold
ApoE	-11.6 fold
Basic fibroblast growth factor (FGF)	+3.4 fold
FGF-receptor activating protein	+6.1 fold
12-lipoygenase	-8.2 fold
β-nerve growth factor	+2.7 fold
Galanin	-2.7 fold
VGAT	-3.0 fold
GABA-A receptor delta	-2.7 fold

Table 1. Alcohol increases expression of genes associated with adipogenesis and lipid synthesis and storage.

In order to identify key metabolic pathways impacted by alcohol on bone marrow fat, we analyzed the effects of chronic alcohol consumption on global gene expression (Affymetrix and Research Genetics rat chips) in the distal femur metaphysis (bone and marrow). In these studies, RNA isolated from individual animals (n=3/group) was analyzed. Alcohol significantly increased expression of key genes associated with fat storage and decreased expression of genes associated with lypolysis (Table 1). In addition, alcohol significantly increased expression of genes associated with adipogenesis. Many of the latter genes are differentially regulated by TNF-α and IGF-I. Importantly, we have verified that alcohol results in rapid increases and decreases in TNF-α and IGF-I gene expression, respectively (Turner et al. 1998). These results are consistent with the hypothesis that alcohol alters energy metabolism in bone marrow in a manner that promotes adipocyte formation and deposition of fat in the bone marrow, potentially at the expense of osteoblast formation. The results do not, however, provide a specific mechanism for the changes.

9. Growth hormone signaling is required for normal bone growth and remodeling

Growth hormone is the most important regulator of postnatal growth and has actions that overlap with leptin. Growth hormone plays multiple important direct and indirect roles in coupling energy expenditure to growth, including the growth of bone. Growth hormone deficiency in humans and animals is associated with decreased bone growth and osteopenia (Nilsson et al. 1995; Kasukawa et al. 2004). Osteoblasts and chondrocytes have receptors for growth hormone and the hormone elicits rapid effects on these cells in culture (Ohlsson et al. 1998). As discussed below, there is evidence that alcohol disrupts growth hormone signaling.

9.1 Alcohol results in skeletal resistance to growth hormone

Hypophysectomy prevented body weight gain and this effect was reversed by growth hormone treatment in rats regardless of dietary alcohol. Compared to normal rats, hypophysectomized rats had less cancellous bone, and lower rates of longitudinal growth and bone formation but higher bone marrow adiposity (Figure 5). Short duration (8 d) treatment of hypophysectomized rats with growth hormone increased cancellous bone formation and longitudinal growth rates, and decreased bone marrow adiposity. Alcohol consumption, however, blunted the effects of growth hormone on bone elongation, cancellous bone formation and bone marrow adiposity. These findings suggest that alcohol induces skeletal resistance to growth hormone at the level of the growth hormone receptor.

There is precedence for skeletal resistance to growth hormone in rats. Skeletal resistance to growth hormone was reported in rat models for disuse (Bikle et al. 1995; Kostenuik et al. 1999; Sakata et al. 2003; Sakata et al. 2004) and senescence (Ren et al. 1999). In regard to the former, alcohol has been shown to accentuate the detrimental skeletal effects of disuse (Hefferan et al. 2003). Further studies, however, are required to determine whether the putative resistance to growth hormone is due to reduced receptor number or impaired post-receptor signaling.

Osteoblasts, chondrocytes, and adipocytes have receptors for growth hormone, as do their stromal cell precursors, and the hormone elicits rapid effects on these cells in culture (Ohlsson et al. 1998). Growth hormone increases stromal cell number and differentiation of stromal cells to osteoblasts. However, growth hormone suppresses adipocyte differentiation. As discussed below, alcohol-induced reductions in growth hormone signaling could be responsible for the observed changes in the balance between adipocyte and osteoblast differentiation.

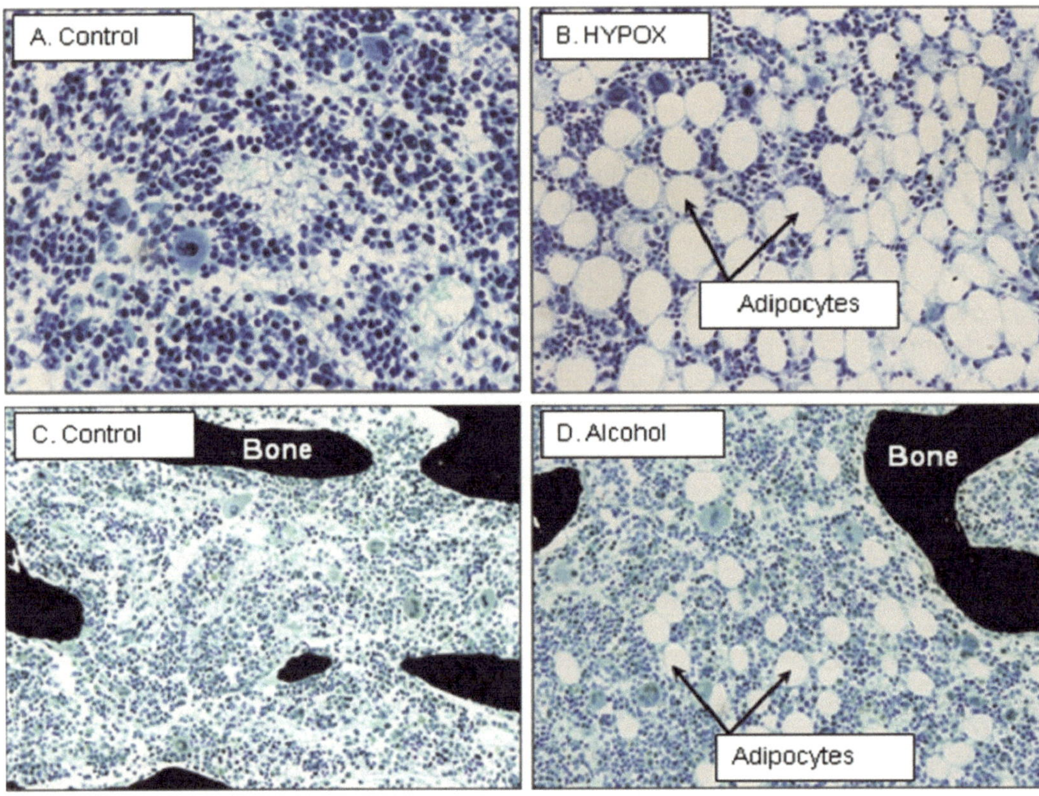

Fig. 5. Effects of hypophysectomy (panels A and B, proximal tibia, 36X objective) and alcohol consumption (panels C and D, lumbar vertebra, 20X objective) on bone marrow adiposity in growing male rats. Severe growth hormone deficiency induced by hypophysectomy resulted in very rapid (within days) increase in bone marrow adiposity in growing rats. An increase in adiposity is also observed in adolescent rats following 6 weeks of consuming alcohol. As described in the text, the increase in bone marrow fat in rats fed a diet containing alcohol is associated with skeletal resistance to growth hormone.

Hypophysectomized animals are deficient in several hormones known to influence bone metabolism; including growth hormone, leptin, sex steroids, and adrenal and thyroid hormones. Thus, the profound skeletal changes resulting from hypophysectomy need not be exclusively due to growth hormone deficiency. However, we have shown that growth hormone replacement is sufficient to increase bone formation and decrease bone marrow adiposity to pituitary-intact control values. In contrast, administration of thyroxine, cortisol or 17β-estradiol to hypophysectomized rats was ineffective in normalizing either bone formation or bone marrow adiposity (Menagh et al. 2010). Also, short duration treatment with growth hormone did not restore white adipose tissue mass or serum leptin levels to normal. These findings suggest that the profound changes in leptin levels following hypophysectomy are not essential for the actions of growth hormone on bone growth, turnover or adiposity. Thus, growth hormone appears to be sufficient to increase bone formation and reduce bone marrow adiposity in hypophysectomized rats. However, pharmacological replacement with growth hormone may obscure the role of leptin deficiency as a regulator of bone metabolism. Physiologically, low leptin levels are associated with impaired growth hormone signaling. Thus, it is likely that leptin and growth hormone have overlapping effects on bone growth and turnover.

9.2 Alcohol impairs IGF-I signaling in bone

IGF-I mediates most, if not all, of the actions of growth hormone on bone and multiple lines of evidence indicate that IGF-I is essential for normal bone growth and remodeling. The activity of IGFs depends upon specific receptors, whose numbers are regulated, on target cells (Brown-Borg 2003). IGF-I, in addition to stimulating osteoblast differentiation, acts as an autocrine growth and survival factor for osteoblasts and may be essential for these cells to maintain their fully differentiated phenotype. Studies in mice and humans have confirmed the important actions of IGF-I on bone metabolism. IGF-I knockout mice are severely osteopenic and have reduced bone formation, despite the ability to produce growth hormone (Stabnov et al. 2002). The liver is the principal source of circulating IGFs. However, IGF-I is produced locally by osteoblasts, adipocytes and cartilage cells. The relative importance of locally produced versus systemic IGF-I on bone metabolism is under investigation.

Compelling data support a role for locally produced IGF-I in regulation of bone metabolism. Targeted over-expression of IGF-I in mouse osteoblasts resulted in increased bone formation (Zhao et al. 2000), and osteoblast-derived IGF-I is required for the bone anabolic response to parathyroid hormone (Bikle et al. 2002; Wang et al. 2007). We have shown that parathyroid hormone increases bone formation in hypophysectomized rats. This response is accompanied by an increase in skeletal IGF-I mRNA levels with no rise in circulating IGF-I, illustrating the important role of locally produced IGF-I. However, equally compelling data support a role for circulating IGF-I in the regulation of bone metabolism. IGFs circulate bound to binding proteins which either potentiate or antagonize IGF-I activity in specific tissues, and the circulating levels of these binding proteins are regulated by a variety of factors (Jones & Clemmons 1995) Liver IGF-I-deficient (Lid) mice and acid labile subunit (a key component in the IGF-I serum transport complex) knockout (Alsko) mice exhibited relatively normal growth and development, despite having 75% and 65% reductions in serum IGF-I levels, respectively. The double knockout mice (LA), however, exhibited growth inhibitions and osteopenia that were reversed by IGF-I treatment (Yakar et al. 2002). More recent findings using a variety of model systems support a regulatory role for systemic IGF-I on bone metabolism (Yakar et al. 2002; Mohan et al. 2003; Wang et al. 2004; Mohan & Baylink 2005). Taken together, the above findings suggest that locally produced as well as circulating IGF-I are both important to skeletal growth and remodeling and are likely to have overlapping but not identical actions.

There is mounting evidence that the skeletal effects of growth hormone, via IGF-I signaling, are impaired by alcohol consumption. Chronic alcohol abuse results in decreased serum IGF levels, reduced mRNA levels for IGF-I in liver and altered hepatic synthesis of IGF binding proteins (Turner et al. 1998; Lang et al. 2000). Locally, alcohol decreases IGF-I gene expression in bone (Turner et al. 1998). Alcohol may also reduce IGF receptor number in target cells (Lang et al. 2000). Thus, the numerous ways that alcohol could disrupt IGF-I signaling fall into two general non-mutually exclusive classes of action: 1) decreased IGF-I bioavailability and 2) target organ resistance to GH. Exposure to alcohol rapidly (within 8 hours) decreases mRNA levels for IGF-I in bone tissue (Figure 6). This decline precedes decreases in mRNA expression for bone matrix proteins and subsequent bone matrix synthesis (Turner et al. 1998). Thus, decreased production of IGF-I may play a causative role in mediating the inhibitory effects of alcohol on bone formation. Osteoblasts generate IGF-I and the growth factor is deposited into bone matrix where it is retained until released by osteoclast-mediated bone resorption. IGF-I located in bone matrix is thought to be osteoblast-derived but its origin has not been rigorously investigated. IGF-I in bone matrix, irrespective of origin, helps couple bone formation to bone resorption during bone remodeling; IGF-I released from the matrix during bone resorption acts in concert with other matrix-derived growth factors (e.g., TGF-ß) to induce renewed bone formation (Centrella et al. 1991; Mohan & Baylink 1991). Additionally, IGF-I incorporated into bone matrix plays a role in mediating bone healing when released following a fracture (Okazaki et al. 2003).

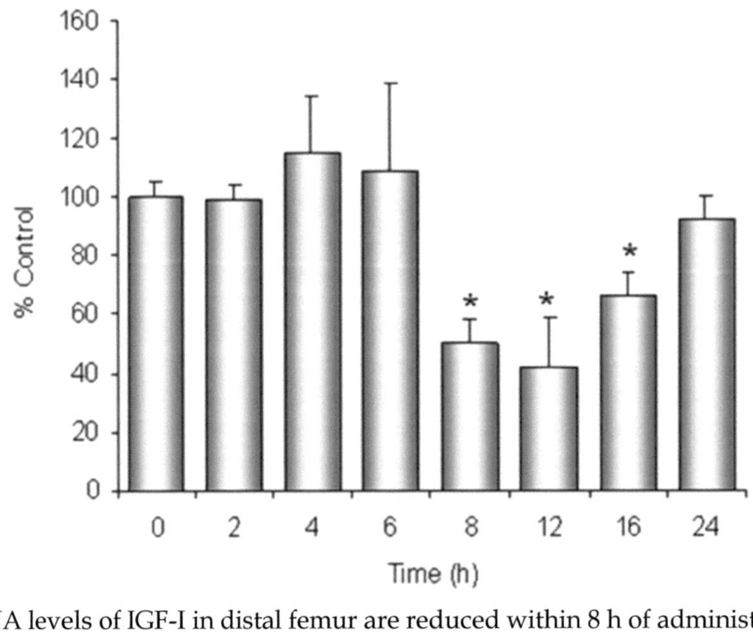

Fig. 6. mRNA levels of IGF-I in distal femur are reduced within 8 h of administration of alcohol (1 g/kg) and return to normal by 24 hours. Values are man ± SE, n=4-5/group. *p <0.05 compared to time 0.

9.3 Parathyroid hormone may reverse alcohol-induced inhibition of bone formation by increasing IGF-I gene expression in skeletal tissues

The molecular mechanisms that mediate the bone anabolic response to parathyroid hormone are incompletely understood but appear to require IGF-I signaling. As mentioned, animals with low circulating levels of IGF-I have deficient bone formation (Yakar et al. 2005). Also, bone in IGF-I knockout mice is insensitive to parathyroid hormone, suggesting that IGF-I is essential for the bone anabolic effects of the hormone (Miyakoshi et al. 2001;

Bikle et al. 2002). Acute administration of alcohol decreases IGF-I mRNA levels in liver and bone (Lang et al. 1998). Alcohol also reduces the circulating level of IGF-I. Thus, alcohol abuse could decrease the skeletal response to parathyroid hormone by reducing systemic and/or locally produced IGF-I or, alternatively, by inducing a target organ resistance to IGF-I signaling (Wang et al. 2007). Parathyroid hormone increases mRNA levels for IGF-I in skeletal tissue in rats (Watson et al. 1995) and the hormone has been shown to be effective in increasing cancellous bone formation in severely growth hormone-deficient hypophysectomized rats (Schmidt et al. 1995). Since hypophysectomized rats have very low serum IGF-I levels, locally generated IGF-I may be sufficient for the bone anabolic effects of parathyroid hormone (Fielder et al. 1996). However, other studies suggest that systemic IGF-I is critically important for the bone anabolic response to the hormone (Yakar et al. 2006). Thus, parathyroid hormone-induced IGF-I in bone cells may compensate for the reduced circulating levels of the growth factor in alcohol-fed rats. Regardless of the relative importance of locally generated versus systemically derived IGF-I, parathyroid hormone increases cancellous bone formation in alcohol-fed rats without the requirement for restoring normal serum IGF-I levels. Taken together, these findings suggest that alcohol consumption results in a defect in growth hormone signaling that leads to impaired production of IGF-I by bone cells. Parathyroid hormone reverses this defect by its ability to increase IGF-I expression in bone cells by a growth hormone-independent mechanism. These findings provide a mechanistic explanation for the observed ability of parathyroid hormone to maintain normal bone formation in alcohol-fed rats and to reverse bone loss in a rat model for chronic alcohol abuse, whether or not alcohol is removed from the diet (Turner et al. 2001; Sibonga et al. 2007; Iwaniec et al. 2008; Howe et al. 2011).

10. Alcohol may disturb estrogen signaling

Although the skeletal changes in alcohol-fed rats are similar to those observed in growth hormone-deficient and leptin-deficient mice and rats, disruption of growth hormone and leptin signaling may represent only two of numerous mechanisms by which alcohol negatively impacts the growing skeleton. Disruption of estrogen signaling is another potential mechanism. We have already discussed estrogen as an important regulator of energy metabolism. In addition, estrogen is an important regulator of bone growth where the hormone plays an essential role in the sexual dimorphism of the skeleton (Turner et al. 1994).

The possible mechanisms by which alcohol could influence the skeletal response to estrogen on bone have been reviewed (Turner & Sibonga 2001). More recent *in vitro* studies suggest that very high concentrations of alcohol increase estrogen receptor levels but disrupt normal estrogen receptor signaling in cultured osteosarcoma cells (Chen et al. 2006; Chen et al. 2009). It is not clear, however, whether the much lower levels of alcohol exposure experienced by most adolescent drinkers would have this effect. Also, alcohol consumption results in similar skeletal abnormalities in male and female growing rats. In contrast, whereas estrogen receptor blockade by the potent estrogen receptor antagonist ICI 182,780 largely recapitulates the skeletal response to ovariectomy, the antagonist had no effect on bone growth and turnover in growing male rats (Sibonga et al. 1998; Turner et al. 2000). Therefore, alterations of estrogen receptor signaling may contribute to but are unlikely to be the major cause for the detrimental effects of alcohol consumption on the growing skeleton.

11. Summary

The skeletal changes in growing rats consuming alcohol are similar to the skeletal changes observed in growth hormone-deficient rats; decreased bone elongation, decreased cortical and cancellous bone mass, decreased bone formation and resorption, and increased bone marrow adiposity. Studies performed in hypophysectomized rats suggest that growth

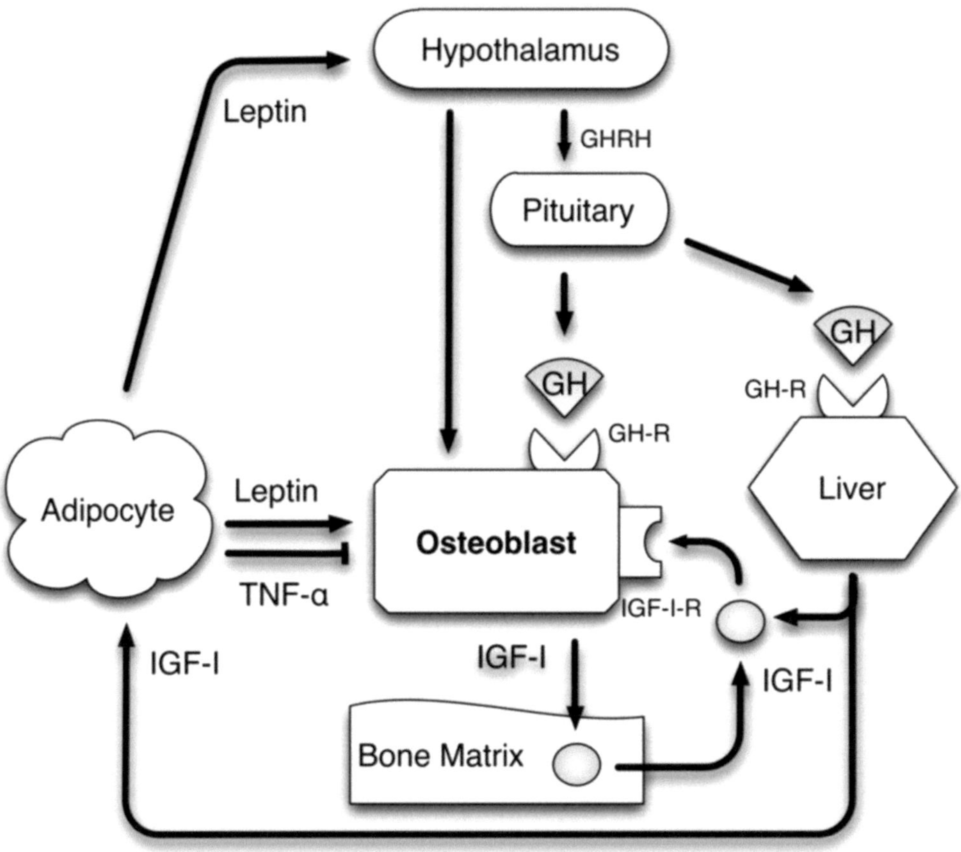

Fig. 7. A simplified model for the coupling of bone growth and turnover to energy metabolism. Systemic and osteoblast-generated IGF-I are bone anabolic whereas leptin has direct and indirect hypothalamic effects on cancellous bone. We hypothesize that the detrimental effects of alcohol on bone metabolism are mediated through changes in key hormones involved in the tight coupling between energy homeostasis and bone growth. Alcohol-impaired IGF-I and leptin signaling results in depressed bone growth, depressed osteoblast differentiation and increased bone marrow adiposity. Finally, the alcohol-induced increase in bone marrow adiposity results in increased local levels of TNF-α and other inhibitory adipokines which further inhibits osteoblastogenesis. Other factors that may contribute to the detrimental effects of alcohol on bone metabolism include: impaired growth hormone (GH)-growth hormone receptor (GH-R) interactions, impaired IGF-I-IGF-I receptor (IGF-I-R) interactions, impaired growth hormone releasing hormone (GHRH) secretion from the hypothalamus and/or decreased deposition of IGF-I into bone matrix.

hormone is essential to maintain a mature osteoblast phenotype and suppress excessive adipogenesis. We have also shown that alcohol impairs the action of growth hormone to increase bone growth and turnover, and decrease bone marrow adiposity in hypophysectomized rats. These results are consistent with skeletal resistance to growth hormone as a contributing mechanism for the detrimental skeletal effects of chronic alcohol consumption. Other studies suggest that heavy drinking decreases energy intake and in some situations can increase energy expenditure. It is likely that reduced leptin signaling is, at least in part, responsible for changes in energy homeostasis. Reduced leptin levels may also contribute to the alcohol-induced inhibition of bone growth and turnover, and increase in bone marrow adiposity. Thus impairments in growth hormone and leptin signaling may act in consort to mediate the reduced peak bone mass in rats fed a diet containing alcohol. Although our work to date has focused on leptin and growth hormone, it does not preclude an important role for other factors, such as estrogen, that facilitate the coupling of bone growth to energy metabolism. As depicted in our working model (Figure 7), alcohol consumption may also decrease the deposition of growth factors into bone matrix prior to its mineralization. Thus, heavy underage drinking, in addition to an immediate increase in the likelihood of a fracture, may have serious long-term consequences to bone health. By decreasing peak bone mass, heavy alcohol consumption may increase the risk for premature osteoporosis and by decreasing the incorporation of skeletal growth factors into bone during formation, alcohol may increase the risk for impaired healing should a fracture occur.

12. References

Akune, T., S. Ohba, et al. (2004). Ppargamma insuffICIency enhances osteogenesis throuGH osteoblast formation from bone marrow progenitors. *J Clin Invest*, Vol. 113, No. 6, pp.(846-55).

Bartell, S. M., S. Rayalam, et al. (2011). Central (icv) leptin injection increases bone formation, bone mineral density, muscle mass, serum IGF-I, and the expression of osteogenic genes in leptin-defICIent ob/ob mice. *J Bone Miner Res*, Vol. 26, No. 8, pp.(1710-20).

Bergmann, P., J. J. Body, et al. (2010). Loading and skeletal development and maintenance. *J Osteoporos*, Vol. 2011, No., pp.(786752).

Bikle, D. D., J. Harris, et al. (1995). The molecular response of bone to growth hormone during skeletal unloading: Regional differences. *Endocrinology*, Vol. 136, No. 5, pp.(2099-109).

Bikle, D. D., T. Sakata, et al. (2002). Insulin-like growth factor-I is required for the anabolic actions of parathyroid hormone on mouse bone. *J Bone Miner Res*, Vol. 17, No. 9, pp.(1570-8).

Bikle, D. D., A. Stesin, et al. (1993). Alcohol-induced bone disease: Relationship to age and parathyroid hormone levels. *Alcohol Clin Exp Res*, Vol. 17, No. 3, pp.(690-5).

Brown-Borg, H. M. (2003). Hormonal regulation of aging and life span. *Trends Endocrinol Metab*, Vol. 14, No. 4, pp.(151-3).

Burguera, B., L. C. Hofbauer, et al. (2001). Leptin reduces ovariectomy-induced bone loss in rats. *Endocrinology*, Vol. 142, No. 8, pp.(3546-53).

Calissendorff, J., K. Brismar, et al. (2004). Is decreased leptin secretion after alcohol ingestion catecholamine-mediated? *Alcohol Alcohol*, Vol. 39, No. 4, pp.(281-6).

Centrella, M., T. L. McCarthy, et al. (1991). Transforming growth factor-beta and remodeling of bone. *J Bone Joint Surg Am*, Vol. 73, No. 9, pp.(1418-28).

Chakkalakal, D. A., J. R. Novak, et al. (2005). Inhibition of bone repair in a rat model for chronic and excessive alcohol consumption. *Alcohol*, Vol. 36, No. 3, pp.(201-14).

Chen, J. R., R. L. Haley, et al. (2006). Estradiol protects against ethanol-induced bone loss by inhibiting up-regulation of receptor activator of nuclear factor-kappaβ ligand in osteoblasts. *J Pharmacol Exp Ther*, Vol. 319, No. 3, pp.(1182-90).

Chen, J. R., O. P. Lazarenko, et al. (2009). Ethanol impairs estrogen receptor signaling resulting in accelerated activation of senescence pathways, whereas estradiol attenuates the effects of ethanol in osteoblasts. *J Bone Miner Res*, Vol. 24, No. 2, pp.(221-30).

Cooper, C., S. Westlake, et al. (2006). Review: Developmental origins of osteoporotic fracture. *Osteoporos Int*, Vol. 17, No. 3, pp.(337-47).

Department of Health and Human Services (2010). Results from the 2009 national survey on drug use and health. SMA 10-456, Available at: <http://oas.samhsa.gov/nsduh/2k9nsduh/2k9resultsp.pdf>.

Devlin, M. J., A. M. Cloutier, et al. (2010). Caloric restriction leads to hiGH marrow adiposity and low bone mass in growing mice. *J Bone Miner Res*, Vol. 25, No. 9, pp.(2078-88).

Diamond, T., D. Stiel, et al. (1989). Ethanol reduces bone formation and may cause osteoporosis. *Am J Med*, Vol. 86, No. 3, pp.(282-8).

Ducy, P., M. Amling, et al. (2000). Leptin inhibits bone formation throuGH a hypothalamic relay: A central control of bone mass. *Cell*, Vol. 100, No. 2, pp.(197-207).

Dumitrescu, R. G. & P. G. Shields. (2005). The etiology of alcohol-induced breast cancer. *Alcohol*, Vol. 35, No. 3, pp.(213-25).

Dyer, S. A., P. Buckendahl, et al. (1998). Alcohol consumption inhibits osteoblastic cell proliferation and activity in vivo. *Alcohol*, Vol. 16, No. 4, pp.(337-41).

Eisman, J. A. (1999). Genetics of osteoporosis. *Endocr Rev*, Vol. 20, No. 6, pp.(788-804).

Fielder, P. J., D. L. Mortensen, et al. (1996). Differential long-term effects of insulin-like growth factor-I (IGF-I) growth hormone (GH), and IGF-I plus GH on body growth and IGF binding proteins in hypophysectomized rats. *Endocrinology*, Vol. 137, No. 5, pp.(1913-20).

French, S. W. (2001). Intragastric ethanol infusion model for cellular and molecular studies of alcoholic liver disease. *J Biomed Sci*, Vol. 8, No. 1, pp.(20-7).

Gimble, J. M., S. Zvonic, et al. (2006). Playing with bone and fat. *J Cell Biochem*, Vol. 98, No. 2, pp.(251-66).

Giuliani, N., G. Girasole, et al. (1999). Ethanol and acetaldehyde inhibit the formation of early osteoblast progenitors in murine and human bone marrow cultures. *Alcohol Clin Exp Res*, Vol. 23, No. 2, pp.(381-5).

Gordeladze, J. O., C. A. Drevon, et al. (2002). Leptin stimulates human osteoblastic cell proliferation, de novo collagen synthesis, and mineralization: Impact on differentiation markers, apoptosis, and osteoclastic signaling. *J Cell Biochem*, Vol. 85, No. 4, pp.(825-36).

Goulding, A. (2007). Risk factors for fractures in normally active children and adolescents. *Med Sport Sci*, Vol. 51, No., pp.(102-20).

Hamrick, M. W., M. A. Della-Fera, et al. (2005). Leptin treatment induces loss of bone marrow adipocytes and increases bone formation in leptin-deflClent ob/ob mice. *J Bone Miner Res*, Vol. 20, No. 6, pp.(994-1001).

Hamrick, M. W. & S. L. Ferrari. (2008). Leptin and the sympathetic connection of fat to bone. *Osteoporos Int*, Vol. 19, No. 7, pp.(905-12).

Hamrick, M. W., C. Pennington, et al. (2004). Leptin deflClency produces contrasting phenotypes in bones of the limb and spine. *Bone*, Vol. 34, No. 3, pp.(376-83).

Hefferan, T. E., A. M. Kennedy, et al. (2003). Disuse exaggerates the detrimental effects of alcohol on cortical bone. *Alcohol Clin Exp Res*, Vol. 27, No. 1, pp.(111-7).

Henry, Y. M., D. Fatayerji, et al. (2004). Attainment of peak bone mass at the lumbar spine, femoral neck and radius in men and women: Relative contributions of bone size and volumetric bone mineral density. *Osteoporos Int*, Vol. 15, No. 4, pp.(263-73).

Hibell, B., U. Guttormsson, et al. (2009). The 2007 ESPAD report: Substance use among students in 35 European countries. Available at: <http://www.espad.org/documents/Espad/ESPAD_reports/2007/The_2007_ESPAD_Report-FULL_091006.pdf>.

Hogan, H. A., F. Argueta, et al. (2001). Adult-onset alcohol consumption induces osteopenia in female rats. *Alcohol Clin Exp Res*, Vol. 25, No. 5, pp.(746-54).

Hogan, H. A., H. W. Sampson, et al. (1997). Alcohol consumption by young actively growing rats: A study of cortical bone histomorphometry and mechanical properties. *Alcohol Clin Exp Res*, Vol. 21, No. 5, pp.(809-16).

Howe, K. S., U. T. Iwaniec, et al. (2011). The effects of low dose parathyroid hormone on lumbar vertebrae in a rat model for chronic alcohol abuse. *Osteoporos Int*, Vol. 22, No. 4, pp.(1175-81).

Iwaniec, U. & R. Turner (2008). Animal models for osteoporosis. *Osteoporosis*. R. Marcus, D. Feldman, D. Nelson and C. Rosen. New York, Elsevier Academic Press.

Iwaniec, U. T., S. BoGHossian, et al. (2007). Central leptin gene therapy corrects skeletal abnormalities in leptin-deflClent ob/ob mice. *Peptides*, Vol. 28, No. 5, pp.(1012-9).

Iwaniec, U. T., C. H. Trevisiol, et al. (2008). Effects of low-dose parathyroid hormone on bone mass, turnover, and ectopic osteoinduction in a rat model for chronic alcohol abuse. *Bone*, Vol. 42, No. 4, pp.(695-701).

Jones, J. I. & D. R. Clemmons. (1995). Insulin-like growth factors and their binding proteins: Biological actions. *Endocr Rev*, Vol. 16, No. 1, pp.(3-34).

Kasukawa, Y., N. Miyakoshi, et al. (2004). The anabolic effects of GH/IGF system on bone. *Curr Pharm Des*, Vol. 10, No. 21, pp.(2577-92).

Kidder, L. S. & R. T. Turner. (1998). Dietary ethanol does not accelerate bone loss in ovariectomized rats. *Alcohol Clin Exp Res*, Vol. 22, No. 9, pp.(2159-64).

Kontulainen, S. A., J. M. HuGHes, et al. (2007). The biomechanical basis of bone strength development during growth. *Med Sport Sci*, Vol. 51, No., pp.(13-32).

Kostenuik, P. J., J. Harris, et al. (1999). Skeletal unloading causes resistance of osteoprogenitor cells to parathyroid hormone and to insulin-like growth factor-I. *J Bone Miner Res*, Vol. 14, No. 1, pp.(21-31).

Lang, C. H., J. Fan, et al. (1998). Modulation of the insulin-like growth factor system by chronic alcohol feeding. *Alcohol Clin Exp Res*, Vol. 22, No. 4, pp.(823-9).

Lang, C. H., X. Liu, et al. (2000). Acute effects of growth hormone in alcohol-fed rats. *Alcohol Alcohol*, Vol. 35, No. 2, pp.(148-58).
Leibowitz, S. F. (2005). Regulation and effects of hypothalamic galanin: Relation to dietary fat, alcohol ingestion, circulating lipids and energy homeostasis. *Neuropeptides*, Vol. 39, No. 3, pp.(327-32).
Liangpunsakul, S., D. W. Crabb, et al. (2010). Relationship among alcohol intake, body fat, and physical activity: A population-based study. *Ann Epidemiol*, Vol. 20, No. 9, pp.(670-5).
Lieber, C. S., L. M. DeCarli, et al. (1989). Experimental methods of ethanol administration. *Hepatology*, Vol. 10, No. 4, pp.(501-10).
Lin, Y. C., R. M. Lyle, et al. (2003). Peak spine and femoral neck bone mass in young women. *Bone*, Vol. 32, No. 5, pp.(546-53).
Maddalozzo, G. F., R. T. Turner, et al. (2009). Alcohol alters whole body composition, inhibits bone formation, and increases bone marrow adiposity in rats. *Osteoporos Int*, Vol. 20, No. 9, pp.(1529-38).
Maran, A., M. Zhang, et al. (2001). The dose-response effects of ethanol on the human fetal osteoblastic cell line. *J Bone Miner Res*, Vol. 16, No. 2, pp.(270-6).
Martin, E. A., E. L. Ritman, et al. (2003). Time course of epiphyseal growth plate fusion in rat tibiae. *Bone*, Vol. 32, No. 3, pp.(261-7).
MenaGH, P. J., R. T. Turner, et al. (2010). Growth hormone regulates the balance between bone formation and bone marrow adiposity. *J Bone Miner Res*, Vol. 25, No. 4, pp.(757-68).
Miyakoshi, N., Y. Kasukawa, et al. (2001). Evidence that anabolic effects of PTH on bone require IGF-I in growing mice. *Endocrinology*, Vol. 142, No. 10, pp.(4349-56).
Mohan, S. & D. J. Baylink. (1991). Bone growth factors. *Clin Orthop Relat Res*, Vol., No. 263, pp.(30-48).
Mohan, S. & D. J. Baylink. (2005). Impaired skeletal growth in mice with haploinsuffICIency of IGF-I: Genetic evidence that differences in IGF-I expression could contribute to peak bone mineral density differences. *J Endocrinol*, Vol. 185, No. 3, pp.(415-20).
Mohan, S., C. Richman, et al. (2003). Insulin-like growth factor regulates peak bone mineral density in mice by both growth hormone-dependent and -independent mechanisms. *Endocrinology*, Vol. 144, No. 3, pp.(929-36).
Morita, Y., I. Iwamoto, et al. (2006). Precedence of the shift of body-fat distribution over the change in body composition after menopause. *J Obstet Gynaecol Res*, Vol. 32, No. 5, pp.(513-6).
Nicolas, J. M., J. Fernandez-Sola, et al. (2001). Increased circulating leptin levels in chronic alcoholism. *Alcohol Clin Exp Res*, Vol. 25, No. 1, pp.(83-8).
Nilsson, A., D. Swolin, et al. (1995). Expression of functional growth hormone receptors in cultured human osteoblast-like cells. *J Clin Endocrinol Metab*, Vol. 80, No. 12, pp.(3483-8).
Odvina, C. V., I. Safi, et al. (1995). Effect of heavy alcohol intake in the absence of liver disease on bone mass in black and white men. *J Clin Endocrinol Metab*, Vol. 80, No. 8, pp.(2499-503).
Ohlsson, C., B. A. Bengtsson, et al. (1998). Growth hormone and bone. *Endocr Rev*, Vol. 19, No. 1, pp.(55-79).

Ohlsson, C., A. Darelid, et al. (2011). Cortical consolidation due to increased mineralization and endosteal contraction in young adult men: A five-year longitudinal study. *J Clin Endocrinol Metab*, Vol. 96, No. 7, pp.(2262-9).

Okazaki, K., S. Jingushi, et al. (2003). Expression of parathyroid hormone-related peptide and insulin-like growth factor I during rat fracture healing. *J Orthop Res*, Vol. 21, No. 3, pp.(511-20).

Otaka, M., N. Konishi, et al. (2007). Effect of alcohol consumption on leptin level in serum, adipose tissue, and gastric mucosa. *Dig Dis Sci*, Vol. 52, No. 11, pp.(3066-9).

Pei, L. & P. Tontonoz. (2004). Fat's loss is bone's gain. *J Clin Invest*, Vol. 113, No. 6, pp.(805-6).

Pravdova, E. & M. Fickova. (2006). Alcohol intake modulates hormonal activity of adipose tissue. *Endocr Regul*, Vol. 40, No. 3, pp.(91-104).

Pumarino, H., P. Gonzalez, et al. (1996). Assessment of bone status in intermittent and continuous alcoholics, without evidence of liver damage. *Rev Med Chil*, Vol. 124, No. 4, pp.(423-30).

Recker, R. R., K. M. Davies, et al. (1992). Bone gain in young adult women. *JAMA*, Vol. 268, No. 17, pp.(2403-8).

Ren, J., L. Jefferson, et al. (1999). Influence of age on contractile response to insulin-like growth factor I in ventricular myocytes from spontaneously hypertensive rats. *Hypertension*, Vol. 34, No. 6, pp.(1215-22).

Reseland, J. E., U. Syversen, et al. (2001). Leptin is expressed in and secreted from primary cultures of human osteoblasts and promotes bone mineralization. *J Bone Miner Res*, Vol. 16, No. 8, pp.(1426-33).

Ronis, M. J., J. R. Wands, et al. (2007). Alcohol-induced disruption of endocrine signaling. *Alcohol Clin Exp Res*, Vol. 31, No. 8, pp.(1269-85).

Rosa, M. L., M. M. Beloti, et al. (2008). Chronic ethanol intake inhibits in vitro osteogenesis induced by osteoblasts differentiated from stem cells. *J Appl Toxicol*, Vol. 28, No. 2, pp.(205-11).

Sakata, T., B. P. Halloran, et al. (2003). Skeletal unloading induces resistance to insulin-like growth factor I on bone formation. *Bone*, Vol. 32, No. 6, pp.(669-80).

Sakata, T., Y. Wang, et al. (2004). Skeletal unloading induces resistance to insulin-like growth factor-I (IGF-I) by inhibiting activation of the IGF-I signaling pathways. *J Bone Miner Res*, Vol. 19, No. 3, pp.(436-46).

Sampson, H. W., C. Chaffin, et al. (1997). Alcohol consumption by young actively growing rats: A histomorphometric study of cancellous bone. *Alcohol Clin Exp Res*, Vol. 21, No. 2, pp.(352-9).

Sampson, H. W., S. Gallager, et al. (1999). Binge drinking and bone metabolism in a young actively growing rat model. *Alcohol Clin Exp Res*, Vol. 23, No. 7, pp.(1228-31).

Sampson, H. W., N. Perks, et al. (1996). Alcohol consumption inhibits bone growth and development in young actively growing rats. *Alcohol Clin Exp Res*, Vol. 20, No. 8, pp.(1375-84).

Sampson, H. W. & H. Spears. (1999). Osteopenia due to chronic alcohol consumption by young actively growing rats is not completely reversible. *Alcohol Clin Exp Res*, Vol. 23, No. 2, pp.(324-7).

Santolaria, F., A. Perez-Cejas, et al. (2003). Low serum leptin levels and malnutrition in chronic alcohol misusers hospitalized by somatic complications. *Alcohol Alcohol,* Vol. 38, No. 1, pp.(60-6).
Schmidt, I. U., H. Dobnig, et al. (1995). Intermittent parathyroid hormone treatment increases osteoblast number, steady state messenger ribonucleic acid levels for osteocalcin, and bone formation in tibial metaphysis of hypophysectomized female rats. *Endocrinology,* Vol. 136, No. 11, pp.(5127-34).
Schnitzler, C. M., A. P. Macphail, et al. (1994). Osteoporosis in African hemosiderosis: Role of alcohol and iron. *J Bone Miner Res,* Vol. 9, No. 12, pp.(1865-73).
Schnitzler, C. M. & L. Solomon. (1984). Bone changes after alcohol abuse. *S Afr Med J,* Vol. 66, No. 19, pp.(730-4).
Sibonga, J. D., H. Dobnig, et al. (1998). Effect of the hiGH-affinity estrogen receptor ligand ICI 182,780 on the rat tibia. *Endocrinology,* Vol. 139, No. 9, pp.(3736-42).
Sibonga, J. D., U. T. Iwaniec, et al. (2007). Effects of parathyroid hormone (1-34) on tibia in an adult rat model for chronic alcohol abuse. *Bone,* Vol. 40, No. 4, pp.(1013-20).
Stabnov, L., Y. Kasukawa, et al. (2002). Effect of insulin-like growth factor-I (IGF-I) plus alendronate on bone density during puberty in IGF-I-defICIent midi mice. *Bone,* Vol. 30, No. 6, pp.(909-16).
Steppan, C. M., D. T. Crawford, et al. (2000). Leptin is a potent stimulator of bone growth in ob/ob mice. *Regul Pept,* Vol. 92, No. 1-3, pp.(73-8).
Thomas, T. (2004). The complex effects of leptin on bone metabolism throuGH multiple pathways. *Curr Opin Pharmacol,* Vol. 4, No. 3, pp.(295-300).
Trevisiol, C. H., R. T. Turner, et al. (2007). Impaired osteoinduction in a rat model for chronic alcohol abuse. *Bone,* Vol. 41, No. 2, pp.(175-80).
Turner, R. T. (2000). Skeletal response to alcohol. *Alcohol Clin Exp Res,* Vol. 24, No. 11, pp.(1693-701).
Turner, R. T., R. C. Aloia, et al. (1988). Chronic alcohol treatment results in disturbed vitamin d metabolism and skeletal abnormalities in rats. *Alcohol Clin Exp Res,* Vol. 12, No. 1, pp.(159-62).
Turner, R. T., G. L. Evans, et al. (2000). The hiGH-affinity estrogen receptor antagonist ICI 182,780 has no effect on bone growth in young male rats. *Calcif Tissue Int,* Vol. 66, No. 6, pp.(461-4).
Turner, R. T., G. L. Evans, et al. (2001). Effects of parathyroid hormone on bone formation in a rat model for chronic alcohol abuse. *Alcohol Clin Exp Res,* Vol. 25, No. 5, pp.(667-71).
Turner, R. T., V. S. Greene, et al. (1987). Demonstration that ethanol inhibits bone matrix synthesis and mineralization in the rat. *J Bone Miner Res,* Vol. 2, No. 1, pp.(61-6).
Turner, R. T. & U. T. Iwaniec. (2010). Moderate weiGHt gain does not influence bone metabolism in skeletally mature female rats. *Bone,* Vol. 47, No. 3, pp.(631-5).
Turner, R. T. & U. T. Iwaniec. (2011). Low dose parathyroid hormone maintains normal bone formation in adult male rats during rapid weiGHt loss. *Bone,* Vol. 48, No. 4, pp.(726-32).
Turner, R. T., L. S. Kidder, et al. (2001). Moderate alcohol consumption suppresses bone turnover in adult female rats. *J Bone Miner Res,* Vol. 16, No. 3, pp.(589-94).

Turner, R. T., B. L. Riggs, et al. (1994). Skeletal effects of estrogen. *Endocr Rev*, Vol. 15, No. 3, pp.(275-300).

Turner, R. T. & J. D. Sibonga. (2001). Effects of alcohol use and estrogen on bone. *Alcohol Res Health*, Vol. 25, No. 4, pp.(276-81).

Turner, R. T., T. J. Wronski, et al. (1998). Effects of ethanol on gene expression in rat bone: Transient dose-dependent changes in mRNA levels for matrix proteins, skeletal growth factors, and cytokines are followed by reductions in bone formation. *Alcohol Clin Exp Res*, Vol. 22, No. 7, pp.(1591-9).

Vaananen, H. K. (2005). Mesenchymal stem cells. *Ann Med*, Vol. 37, No. 7, pp.(469-79).

Vignesh, R. C., S. Sitta Djody, et al. (2006). Effect of ethanol on human osteosarcoma cell proliferation, differentiation and mineralization. *Toxicology*, Vol. 220, No. 1, pp.(63-70).

Vikman, K., J. Isgaard, et al. (1991). Growth hormone regulation of insulin-like growth factor-I mRNA in rat adipose tissue and isolated rat adipocytes. *J Endocrinol*, Vol. 131, No. 1, pp.(139-45).

Wahl, E. C., D. S. Perrien, et al. (2005). Ethanol-induced inhibition of bone formation in a rat model of distraction osteogenesis: A role for the tumor necrosis factor signaling axis. *Alcohol Clin Exp Res*, Vol. 29, No. 8, pp.(1466-72).

Wang, J., J. Zhou, et al. (2004). Evidence supporting dual, IGF-I-independent and IGF-I-dependent, roles for GH in promoting longitudinal bone growth. *J Endocrinol*, Vol. 180, No. 2, pp.(247-55).

Wang, Y., S. Nishida, et al. (2007). IGF-I receptor is required for the anabolic actions of parathyroid hormone on bone. *J Bone Miner Res*, Vol. 22, No. 9, pp.(1329-37).

Watson, P., D. Lazowski, et al. (1995). Parathyroid hormone restores bone mass and enhances osteoblast insulin-like growth factor I gene expression in ovariectomized rats. *Bone*, Vol. 16, No. 3, pp.(357-65).

Wezeman, F. H. & Z. Gong. (2004). Adipogenic effect of alcohol on human bone marrow-derived mesenchymal stem cells. *Alcohol Clin Exp Res*, Vol. 28, No. 7, pp.(1091-101).

White, V. & G. Smith (2009). Report on australian secondary school students' use of tobacco, alcohol, and over-the-counter and illICIt substances, 2008. Available at: <http://www.nationaldrugstrategy.gov.au/internet/drugstrategy/publishing.nsf/Content/school08>.

Whiting, S. J., H. Vatanparast, et al. (2004). Factors that affect bone mineral accrual in the adolescent growth spurt. *J Nutr*, Vol. 134, No. 3, pp.(696S-700S).

World Health Organization (2011). Global status report on alcohol and health. Available at: <http://www.who.int/substance_abuse/publications/global_alcohol_report/msbgsruprofiles.pdf>.

Xu, L., Q. Wang, et al. (2011). Concerted actions of insulin-like growth factor-I, testosterone and estradiol on peripubertal bone growth - a 7-year longitudinal study. *J Bone Miner Res*, Vol., No.

Yakar, S., M. L. Bouxsein, et al. (2006). The ternary IGF complex influences postnatal bone acquisition and the skeletal response to intermittent parathyroid hormone. *J Endocrinol*, Vol. 189, No. 2, pp.(289-99).

Yakar, S., H. Kim, et al. (2005). The growth hormone-insulin like growth factor axis revisited: Lessons from IGF-I and IGF-I receptor gene targeting. *Pediatr Nephrol*, Vol. 20, No. 3, pp.(251-4).

Yakar, S., C. J. Rosen, et al. (2002). Circulating levels of IGF-I directly regulate bone growth and density. *J Clin Invest*, Vol. 110, No. 6, pp.(771-81).

Zhao, G., M. C. Monier-Faugere, et al. (2000). Targeted overexpression of insulin-like growth factor I to osteoblasts of transgenic mice: Increased trabecular bone volume without increased osteoblast proliferation. *Endocrinology*, Vol. 141, No. 7, pp.(2674-82).

4

Scaffold Materials Based on Fluorocarbon Composites Modified with RF Magnetron Sputtering

S. I. Tverdokhlebov, E. N. Bolbasov and E. V. Shesterikov
Tomsk Polytechnic University, Russia

1. Introduction

A bone is a remarkable organ, which plays the key role in performing of such critical functions in human physiology, as protection, movement and support of other organs, blood production, accumulation and homeostasis of minerals, regulation of blood pH, and location of many cells - progenitors (mesenchimal and hemopoetic). The importance of a bone becomes clear in the case of such diseases, as osteogenesis imperfecta, osteoarthritis, osteomielitis and osteoporosis when a bone is not functioned by proper way. These diseases together with traumatic injuries, orthopaedic operations (total joint replacement, spine arthrodesis, implant fixation and other) and the first tumor resection lead to formation of bone defects. Clinical and economical aspects, accompanying treatment of bone defects are bemusing (Porter et al., 2009). For example, quantity of total joint arthroplastics (TJA) and revision operation only in USA increased from 700 000 in 1998 up to over 1.1 million in 2005 (American Academy of Orthopedic Surgeons, Web Site). According to estimations of specialists medical expenses connected with fractures, reimplantations, and replacement of hip and knee joints to 2003 exceeded $ 20 billions and to 2015 will exceed $ 74 billions (American Academy of Orthopedic Surgeons, Web Site; Kurtz et al., 2007). Traumatic bone fracture caused about 8.5 million doctor's appointments and led to about 1 million hospitalizing (American Academy of Orthopedic Surgeons, Web Site). Also, in 2005 there were performed more than 3000 pediatric hospitalizations connected with cancer with cost more than $ 70 million (US Department of Health and Human Services, Web Site).

In the cases of non-union or defects of critic sizes it is necessary to use replacing materials for filling of bone defects. Actual gold standard of treatment of bone defects of critical sizes is transplantation of autogenous bone. At such treatment the host bone is removed from other part (usually from pelvis or ilium crest) and used to fill the defect. However, complication rates at transplantation of autogenous bone exceeds 30 % and can include morbidness of a donor site, pain, parestesie, long hospitalization and rehabilitation, higher danger of depth infection, heamatoma, inflammation and limited legal capacity (Silber et al., 2003). Other rational version for patients and surgeons is use of bone tissue of other people (usually cadavers) named allograft which can be obtained both from viable and sterilized nonviable sources. During last years many orthopaedic procedures connected with use of allografts have been performed in various countries. Success of autograft and allograft procedures is described to physical and biological similarity of donor and host tissue. However, orhopaedic allografts bears danger for a donor to obtain infection (case rate is more than 3 %) (Mankin et al., 2005) and for a host – transferring of diseases and immune responses (Nishida & Shimamura, 2008). It is possible to consider as acceptable option for patients demanding restoration or replacement of bone use of xenografts or un-human tissues. Each success in xenotransplantation of various cells, tissues and organs, caused optimism and social acceptance of this growing technology (Lanza et al., 1991). However, results of clinical investigations, being performed during more than 20 years, led scientists to conclusion about unsuitability of xenografts for restoring surgeries owing to real and recognizable danger of transfer diseases or viruses, infections, toxicity, connected with sterilization, immunogeneity and final rejection by the host (Laurencin & El-Amin, 2008).

To solve these problems, it has been proposed so-called tissue engineering approach, which became usable alternative allowing stimulating regenerative ability of the organism – host (Kanczler & Oreffo, 2008). To realize this approach on practice many investigators are developing various complicated synthetic construction, named bone scaffolds which simulate complicated physical-chemical properties of bone. Use of such synthetic bone scaffolds is connected with such qualities as wide availability of materials for their manufacturing, elimination of the danger of transfer diseases, decrease of quantity of surgery procedures and reduction of infection danger or immunogenicity.

Basic conception, laying in the basis of tissue engineering is use of natural biologic response on tissue damage with high technological principles. Since role of cell signalizing and functionality are displayed in tissue engineering with great clearness, specialists in the field of tissue engineering develop multifunctional bioactive scaffolds. Ideal synthetic scaffolds have to provide certain physical – chemical milieu in the time of biodegradation, while stimulating actively desirable physiological response and preventing undesirable one (Lee & Shin, 2007).

To fulfill these biomimetic requirements a synthetic bone scaffold must:

1. provide temporary mechanic support for affected area,
2. act as substrate for deposition of osteoids,
3. have architecture which allows flowing processes of vascularization and in-growth of bone,
4. promote migration of bone cells in a scaffold,
5. support and promote osteogenous differentiation in a non-bone synthetic scaffold (osteoinduction),
6. enforce cellular activity in direction of scaffold – tissue host integration (osteointegration),
7. degrade by controlled way to easy load transfer to developing bone,
8. generate non-toxic degradation products,
9. not provoke active confirmed inflammation response,
10. survive sterilization without loss of bioactivity,
11. deliver bioactive molecules or drugs by controlled way to accelerate healing and prevent pathology.

To satisfy above mentioned criteria such various strategies of tissue engineering, as cell transplantation, cell-less scaffolds, gene therapy, stem cell therapy and growth factor delivery were applicated (Ki et al., 2008; Leeuwenburgh et al., 2006; Kumar et al., 2003; Schneider & Decher, 2008; Kim & Mooney, 1998). On practice majority of bone tissue engineering approaches uses combination of these strategies. However, following two main strategies of cell engineering are considered as the most perspective (Langer & Vacanti, 1993):

the first one - mesenchimal stem cells (MSC) are isolated (usually from a patient) before implantation, in following they are expanded *ex vivo*, seeded on a synthetic scaffold, where they obtained possibility to produce extracellular matrix (ECM) on the scaffold and finally, implanted in bone defects or cavities in patient tissues (see Fig. 1) (Mistry &Mikos, 2005); the second one - a cell-less scaffold is implanted immediately after damage / resection of bone.

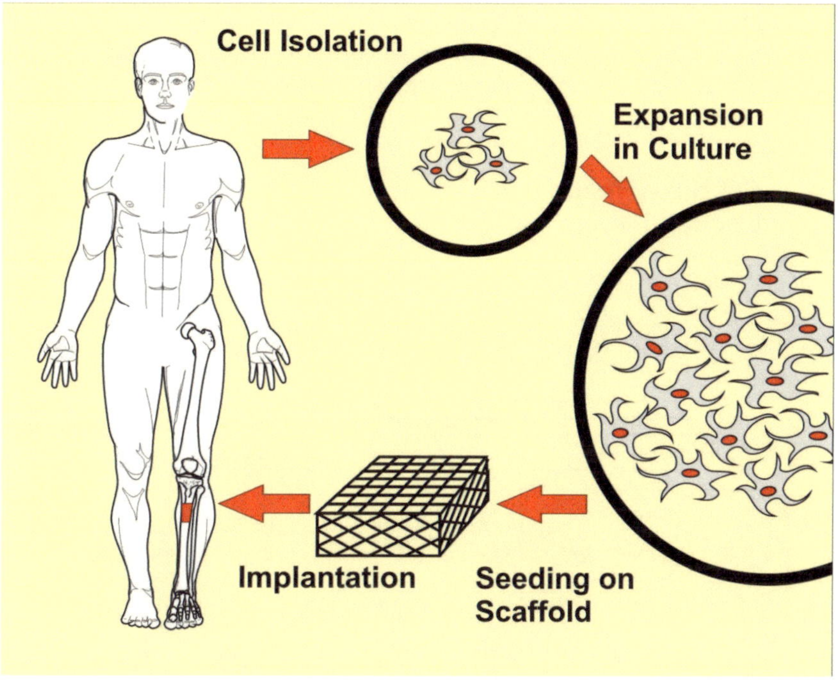

Fig. 1. Scheme of bone tissue engineering by means of scaffolds seeded with cells cultured before implantation *ex vivo*

MSC are pluripotent cells being able to differentiate in cells of various types. Under action of such chemical agents as dexametasone, ascorbic acid, and β-glicerol phosphate differentiation of MSC may be directed in side of bone forming cells or osteoblats, which than produce bone ECM within a scaffold *ex vivo*. It has been shown in many preclinical experiences that MSCs increase osteogenous ability and are integrated with native tissue more quickly than cell-less scaffolds (Service, 2000).

In spite of huge potential of this approach to bone cell engineering, it is necessary to overcome many barriers to transfer it in clinical practice. The first and most considerable one is defined by the fact that in number of investigation it has been shown that MSCs, which were cultured extensively *ex vivo* , being implanted *in vivo*, loss their phenotypical behavior (such as osteodifferentiation and bone forming ability) (Banfi et al., 2000). The second problem appearing at this approach is connected with comparable low concentration of MSCs in bone marrow and their characteristic low proliferative ability and consists in hardship of obtaining of sufficient cell density in a large scaffold (Bruder et al., 1997). In addition to higher risk owing to necessity of the second operation surgeons are facing with necessity to state strict measures of sterilization for scaffolds seeded with cells cultivated *ex vivo* within period up to some weeks.

The second main approach of tissue engineering includes implantation of a cell-less scaffold immediately after trauma/resection of bone (see Fig. 2). Guiding principles of such approach are the same of the first one. However, to provide rapid healing, designing of a scaffold which is built in the native bone tissue and is capable to promote migration of local MSCs in scaffold, to support and promote osteodifferentiation (osteoinduction), while providing formation of biodegradable matrix, which increase production of ECM by MSC and eventually integrates with native tissue and fills cavities or defects (osteointegration) is more critic (Nair & Laurencin, 2006). Obvious values of this approach are that cell-less scaffolds can be sterilized more easy, have large shelf time and lowest potential of infection or immunogenicity.

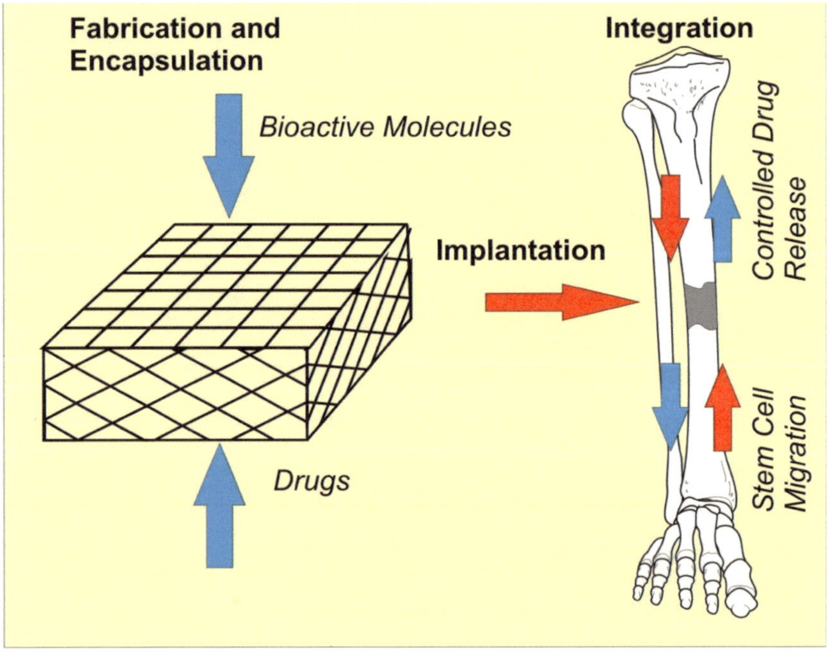

Fig. 2. Schematic description of the second strategy of bone tissue engineering in which biological molecules and pharmaceutical agents are encapsulated in cell-less scaffold to release after implantation

The further development of these strategies is designing of porous scaffolds for bone tissue engineering taking into account not only biomechanics and achievements in the field of material sciences, but and understanding of processes running both in damaged bone on the each stage of its regeneration and on tissue - implant interface. Such constructions must have porous structure, allowing inserting in them pharmacological preparations and cellular materials which will be released from construction while stimulating and controlling osteogenesis processes therefore they can be named biochips. Preliminary consideration of concepts for use of biochips for tissue engineering it is possible to find in papers (Santini et al., 1999, 2000).

2. Methods of scaffold manufacturing

By their essence a biochip is a porous scaffold loaded with bioactive agents (such as various growth factors, DNA, bone morphogenetic proteins etc.) with programmable time and space patterns (principles) of releasing of these components allowing stimulating purposefully osteogenesis process in the implantation place. Taking into account this fact, a biochip performs, in certain degree, function of a drug delivery system with scaffold as basis of his construction.

2.1 The role of physical impetus in synthetic bone scaffolds

Hierarchic geometrical structure of bone, shown in Figure 3 are critical not only for macroscopic mechanical properties, but and for survival of bone cells and functionality in micro- and nanoscale. Owing to directs deposition and bounding of extracellular matrix (ECM) proteins and cell cytoskeleton through cell receptors cells sense and respond to matrix physical properties converting mechanical impetuses in intracellular chemical signals which initiate such activity as gene expression, protein production, and general phenotypical behavior (Vallet-Regır et al., 2006).

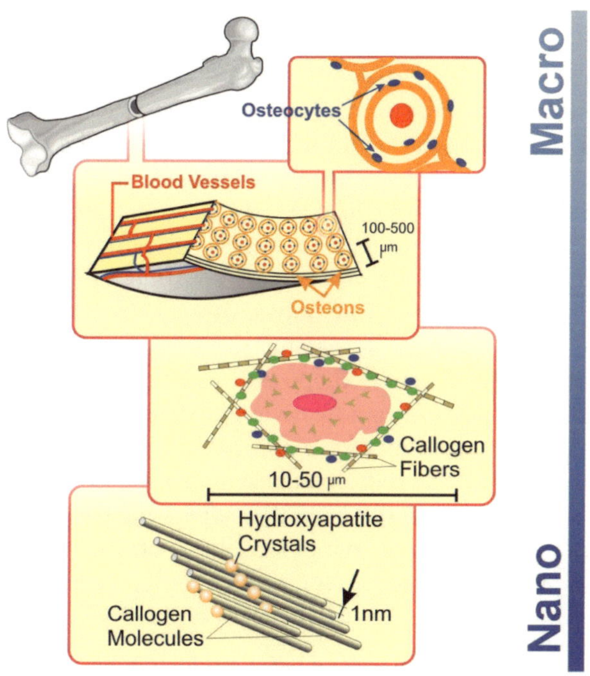

Fig. 3. Scheme of sophisticated hierarchical structure of bone

Therefore the main aim of bone scaffold designing is simulation of unique bone micro- and nanoscale characteristics. It is shown in literature that bone cells are influenced considerably by topography *in vitro* (Desai, 2000). Such, Vagaska found that osteoblasts grown on the microrough surfaces have been stimulated to differentiation as it is shown by expression of their genes and higher mineralization level in comparison with cells growing on smooth surfaces (Vagaska et al., 2010).

Microscale bone peculiarities provide channel for vascularization, nutrient delivery, and cell migration. Some investigators supposed that to assure migration of bone cells and nutrients in a scaffold it is necessary to have pores with sizes closed to cell sizes (Mo et al., 2004). High porous microscale scaffolds also allow more high levels of nutrient diffusion, vascularization, and improved spatial organization for cell growth and ECM production (Woodard et al., 2007). However, some ambiguousness remains in relation to optimal porosity and pore sizes for 3D bone scaffold. Review of literature sources shows that pore sizes in range of (10 – 400) μm can provide sufficient intake of nutrients and osteoblast cells while keeping structural integrality (Walsh et al., 2003). The wide variety of methods of manufacturing of biochip matrix frameworks was investigated to recreate microscale porosity and special organization of native bone. Some examples of good developed methods include: microfabrication, photolitography, calcium phosphate sintering, rapid prototyping, mold extrusion, salt leaching, phase separation, fiber bounding, membrane and polymer delamination. Surprising result is that the most successful methods of fabrication include emulsion and sintering of calcium phosphate materials. Synthetic bone scaffolds with porosity up to 70 % have been prepared using these methods. These scaffolds have demonstrated excellent bioactivity *in vitro* and in-growth of bone *in vivo* (Christenson et al., 2007).

However, microscale porosity plays a key role in scaffold osteoconductivity, nanoscale architectonics of material acts basic physical influence on osteoinductivity and osteointegration of a scaffold. Up to now majority of methods of manufacturing of synthetic bone scaffolds were limited macro- and microscale and were impossible to recreate sophisticated bone nanoarchitectonics. However, in the last decade some successes have been achieved in nanofabrication and, consequently, in control of cell behavior by means of nanomanipulation. Bone cell in native tissue interact with nanoscale proteins and minerals. It is stated authentically, that all living systems are controlled by molecular interactions in nanometer scale. Unique properties of all molecular constructive blocks of life, such as proteins, lipids, carbohydrates and nucleic acid, are controlled by their nanoscale sizes and patterns. Consequently, bone cells are predisposed to adhere, grow, proliferate, differentiate and to product ECM on the basis of nanoscale interactions (Horbett, 1994.). In addition to increase cellular activity nanoscale materials can have regulable surface area and surface energy which, as it was shown, influence on adhesive protein adsorption. The wide range of methods of scaffolds nanofabrication has been developed likewise to microscale fabrication. Examples of successful methods of nanofabrication of 2D and 3D objects include electrospinning (Ki et al., 2008) electrostatic spraying deposition (Leeuwenburgh et al., 2006), RF plasma spraying /deposition (Kumar et al., 2003), molecular self assembling (Schneider & Decher, 2008).

2.2 Methods of 3D- porous scaffold fabrication

Porous ceramic degradable scaffolds are used mainly for correction of bone tissue defects, both gained, as result of trauma of operation, and inherent. Taking into account low mechanical strength of porous ceramics matrices, they are used in areas not bearing load, for example, in maxillofacial surgery. The basis for creation of porous ceramic degradable matrix is hydroxyapatite (HA), obtained both from clear reagents, and by means of hydrothermal treatment of aragonite.

2.2.1 Coral scaffolds

Aragonite is a skeleton of sea reef-forming corals Porites, from which porous scaffolds are manufactured by means of hydrothermal treatment in presence of ammonium phosphate at temperature about 275 °C and pressure of 1200 psi by reaction (Kim & Mooney, 1998):

$$10\ CaCO_3 + 6\ (NH_4)_2HPO_4 + 2\ H_2O \rightarrow Ca_{10}(PO_4)_6(OH)_2 + 6(NH_2)CO_3 + 4H_2CO_3.$$

The carried out investigations revealed two coral kinds having pore size suitable for transformation in hydroxyapatite and following use as matrices for tissue engineering (Ki et al., 2008). It has been found that porosity characteristics of sea invertebrates depend on type and kind. Within kinds and between members of these kinds mean pore diameters are quite uniform with low variation range by a structure.

Before exchange reaction organic component of these corals are removed by sodium hypochlorite. Extreme chemical and thermal conditions of exchange reaction destroy any remnant organic material. Structure of obtained hydroxyapatite is almost accurate replica of porous skeleton of sea animals including their interconnecting porosity with pore diameter 150 – 500 μm resembling the system of haversian channels of compact human bone, that promotes growth and differentiation of cells leading to rapid ingrowth of bone tissue at implantation (Jones & Hench, 2003). Ingrowth of connective and bone tissue in such matrix is accompanied with moderate inflammation and giant-cells reactions (Massry & Holds, 1995), minimal capsule formation about matrix (Dutton, 1991) and osteogenesis in coral depth (Holmes, 1979). The mechanism of osteoinducing action of HA is not revealed decisively.

Ingrowth of bone tissue also depends on pore size and porosity which determine total contact area of porous matrix surface with surrounding tissues. This index determines not only velocity of penetration of biologic liquids and biodegradation of material, but is important element determining ability of bone cells to seed an implant. So, work surface area of dense and porous HA was from 0.01 to 1.0 m^2/g, accordingly (Tofe et al., 1993).

In macroporous material with pore diameter of 20-200 μm natural liquid convection appears owing to capillary processes. It promotes transportation of substances, biodegradation or dissolving of material (Walsh et al., 2006). So, at using of corals with through porosity, process of cell migration and osteoclast resorption of material lasts about 6 - 8 weeks. If pores are not interconnective, closed cavity appears from which exit of substances is hampered. In these conditions process of biodegradation can delay up to 18 months (Holmes et al., 1984; Hanusiac, PhD Thesis).

To simulate osteon - free stroma of cortical bone one uses the coral Porties skeleton. Solid frameworks and porous network are continuous and interconnective domens. Mean size of solid components of implant framework is 75 μm, mean pore diameter achieves 230 μm and their interconnections 190 μm, volume part of cavities is 65 % (White & Shors, 1986).

To simulate osteon - free stroma of cancellous bone one uses the coral Goniopora skeleton. Mean size of solid components of implant framework is 130 μm, mean pore diameter achieves 600 μm and volume part of cavities is 63 % (Malluche et al., 1982).

Due to high biocompatibility of a coral, a material obtained from coral skeletons has been permitted for clinical use in the USA only in four years after first implantation performed by A. C. Perry in 1985. In period of six years coral spheres have been implanted in 25,000 patients. Wide distribution of the materials is promoted by industrial production of coral apatite matrices by the firm «Interpore Int, California» (USA) under trade names Interpore®

200, ProOsteon®200, ProOsteon® 500, and «BIO-EYE» by the «Integrated orbital implants Inc.» (USA).

2.2.2 Scaffolds from cattle bones

Materials obtained from cattle bones are used for fabrication of matrices, too. They are unsintered (BioOss®, Oxbone®, Lubboc®, Laddec®) or sintered at temperature about 1000 °C (BonAP, Endobon®, Osteograf®). To remove proteins unsintered materials are treated usually in organic solutions or CO_2 supercritical liquids. Remained bone material is mainly carbonated hydroxyapatite (CHA) with little additions of magnesium, sodium and other trace elements. Its chemical composition and crystallinity, naturally, resembles one of a bone with large specific surface area and macroporosity (Thaller, 1993). This material has osteoinductive properties and at implantation in bone defects bone formation takes place on its surface. Antigenic or immugenic inflammation responds are not observed while using of deproteinized cattle bone, however, velocity of its resorption is issue of disputes. In some investigations it has been observed no signs of resorption (Valentini et al., 1998) or only slight resorption (Piatelli et al., 1999). In other animal experiments vats resorption took place (Merkx et al., 1999). To burn organic components and to remain sintered body cancellous cattle bone is heated to temperature about 1000 °C. In dependence on conditions of sintering, temperature and time, porosity (micro/ macroporosity) of initial bone has been kept essentially, but phase composition is changed sharply, when carbonate apatite (CHA) is decomposed at high temperatures on HA and ß-TCP (Le Geros et al., 1991). These materials differ by composition (HA/ ß-TCP ratio) in dependence on stoichiometry of initial cattle bone.

However unique chemical composition and spatial pore structure of above mentioned matrices is combined with such their physical chemical properties as high density and fragility which create many inconveniences at work with them, since hinder hand treatment to model a scaffold. To work with them it is necessary additional equipment of operation room with cutting or milling diamond instruments. Impossibility of suture fixation of tissue to such scaffolds, their coarse rough surface injuring surrounding tissues (Goldberg et al., 1992; Kim et al., 1994), force in certain cases to wrap them with donor or synthetic tissue.

Therefore scaffolds from synthetic calcium phosphate are implemented actively as alternative to natural expensive material (for example, for orbital implants trade marks «FCI ophthalmics» and «LIFECORE»). Implant FCI (French firm Issy-Les-Moulineaux) of the third (last) generation has the same chemical composition and mechanical strength as natural coral, sufficient porosity and suitable for hand treatment.

2.2.3 Scaffolds from synthetic calcium phosphates

Synthetic calcium phosphates are divided on hydroxyapatite (HA), $Ca_{10}(PO_4)_6(OH)_2$ (Cerapatite®, Synatite®); tricalcium phosphate (ß-TCP), $Ca_3(PO_4)_2$ (Biosorb®, Calciresorb®, Chronos®), bi-phase calcium phosphate (BCP) for admixtures HA and ß-TCP (Biosel®, Ceraform®, Eurocer®, MBCP®, Hatric®, Tribone 80®, Triosite®, TricOs®); and unsintered or calcium deficit apatite.

Calcium phosphates have various solubility velocities *in vitro* or velocity of solution in acid buffers that can reflect comparative dissolution or degradation *in vivo* (Le Geros et al., 1995). Comparative solution degree is changed in following order: α-TCP >> ß-TCP >> HA.

Calcium phosphate (CaP) biomaterials are available in various physical forms (particles or blocks, dense or porous). One of the main characteristics is their porosity. Ideal pore size for bioceramics resembles one of cancellous bone. Before sintering at high temperatures macroporosity (pore size > 50 μm) intentionally introduced by means of additions of volatile substances or porogens (naphthalenes, sugars, hydrogen peroxide, polymer pellets, fibers etc.) before sintering at high temperatures (Hubbard, 1974). Macroporosity forms when volatile substances are released. Microporosity is result of sintering process, where temperature and time are critical parameters. It was displayed that microporosity allows circulation of body liquids, while microporosity provides matrix for colonization of bone cells (Daculsi et al., 1990). It was reported, that mean pore size 565 μm is ideal macropore size for in-growth of bone in comparison with one of smaller size (300 μm) (Gauthier et al., 1999). The main difference between commercially available BCP is miroporosity which depends on sintering process. For osteogenic or osteoconductive properties low temperature sintering processes have to conserve or to increase microporosity. Only bi-phase calcium phosphate prepared at low temperature (less than 1100 °C) are both micro- and macroporous.

In spite of that synthetic calcium phosphates are cheaper than their natural analogues, they have essential shortcoming - fragility. Therefore in last decade porous polymers which are elastic, comparatively easy treated and modeled, fixed with suture material became to use as rival material for scaffolds.

2.2.4 3D porous polymer scaffolds

Various methods are used for manufacturing of 3D porous scaffolds. Usual methods include fibrous felt, fibrous bonding, mold casting, solution casting / particle leaching, gas foam forming/ particle leaching, phase separation and high pressure treatment. Examples of porous scaffolds are given in Figure 4.

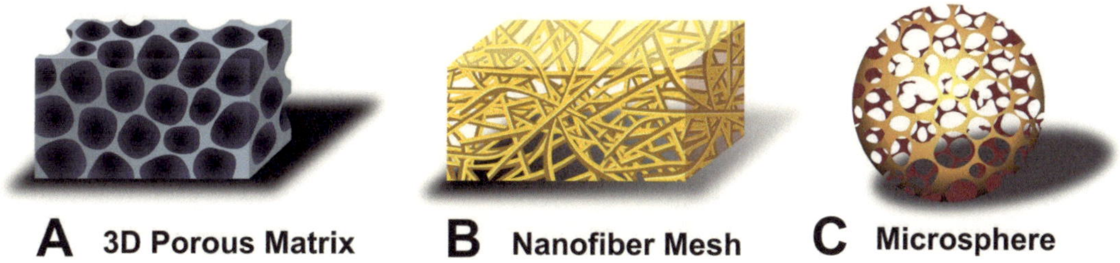

Fig. 4. Various forms of polymer scaffolds for tissue engineering: A - typical 3D - matrix in solid foam form, B - nanofiber matrix, C - porous microspheres

Fibrous bonding

3D porous scaffolds can be fabricated bounding polymer fibers in crossing point using a secondary polymer. For example, fibers of polyglicolic acid (PGA) can be bonded by casting of poly (L-lactic acid) (PLLA), cooling and following removing of PLLA (Whang et al., 1995). However this method faces with difficulties connected with control porosity and solvent selection.

Freeze-drying of emulsion

Freeze-drying of emulsion solution consisted from dispersed water phase and continuous organic phase containing biodegradable polymer can lead to formation of porous scaffolds with various size and interconnectivity of pores. While using this method, Mikos A.G. prepared scaffolds on the basic of poly (lactic-co-glicolic) acid (PLGA) with porosity up to 95 % and pore size up to 200 µm (Mikos et al., 1993).

Solution casting/particle leaching

Solution casting/particle leaching is, probably, the handiest method for preparation of porous scaffolds. It includes casting of mixed solution polymer - salt - organic solvent with following evaporation of solvent and dissolution of salt particles in water solution. However, this method has restrictions, since allows fabricating only thin membranes with dense surface layer as well as may contain remnant particles of the salt used in the time of process. Applied efforts allowed obtaining thin scaffolds with open cellular morphology and porosity higher 93%. To prepare thick 3D scaffolds, PLLA or PLGA porous membranes have been collected in multiple-layer structures of various anatomical forms (Mooney et al., 1996; Harris et al., 1998).

High pressure treatment

High pressure treatment also known as technology of supercritical liquid is performed by means of action on dry polymer with such high pressure gas as carbon dioxide which forms mono-phase solution polymer/ gas. Then pressure is discharge to form thermodynamic instability of dissolved CO_2 that leads to nucleation and growth of gas vesicles, created pores within polymer matrix. Yoon J.J et al. used this method to create high-porous PLGA sponges (Yoon & Park, 2001). Solid PLGA disks, prepared by compressing casting or solution casting, were saturated with CO_2 under high pressure, then pressure was discharged and formed macroporous structure. The main quality of this method is that it eliminates using of organic solvents. Since this method does not include heating process, it is useful for incorporation of thermosensitive bioactive agents. Porous structure is quite uniform since CO_2 - gas uniformly dissolved within polymer as well as acts as softener which induces denser packing of polymer chains that increases mechanical strength. However, this method leads to insufficient interconnectivity of pores within scaffold and in many cases to non-porous surface. To eliminate this shortcoming Nam Y.S. et al. modified this method combining it with method of particle leaching (Nam et al., 2000). Mixture PLGA/NaCl has been casted under pressure in solid disks which were exposed to action of CO_2 gas and submerged in water for leaching of a salt. Described process led to formation of high interconnected mesh without signs of non-porous surface.

Gas foam formation /particle leaching

The method of «gas foam formation» had been developed by Park group, using effervescent salt as gas foaming agent. Double PLA-gel solvent blend containing particles of dispersed salt of bicarbonate ammonium was poured into a mold and then was submerged in hot water. Releasing of gaseous hydrides of nitrogen and carbon dioxide from solidifying polymeric matrix led to the formation of high interconnected pores. Formed scaffolds had open macroporous cellular structure with uniform distribution of pores which size ranged from 100 to 200 µm and without signs of surface layer. Method of gas foam formation / salt releasing had been improved further for preparation of PLGA scaffolds with addition of citric acid in water solution (Kim et al., 2006). In this case the amorphous PLGA dissolved in chloroform was precipitated in ethanol to obtain gel suspension. Particles of ammonium bicarbonate mixed with this gel paste were poured into a mold and semi solidified at room temperature. After that they were submerged in an aqueous solution of citric acid. This method allows obtaining macroporous PLGA scaffolds with porosity more than 90 % and pore size about 200 μm. Porosity and mechanical strength can be controlled by regulating degree of gas forming reactions basic - acid between two salts. These scaffolds were commercialized in Republic Korea under trade mark Innopol-D™ for plastic surgery application. The same principle of gas foam formation allows manufacturing injector PLGA scaffolds - microforms, while using method of evaporation of solvent from double emulsion (Nam & Park, 1999). High opened porous microsphere with size of (200 - 300) μm were prepared by insertion of ammonium bicarbonate in drops of inner water phase, which formed actively gas vesicles in process of removing of solvent. Surface pore size achieved 30 μm, being sufficient for infiltration and seeding that was displayed by culturing of fibroblasts.

Thermally induced phase separation

Method of phase separation is based on thermodynamical separation of uniform polymer - solvent solution on the phase reached with polymer, and the phase depleted with polymer. Usually separation are performed either by action on the solution of other immiscible solvent or cooling of solvent to the point under two node solubility curve (Nam & Park, 1999). In particularly, thermally induced phase separation (TIPS) uses thermal energy as latent solvent to induce phase separation. Polymer solution is quenched under freezing point and than freeze drying forming porous structure, which parameters can be fine controlled, while regulating various thermodynamical and kinetic parameters. The most early scaffold for tissue engineering prepared by TIPS method had microporous structure (1 -10) μm without interconnectivity and open cellularity. Park used TIPS method to obtain scaffolds with macroporous structure and open cellular morphology. To increase size of phase separated drops one used roughness increase process that increased pore size up to 100 μm. Obtained scaffolds had pores with uniform distribution and porosity more than 90 %, too. They also displayed that addition of surfactant (Pluronic F127) increased scaffold pore morphology.

Electrospinning

Owing to its simplicity and efficiency electrospinning is the most wide used method for manufacturing of nanofibrous unwoven matrices which is considered the most prospective strategy to manufacture nanofibrous scaffolds simulating bone. Popularity of electrospinning is stipulated, to all appearance, by simplicity of the experimental plant, ability to include bioactive molecules and plasticity which it provided. Investigation both *in vitro* and in *vivo* has demonstrated that cell osteopredecessors differentiate, proliferate and adhere to synthetic nanofibrous matrices. In electrospinnig process (see Fig. 5) polymer melting or solution in organic solvent are spread out nozzle under action of gravity force and/or mechanical pressure combined with strong electric field created by high voltage (10 - 20) kV. When force acting on electric load of the material exceeds surface tension of polymer solution drop, polymer jet arises from which solid nanofibers are formed at following evaporation of solvent (Li et al., 2002). Electrospinning allows obtaining nanofibers of such materials as biodegradable polymers, for example: PLGA and polycaprolacton (PCL), materials soluble in water, for example poly (ethylenoxide) (PEO), polyvinyl alcohol (PVA) and such natural polymers as collagen, silk protein and other peptide.

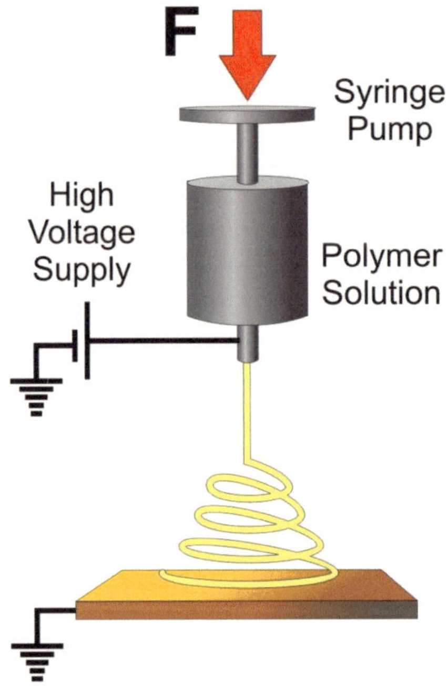

Fig. 5. Typical electrospinning plant consisting of high voltage supply, syringe and syringe pump

Usually electrospinning is used for creation of 2D mesh structure with nanosized pores, which are insufficient for seeding and infiltration of pores. Therefore it is necessary to form macroporous and nanofibrous 3D hybrid scaffolds with required volume and form for application as implantable scaffold for regeneration of tissues.

2.3 Methods of polymer scaffold modification

Although porous scaffolds with good interconnected pores are sufficiently suitable to allow infiltration and in-growth of cells such their surface characteristics as hydrophilicity /hydrophobicity resulting from chemical composition can not be satisfied to induce selective adhesion, migration and proliferation of cell and, as consequence, osteogenesis. In majority of cases specific cellular interactions are required to form required tissue. In general, adsorption behavior of proteins with accompanying determining cellular interactions is determined by implanted biomaterials surface properties. To achieve optimal osteogenesis number of investigators made attempts to simulate natural extracellular matrix by immobilization of naturally obtained biomolecules on polymer scaffold surface. Scaffolds with engineering surface were able to amplify adhesion and growth of cells or prolonged release of growth factors (Wolke et al., 1992), thereby assuring chance to facilitate process of tissue regeneration. Scaffold surface can be functionalized both by physical adsorption and by chemical modification.

Important stage of creation of matrix is modification of its surface with aim to create hydrophilic coatings. As experience shows, in the case of using of matrices for restoration of bone tissue defects the best way to provide it is coating the porous matrices surfaces with calcium phosphates, for example, hydroxyapatite. This coating provides accelerated integration of implants with surrounding bone tissue. Some methods are developed for realization of this process, which are used with large or small success. Possible methods of modification of polymeric scaffolds are given below.

2.3.1 Biomimetic deposition

Biomimetic deposition is process of crystallization, i.e. falling of crystals on matrix surface from oversaturated solutions containing calcium phosphates. Principally, biomimetic coatings are formed from solutions simulated body liquids. Advantage of this method are possibility of applying of high crystalline coatings, absence of complicated technological process, simplicity of technological tools, possibility to apply coatings on complicated geometrical forms at room temperature. It makes the method of biomimetic deposition suitable to apply CaP coatings on scaffolds. As shortcomings of the method it is possible to name low adhesion of CaP coatings, especially to inert polymer substrates, large time (about 8 - 10 days) necessary to apply coatings with thickness about some micrometers (Habibovic et al., 2002).

2.3.2 Plasma spraying

Plasma spraying is the method which is used the most often for application of CaP coatings on orthopaedic implants. The method is based on feeding of CaP particles in gas - carrier through plasma of electric or gas -fired arc. Under action of high temperature gas is ionized and becomes plasma, which is accelerated up to high velocities. CaP particles, transferred by gas - carrier, are heated, melted, than deposited on a substrate. However the method proved its usefulness, its shortcoming is low cohesion of coating, especially at applying of calcium phosphate layers of large thickness. In addition at applying of CaP by method of plasma spraying the substrate temperature increases considerably that makes this method practically unsuitable for applying of CaP ceramic coating on polymer materials, on consequence of their melting and thermal destruction (Chen et al., 1994).

2.3.3 The method of pulsed laser deposition

The method is based on process of rapid melting and evaporation of target material in vacuum under action of high energy laser radiation with following transition of evaporated material from target and its deposition on a substrate. The method of pulsed laser deposition is technologically flexible method since energy source - a laser - is located out the vacuum chamber and can be changed on any other source optimally suitable to evaporate a target of one or another chemical composition.

The method of pulsed laser deposition allows to evaporate practically each material, sequential evaporation of various targets with different chemical composition allows to deposit both mono-phase and multilayer films of various materials. Other advantage of pulsed laser deposition is keeping in coating of stoichiometric composition of target to be evaporated. Controlling laser generation mode, it is possible to regulate very accurately thickness of the deposited film (Fernández-Parada et al., 1998). As shortcomings of the method it is possible to name impossibility to obtain coatings of uniform thickness on spatial porous structures presented by scaffolds for tissue regeneration and low velocity of coating growth.

2.3.4 Pulse ion deposition method (deposition from ablation plasma formed by powerful ion beam)

The method of power ion beams (PIB) is based on process of rapid melting and evaporation of target material at its irradiation by power ion beams with energy of some hundred keV and following deposition of coating from formed ablation plasma.

The PIB method is characterized by high values of material coefficient of energy adsorption (for PIB coefficient of energy adsorption is about 1, for laser radiation ~ 0.1). Power efficiency of ion pulsed accelerators is (20 - 40) %, that exceeds considerably power efficiency of laser plants which does not achieve 3 %. The method allows obtaining nanosized multilayer coating on various materials: metal, alloys and ceramics. Coating, obtained by PIB method are amorphous, characterized low inner stresses and good adhesion to a substrate being (10 - 60) MPa (Saltymakov et al., 2010; Struts et al., 2011).

However it is necessary to note that the method requires certain improvement and at the present this circumstance hinders wide use for formation of coatings on polymer scaffold.

2.3.5 The method of explosive evaporation

We proposed to use the method of explosive evaporation for applying of coating on metallic and ceramic implants. This method is based on phenomenon of instant evaporation of powdery material at its hit on the high temperature evaporator. Appearance of vacuum work chamber in process of coating applying is given in Figure 6. Structurally devices for explosive evaporation are manufactured by such way, that material particles would fed with velocity equal to velocity of its evaporation. In this case at steady conditions there are all components of material of complex composition will be in vaporous form in the same ratio as in initial material and the film of specified composition will be obtained on matrix surface. Advantage of the method is high velocity of calcium phosphate coating applying being about 5 μm/h (Tverdokhlebov et al., 2010).

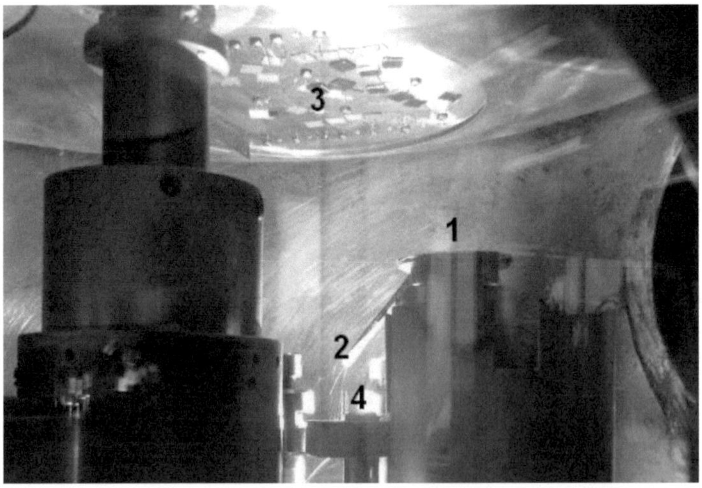

Fig. 6. Appearance of vacuum chamber of explosive evaporation plant: 1 - vibrating bin, 2 - device for feeding of materials, 3 - sample, 4 - evaporator

To estimate ability of application of the explosive evaporation method for applying of calcium phosphate coatings on polymer materials is necessary additional investigations.

2.3.6 The method of radio-frequency magnetron sputtering

Radio-frequency magnetron sputtering (RFMS) is used widely in microelectronics to apply films of complex chemical composition without change of their stoichiometry. The method is based on sputtering of material in vacuum owing to bombardment of target surface with work gas (mainly argon) ions, forming in plasma of anomalous glow discharge at applying of magnetic field.

Principal electric circuit of RF magnetron sputtering system is given in Figure 7. For applying of calcium phosphate coating one uses RFMS plants with work frequency, as rule, 13.56 MHz, allowing obtain high homogeneity of plasma and, as result, to achieve even applying of coating with growth rate of dielectric fields (0.2 - 0.8) μm/h.

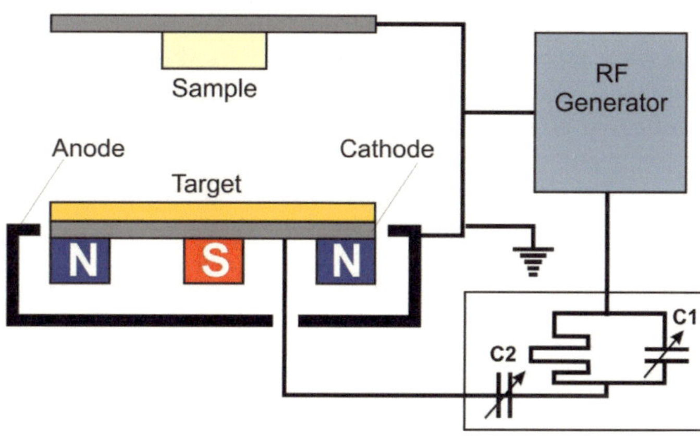

Fig. 7. Principle electric circuit of RFMS

RFMS technology allows to form elastic CaP coating with regulated chemical composition with thickness about 1-2 μm, low porosity, high adhesion to matrix material. Magnetron coating applied on polymer materials are able to withstand essential mechanical deformation without destruction. Microscopic investigation show that coating obtained by the RFMS method are solid, able to repeat initial matrix surface morphology, have no own macro- and microporous structure that is explained by mechanism of their atomic growth (Pichugin et al., 2008; Aronov et al., 2008). At the present the method of RF magnetron sputtering of calcium phosphate on polymer materials is developed by us in the maximal degree therefore it was used in this work for modification of scaffold surface.

3. Fluorocarbon composites modified with rf magnetron sputtering

As it has been shown above up to now treatment of diseases and injuries of loco-motor apparatus is the complicated clinical problem. Traditional methods and ways based on the use of inner and external osteosynthesis with application of fixators achieved limits of their biomechanical abilities.

For effective treatment of loco-motor apparatus injuries it is necessary to act actively on bone tissue and to control processes of its regeneration and mineralization. With this aim some scientific collectives proposed concept, based on active influence on processes of reparative osteogenesis by means of application of osteoplastic materials (in the first time - calcium phosphates, for example, hydroxyapatite (HA) and tricalcium phosphate (TCP)) and various growth factors (bone morphogenetic protein, fibroblast growth factor, transforming factor, platelet factor, insulin-like factors and others) which jointly promote processes of remodeling and regeneration of bone tissue (Karlov & Shachov, 2001; Barinov & Komlev, 2005).

It is necessary to note that variety of clinical problems to be solved with help of scaffolds stipulates various action on a scaffold and biomechanical characteristics of adjoining bone tissue (density, elasticity modulus and rigidity) and determines various requirements put to physical - mechanical characteristics of coating (thickness, porosity, crystalline structure, chemical composition, solubility etc.). By these causes for successful restoration of loco-motor apparatus functions in various clinical cases traumatologists must have in their arsenal wide line of scaffolds with various surface characteristics which are suitable by optimal way for treatment of concrete patient.

However it is necessary to understand clearly that at the present it is impossible to manufacture, while using any one technology, a material which would totally satisfy the various and contradictory requirements put forward to scaffolds. It is evidently that to manufacture really efficient devices it is necessary to integrate various technologies of manufacturing of scaffolds with technologies of their surface modification. The paper is devoted to technology of hybrid scaffolds fabrication developed by our scientific collective in the Tomsk Polytechnic University (TPU).

3.1 Materials and methods of investigation

As binding material for manufacturing of composite scaffolds we selected copolymer tetrafluorpolyethylene with vinilidenfluoride (TFE/VDF). Our selection was stipulated by its high chemical resistance, good physical-mechanical characteristics, and temperature stability (Kataeva et al., 1975), and biological inertness (Grafskaya, 1967). Such polymers can be processed from solution that simplifies apparatus realization of framework manufacturing process.

As biologically active filler which assures realization of processes of osteoinduction and osteoconduction, we selected hydroxyapatite obtained by means of high temperature processing of biological raw materials. Selection of hydroxyapatite as biological active filler is not occasional but is stipulated by its high ability to bind various molecules including proteins, enzymes, antibody fragments, nucleic acids and others.

It is stated that level of protein bounding depends on phase composition of hydroxyapatite. So, high crystalline hydroxyapatite (crystallinity more than 90%) adsorbs about 90 ng/ml of protein and low crystalline (up to 60%) - 60 ng/ml. It is stated also that high crystalline CaP has more high ability to support growth of osteoblast cells in comparison with more amorphous form as well as control plastic surface in the *in vitro* system (Melican et al., 1998). Consequently, osteoinductive properties of hydroxyapatite in a large extent depend on its crystallinity, therefore task to obtain hydroxyapatite with set phase composition is urgent.

One of the ways to control crystallinity of calcium phosphates and, particularly, hydroxyapatite is method of high temperature burning of biologic raw materials, for example, cattle bones. Hydroxyapatite, obtained in process of such high temperature treatment after multiple washings is non toxic, apirogenic and sterile that makes possible to use it as filler to manufacture composite scaffolds. Other considerable advantage of the high temperature treatment method is keeping of microelement composition of processed biological raw materials.

The main task of this stage of investigation was study of action of temperature of biological raw material treatment on phase composition and parameters of crystalline lattice of hydroxyapatite by method of X-ray phase analysis. Investigations have been carried out with a Shimadzu XRD 6000 diffractometer using CuKα radiation. Analysis of phase composition, sizes of coherent scattering areas, inner elastic stresses has been performed while using PCPDFWIN date bases, as well as program of total profile analysis POWDER CELL 2.4.

Process of manufacturing of hybrid scaffold conditionally can be divided on 2 stages: manufacturing of frameworks and modification of its surface. Framework material was prepared on the first stage as solution of TFE/VDF copolymer in acetone at continuous stirring and constant temperature about 70 °C. Biologically active filler presenting HA dispersion was prepared by means of agitation of HA powder in ethyl acetate in a ball mill at 30 °C during 2 hours. After obtaining of TFE/BDF copolymer solution HA dispersion was added to it at continuous stirring up to achievement of necessary viscosity. Framework material was formed by the method of thermally induced phase separation, while using thermal energy as latent solvent to form porous structure of scaffold. After forming scaffolds specimens were placed in the cabinet dryer with temperature of 130 °C for 12 hours to remove solvent remnants. Selected modes allows to obtain homogenous and flexible (elastic) frameworks TFE/VDF-HA from components prepared with mass ratio of TFE/VDF polymer to HA filler being equal 30:70.

Surface morphology of TFE/VDF-HA frameworks are studied by means of optical microscopy with the «Motic» microscope with following computer processing of data with help of the Motic Image Life plus program package, which allows to determine morphometric characteristics of composite surface: total surface porosity, area and perimeter of pores.

Surface of TFE/VDF-HA framework was investigated with a Philips SEM 515 scanning electron microscope. Framework surface was coated with thin carbon layer to reflux load and to obtain qualitative images of the framework.

Inner structure of framework micropores was investigated by the method of atomic force microscopy using a «C3M Solver HV» device. Investigations were carried out in the contact mode of microscope work.

Chemical composition of the framework was investigated by means of X-ray fluorescent analysis with the Shimadzu XRF 1800 plant. Specimens (samples) for investigation in form of discs with diameter of 5 mm were fabricated by method of cold pressing of material.

Modification of various substrate surface were performed by the method of RF magnetron sputtering of thin calcium phosphate films with aim to study influence of CaP coatings on properties of these materials. Influence of surface modification by the RFMS was investigated using a «Solver-HV» (NT-MDT) atomic force microscope (AFM), allowing to measure surface relief, its phase contrast, surface potential distribution by Kelvin method (Mironov V.L., 2004; McCaig et al., 2005). Measurements were carried out on air in standard conditions in semicontact work mode with the use of two-pass technique. For working in semicontact mode we used cantilevers of grade NSG11 with needle rounding radius of 10 nm and alloying admixture concentration of 5×10^{20} cm^{-3}. Let`s note that this kind of investigations required high cleanness of the surface to be investigated therefore to execute these requirements we prepared some types of reference specimen conditionally divided on groups: I, II, III, IV. Results of influence of RFMS Ca-P coating on reference specimen allow extrapolating obtained data on composite scaffolds.

Specimen of the I group presented plates manufactured from titanium alloy of grade BT – 6 with sizes 20×20×3 mm, which preliminary were polished by mechanical way using GOI paste.

Specimens of the II group were prepared in the same way that specimens of the I group, at this on one side of specimen was applied Ca-P coating formed by method of radio frequency magnetron sputtering (RFMS) of hydroxyapatite target. To apply CaP coating we used the industrial plant «Katod 1M», which vacuum chamber contains standard high frequency magnetron source supplied by HF generator with maximal power 4 kW and work frequency 13.56 MHz. The following technological modes have been selected to apply CaP coating: preliminary pressure in chamber - $5{\cdot}10^{-5}$ Pa, work pressure of Ar – $3{\cdot}10^{-1}$ Pa; specific HF power ~ 20 W/cm^2; time of applying - 2 hours. Specimens – witnesses (polished silicon plates with masked part) were used to determine coating thickness, which was determined with a Talysurf 5 (Tyler-Hobson, England) mechanical profilometer by "step" method. With selected sputtering parameters thickness of formed CaP coating was 0.8 ± 0.02 µm.

Specimens of the III group were prepared in the same way that specimens of the I group, at this on one side of specimen was coated with solution of copolymer of tetrafluorethylene with viniliden fluoride (TFE/VDF) in acetone by the method of pneumatic spraying. Part of a specimen has been masked to obtain coating – substrate interface. Then, specimens with applied polymer coating were places in the ИТМ 50.1100 (ИТМ, Tomsk, Russian Federation) furnace of chamber type, where they were heated up to temperature 200 °C to remove solvent remnants and finally to form coating. Thickness of coatings was determined with a Talysurf 5 mechanical profilometer with the "step" method. Thickness of formed polymer coatings was 5 ± 0.4 µm.

Specimens of the IV group were prepared in the same way that specimens of the III group, after that surface of formed TFE/VDF polymer was underwent modification by means of forming of calcium phosphate coating by the RFMS method in the same technological modes, as specimens of the II group. At selected sputtering parameters thickness of formed CaP coating was 0.8 ± 0.02 µm.

AFM images of surface relief, phase contrast and surface potential have been built for all studied types of specimens. Processing of obtained AFM images were performed with help of Gwiddion 2.25 program complex. The following parameters of surface roughness have been determined: mean arithmetic deviation of surface profile *Ra*, height of profile irregularities by ten points - *Rz*, maximal height of roughness profile – *Pt*, mean maximal depth of roughness hollows – *Rvm*, mean maximal height of roughness peaks– *Rpm*, mean arithmetic deviation of potential profile φ_a, mean value of surface potential U_m, maximal value of surface potential U_{Max}, minimal value of surface potential U_{min}.

To determine limiting water wetting angle of modified surfaces we used the static method of "laying drop". Measurements of limiting wetting angle have been carried out in 60 seconds after placing of a drop on substrate surface. Limiting wetting angle has been accepted as mean value of 5 measurements, which have been carried out with help of an «EasyDrop DSA-15E» (the firm KRUSS) device for drop form analysis.

Toxicological tests, estimations of local irritant action, hemolytic activity of framework from composite materials have been carried out after its sterilization with ethylene oxide in a AN4000 (Andersen Sterilizers Inc.) sterilizator in accordance with GOST R ISO 10993.

Biocompatibility and bone forming ability of framework have been estimated *in vivo* by means of ectopic bone formation test (US Department of Health and Human Services, Web Site) on 40 mice males of BALB/C line with mass of 18–21 g. Titanium discs from alloy BT-6 with diameter d = 1 mm with framework applied on their surface were implanted in mice subcutaneously. Before implantation the discs with composite framework had been coated with bone marrow column extracted from animal femur (1.5×10^6 cell/ml), in DI-MEM (ISN) medium with 10 % fetal calf serum («Vector», Novosibirsk, Russian Federation). After 1.5 months the animals were sacrificed with ether anesthesia, the discs were explanted, decalcified, after that paraffin sections (thickness of 10 μm) of tissue grown on the discs were prepared for further investigation. The sections were painted with hematoxylin-eosin and subjected to histological analysis.

3.2 Results and discussion

XRD spectra of hydroxyapatite powder obtained by means of high temperature burning of biological raw materials at temperature 800 °C are given in Figure 8. Results of investigations of phase composition, crystalline lattice parameters, mean size of hydroxyapatite particles, obtained at various temperatures are given in the Table 1.

Annealing temperature, °C	Revealed phases	Volume phase content, %	Lattice parameters	Average particle size, nm	$\Delta d/d \cdot 10^{-3}$
600	$Ca_5(PO_4)_3(OH)$ hydroxyapatite	63.43	A=9.4119 C=6.8756	64	0.9
	$Ca_{10}(PO_4)_6(OH)_2$ monoclinic hydroxyapatite	36.57	A=9.5189 B=18.7480 C=6.8903	14	2.5
800	$Ca_5(PO_4)_3(OH)$ hydroxyapatite	83.0	A=9.4126 C=6.8769	67	0.7
	$Ca_{10}(PO_4)_6(OH)_2$ monoclinic hydroxyapatite	17.0	A= 9.3190 B=18.4729 C=6.7840	30	2.2
1000	$Ca_5(PO_4)_3(OH)$ hydroxyapatite	96.96	A=9.4125 C=6.8763	134	0.4
	$Ca_{10}(PO_4)_6(OH)_2$ monoclinic hydroxyapatite	3.04	A=9.4623 B=18.7480 C=6.9641	42	1.1

Table 1. Phase composition of hydroxyapatite in dependence of annealing temperature

It has been stated that temperature of raw material treatment influences on phase composition of obtained hydroxyapatite since the increase of treatment temperature decreases output of hydroxyapatite with monoclinic structure. It is shown that the increase of annealing temperature leads to the increase of grain size of obtained calcium phosphates. Grain size of phase $Ca_5(PO_4)_3(OH)$ increases on 200% at the increase of treatment temperature on 400 °C, and grain size of phase $Ca_{10}(PO_4)_6(OH)_2$ – on 300% (see Table 1).

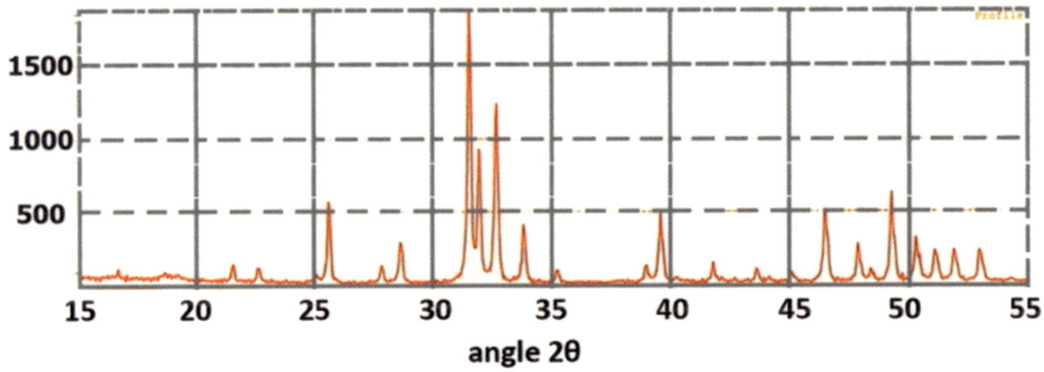

Fig. 8. XRD spectra of hydroxyapatite powder

Images of scaffold obtained in reflected light with help of the "Motic"optical microscope at various amplifications are given in Figure 9.

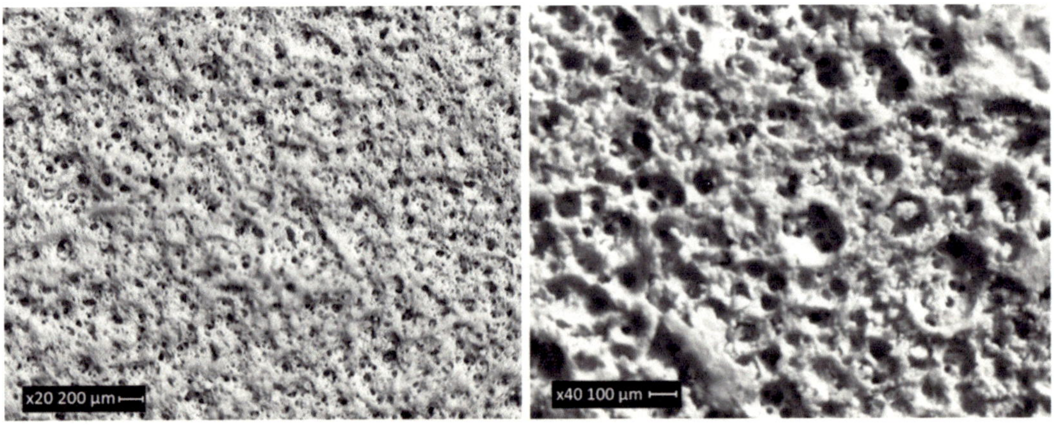

Fig. 9. Image of scaffold surface at various amplifications

The main morphometric characteristics of framework surface obtained by means of computer processing of optical images with help of the Motic Image Life plus program package, are following: total pore area 441280 cm^2, total porosity of the framework 47.79 %, min pore area 0.8 μm^2, max pore area 25379.6 μm^2, mean pore area 190.0 μm^2, min pore perimeter 4.7 µm, max pore perimeter 3393.1 µm, mean pore perimeter 22.7 µm. Histogram of pore distribution by sizes is given in Figure 10.

Analysis of obtained data allows distinguishing at least three conditional levels of TFE/VDF-HA framework: porosity with pore sizes about 10 μm^2, microporosity with pore sizes under 5000 µm and macroporosity with pore sizes more than 8000 μm^2. To our opinion presence of some porosity levels says about presence of some mechanisms of pore formation that will be investigated later. The most contribution on total surface porosity (TSP) is put by micropores with sizes more than 5000 μm^2.

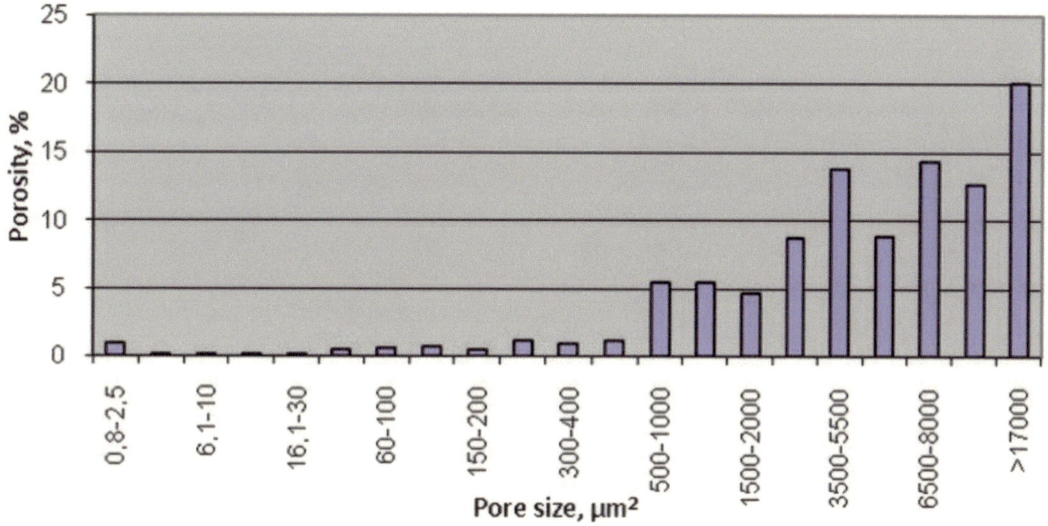

Fig. 10. Histogram of pore distribution

Images of scaffold obtained with the help of scanning electron microscope at various amplifications are presented in Figure 11.

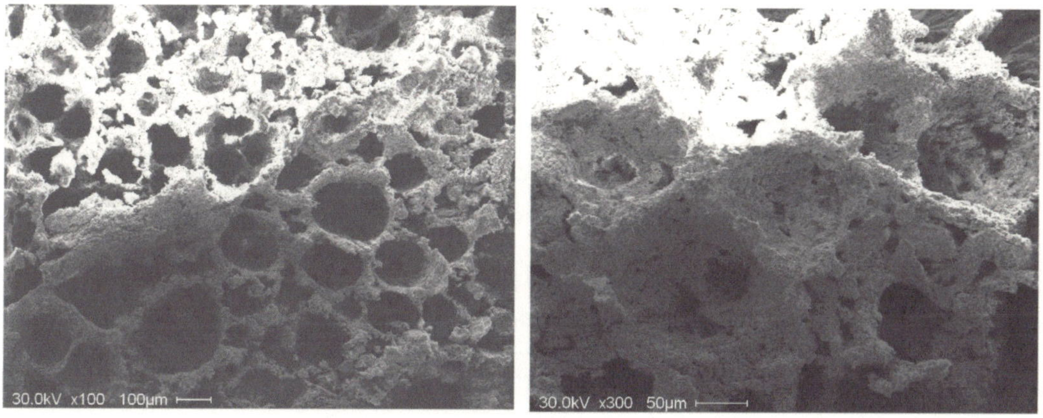

Fig. 11. Scanning electron microscopic (SEM) image of scaffold surface at various amplifications

The analysis of framework surface carried out by scanning electron microscopy had allowed to verify that used obtaining modes made it possible to steadily create porous surface with pore diameter more than 100 μm forming multilevel interpenetrate structures. Sufficient magnification clearly shows that the framework microstructure is a porous system in which particles of HA are interconnected with polymer binding agent.

Images of inner structure of scaffold macropores obtained with the help of a «C3M Solver HV» atomic force microscope are presented in Figure 12. This method allowed determining that macropore walls are penetrated with the system of smaller pores with size approximately 0.5 μm. It can be assumed that the walls and the micropores have a similar structure.

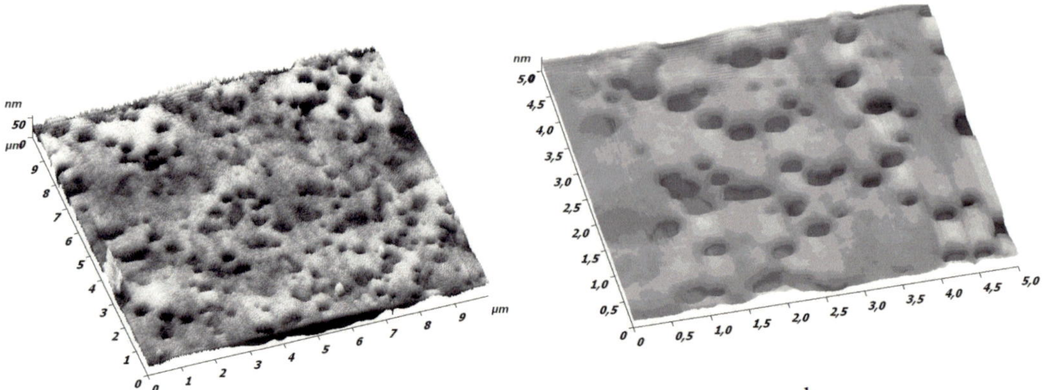

a b

Fig. 12. AFM images of inner structure of scaffold macropores, a - 10×10 µm, b - 5×5 µm

Thus microscopic investigations of scaffold structure show that it is similar to cancellous bone structure. It is the main factor promoting colonization of frameworks with osteoblasts and pullulation of bone tissue in its pores with formation of bone blocks of the "biocomposite - bone tissue" type that leads to increasing of fixation rigidity, for example, of intramedullar implant in medullary channel (Karlov & Shachov, 2001).
Data of scaffold chemical composition obtained by means of X-ray fluorescent analysis are given in the Table 2.

Ca	P	O	F	Mg	K	Na	Ni	others
37.1635	16.3777	32.6303	11.7968	0.6010	0.0444	0.5422	1.9413	0.8441

Table 2. Chemical composition of composite scaffold, mass %

Analysis of element composition shows, that the main composition of composite scaffold is calcium, phosphorous, fluorine and oxygen. Material contains admixtures of magnesium, nickel, potassium, carbon as well as trace quantities of copper, iron and sodium. Presence of admixtures can be explained by the fact that hydroxyapatite obtained by means of burning of biological raw materials has not ideal crystalline lattice with admixtures of various elements (Barinov & Komlev, 2005).

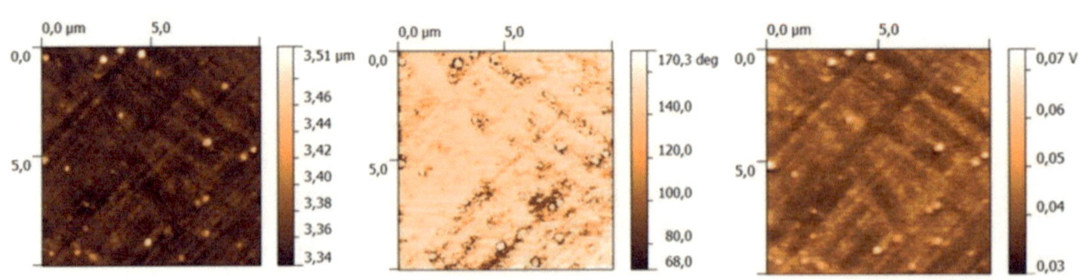

a b c

a - surface relief image, b - phase contrast image, c - surface potential images

Fig. 13. AFM surface images of the I group specimens, scanning field is 10×10 µm,

AFM images of surface of I group specimens - titanium are presented in Figure 13. On the presented images of surface relief (see Fig. 13, a), phase contrast (see Fig. 13, b) and surface potential (see Fig. 3, c) it is possible to separate globular defects being, by all appearance, particles of abrasive, "inserted' in titanium surface in process of its polishing, however detailed investigation of this question is matter of additional investigations.

Results of measurement of polished titanium substrate obtained using a Gwiddion 2.25 program complex of AFM images are presented in the Table 4. Measured parameters of surface roughness of the I group specimens allow to attribute obtained surfaces to the 13th class of roughness (See Table 3). Results of measuring of surface potential parameters of the I group specimens are presented in the Table 4.

Analysis of obtained data allows say about practically zero potential of the I group specimens, unessential changes of potential in our opinion are connected with adsorption of water vapors by a substrate and unessential oxidation of a substrate.

Images of surface relief (a), phase contrast (b) and surface potential relief (c) specimens of polished titanium with CaP coating - the II group are presented in Figure 14. Analysis of obtained images allows making a conclusion that CaP coating applied on a polished titanium substrate by the RFMS method essentially changes surface microrelief, on images of relief and phase contrast it is easily to trace grain boundaries with sized about 0.3 μm and height 0.19 μm that is connected with mechanisms of atomic growth of CaP coatings. Analysis of phase contrast allows to make conclusion that coating covers a substrate totally, isolating it from external action. Investigation of surface potential of CaP coating, gives evidence about its increasing toward positive values that is displayed especially brightly on coating projections presenting centers of crystallization and growth of thin CaP film.

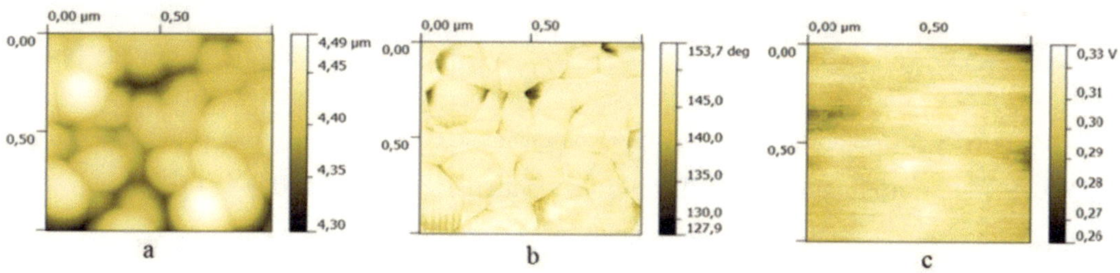

a - surface relief image, b - phase contrast image, c - surface potential images

Fig. 14. AFM surface images of the II group specimens, scanning field is 1×1 μm,

Results of measurements of roughness of the polished titanium substrate with CaP coating are presented in the Table 3. On the basis of this data it is possible to make conclusion that CaP coating changes essentially microrelief of the polished titanium substrate, parameters of its roughness increase; obtained coatings are attributed to the 10th class. Increasing of coating roughness in micro scale can be additional stimulating factor of tissue growth, for example, by means of attachment and proliferation of osteogenic cells on CaP coating surface (Karlov & Khlusov, 2003).

Let's note that CaP coatings formed on a titanium substrate by the RFMS method increase mean values of surface potential on value up to 0.052 V. At this in addition to fields with positive surface load, one found microfields with negative surface potential with value up to -0.395 V in relation to ground.

Specimen group	Mean arithmetic deviation of surface profile *Ra*, nm	Height of profile inequalities by ten points *Rz*, nm	Maximal height of roughness profile *Pt*, nm	Mean maximal depth of roughness holes *Rvm*, nm	Mean maximal height of roughness peaks *Rpm*, nm
I	6.32	96.1	95.97	12.47	38.82
II	152	801	1622	440	429
III	16.2	92.2	231.3	52.5	49.9
IV	47.2	376	918.2	141.2	152.2

Table 3. Roughness parameters of specimens by AFM data

Image of surface relief, phase contrast and surface potential of the III group specimens - titanium with polymeric TFE/VDF coating is given in Figure 15. Analysis of AFM images allows saying that formed surface of polymer TFE/VDF coating is sufficiently uniform film with negative surface potential. TFE/VDF coating film is formed as ordered structure of polymer spherulites presenting polymer parts with various degree of crystallinity that corresponds to modern ideas about structure of TFE/VDF copolymers (Panshin et al., 1978).

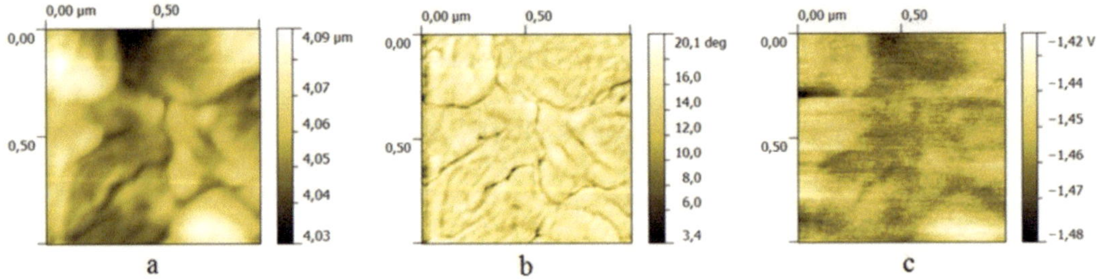

a - surface relief image, b - phase contrast image, c - surface potential images

Fig. 15. AFM surface images of the III group specimens, scanning field is 1×1 µm,

Results of measurements of surface roughness of TFE/VDF polymer coating are presented in the Table 3. Analysis of obtained data testifies that polymer coating allows to level defects appearing in process of mechanical treatment of a titanium substrate, obtained coatings are attributed to the 13th class. Such coatings can be used as biomaterials with low ability to cell adhesion, for example, thromb resistive coatings of vascular stents for which is necessary together with high class of surface cleanness and negative surface potential. It is known that complex of these requirements provides reliable functioning of intravascular stents with minimal percentage of secondary operative interventions (Guidance, 2003).

Results of measurement of surface potential parameters of the III group of specimens are presented in the Table 4.

AFM images of surface relief (a), phase contrast (b) and surface potential relief (c) of the IV group specimens - titanium with TFE/VDF polymer coating modified with RF sputtering of CaP coating are presented in Figure 16. Coating covers totally polymer layer that is proved by distribution of phase contrast. It has been stated that CaP coatings on a polymer substrate formed by RFMS of hydroxyapatite target resemble, in many way, coatings formed on a polished titanium substrate and present uniform conglomerate consisting from separate grains of calcium phosphates with size about 0.3 µm. It is displayed especially well on image of phase contrast of CaP coating. On the basis of above mentioned, it is possible to supposes that substrate material where RFMS coating is formed, does not act essential influence on CaP coating parameters.

Specimen group	Mean arithmetic deviation of potential profile φ_a, V	Mean value of surface potential U_m, V	Minimal value of surface potential U_{min}, V	Maximal value of surface potential U_{Max}, V
I	0.00392	0.03311	-0.0092	0.0655
II	0.133	0.052	-0.395	0.642
III	-0.082	-1.82	-2.178	-1.272
IV	-0.042	-0.526	-1.014	-0.054

Table 4. Surface potential parameters of specimens by AFM data

The analysis of images of surface potential of CaP coating and data of Table 4 demonstrates essential decrease of negative potential of initial polymer substrate after applying of CaP coating. Possibly it is connected with the fact that ceramic-like CaP coatings is semiconductor of p-type with large width of energy band gap equal about 4 eV (Rosenman & Aronov, 2006). This circumstance is stated by the method of exoelectron emission being sensitive to presence of defects in thin surface layer. Using of this method allowed to state that nanostructured calcium-phosphate surface has many defects. Moreover, part of defects are the centers of electron - hole capture bearing electrical charge. Owing to various mobility of electrons and holes these localized charges take part in formation of double electric layer and can change surface potential (Aronov & Rosenman, 2007). In general, we can conclude that CaP coatings formed by the RFMS have positive surface potential that is conformed to article (Khlusov et al., 2011).

Results of measurement of roughness of polymer TFE/VDF coating with CaP coating formed by the RFMS method - the IV group of specimens - are presented in the Table 3.

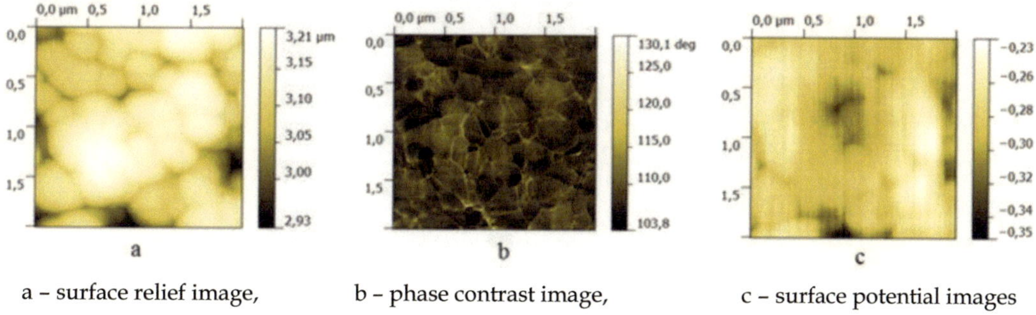

a - surface relief image, b - phase contrast image, c - surface potential images

Fig. 16. AFM surface images of the IV group specimens, scanning field is 2×2 µm,

On the basis of coating roughness data given in the Table3, it is possible to make conclusion that CaP coating changes essentially microrelief of polymer coating as in the case of a polished titanium substrate. Value of mean arithmetic deviation of surface profile *Ra* increases in 2.9 times, at maximal height of roughness surface profile *Pt* increases in 3.9 times. Formed coatings are attributed to the 11th roughness class.

Photo of water drop placed on surface of TEF/VDF coating applied on polished titanium surface is presented in Figure 17. Mean value of limiting wetting angle of TEF/VDF copolymer surface θ measured with the "EasyDrop" device was 95.5° that gives evidence of high hydrophobicity and low surface energy of TEF/VDF copolymer.

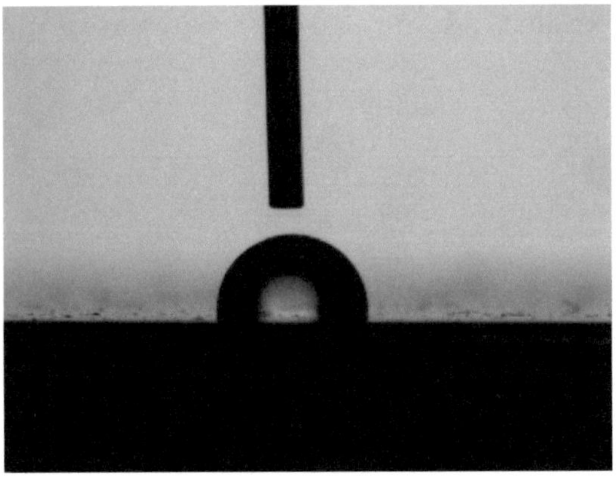

Fig. 17. Water drop form on surface of TFE/VDF copolymer

Photo of water drop placed on surface of TEF/VDF coating modified by means of RFMS of hydroxyapatite target in 2 hours is presented in Figure 18. Mean value of limiting wetting angle of TEF/VDF copolymer with calcium phosphate coating was 55.1° that gives evidence of the increase of the free energy of modified TEF/VDF copolymer surface and the increase of its hydrophilicity.

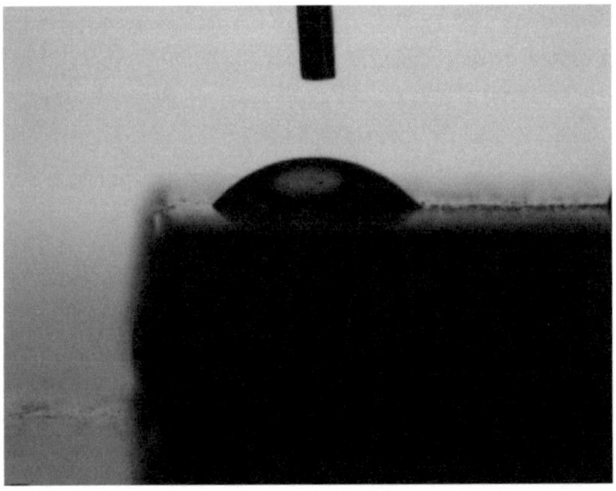

Fig. 18. Water drop form on surface of TFE/VDF copolymer, modified with the RFMS method

Thus modification of polymer TFE/VDF material surface realized by the method of RFMS hydroxyapatite target allows to increase surface energy of TFE/VDF polymer and to put it hydrophilic properties. Extrapolating this conclusion on the scaffold manufactured on the basis of TFE/VDF copolymer and hydroxyapatite we can suppose that modification of scaffold surface by the RFMS method should allow to range limiting wetting angle that must promote its impregnation of various drugs.

Data of toxicity, local irritant action, apirogenity and sterility of composite scaffold obtained in accordance with ISO 10993 are given in the Table 5. In the course of investigation death of laboratory animals did not registered, macroscopic changes of organs and tissues, and changes of weight coefficients of inner organs have not been revealed. Drawings from composite framework did not render local and general irritant action on skin and mucosa membrane of laboratory animals.

№	Index name	Admissible values	Test results	Conclusion of conformity
1.1	Toxicological tests Irritant action on skin and mucosa membranes of animals in balls : Skin Mucosa of rabbit eye	 0 0	 0 0	 Conforms Conforms
1.2	Acute toxicity at abdominal injection: - Mortality rate Clinical symptoms : -Macroscopic changes of organs and tissues; -Weight coefficients of inner organs (presence of trusted changes)	 No No No	 No No No	 Conforms Conforms Conforms
3	Determination of hemolytic activity	Not more than 2%	0.7	Conforms
4	Determination of toxicity index	70-120%	88.4%	Conforms
5	Determination of pyrogenity	Raise of temperature not more than 3°C	0.4 °C	Conforms
6	Microbiological index	Sterile	Sterile	Conforms

Table 5. Results of investigations of composite scaffold cytotoxicity

Results of investigation of composite scaffold *in vivo* after subcutaneous implantation in mice of BALB/C line is presented in the Table 6.

Inflammation in implantation site	Encapsulation of implant	Tissue plate, %	Histological estimation	Efficiency of bone tissue growth, %
No reaction	Low reaction	100	Bone with bone marrow	93

Table 6. Quantitative estimation of biological activity of composite scaffold

In the course of investigation it has been noted that animals endured easily surgery intervention. There were not pointed out natural death of animals, local or general inflammation and toxic reaction on implant, and scaffold biocompatibility was good. Framework surface has thin stromal capsule. Histological section of obtained preparation is presented in Figure 19.

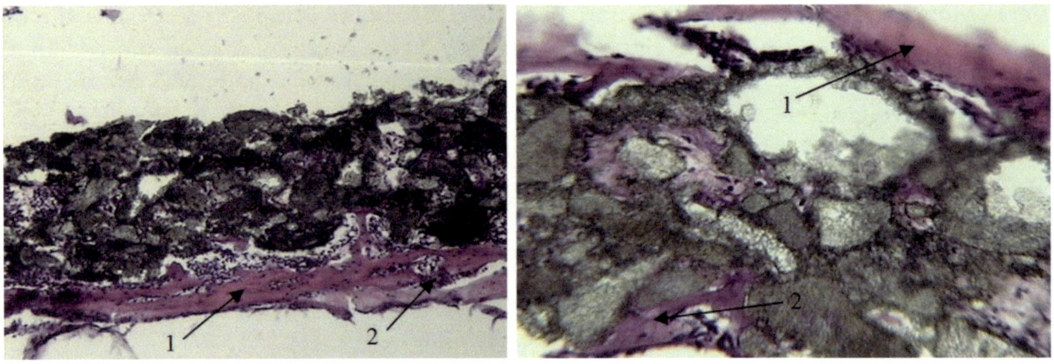

Fig. 19. Histological sections of preparation grown on composite scaffold, painting - hematoxilen - eosin, 1 - bone tissue, 2 - medullary cavity, filled with bone marrow

On histological section (Fig. 19) one can see bone tissue (1) and medullary cavities filled with bone marrow (2). Ingrowth of bone in composite scaffold pores is observed that testifies possibility its application for osteogenesis.

4. Conclusion

Method of thermal induced phase separation allows to obtain high porous scaffolds with interconnected porosity necessary to provide processes of osteoinduction and osteoconduction on the basis of tetrafluorethylene with viniliden fluoride copolymer and hydroxyapatite (TFE/VDF - HA).

The method of high temperature burning of biological raw materials with following multiply washing and drying allows obtaining hydroxyapatite used as biologically active filler for composite scaffolds.

Chemical composition of composite scaffold on the basis of tetrafluorethylene and viniliden fluoride copolymer and hydroxyapatite (TFE/VDF - HA) is presented mainly by calcium, phosphorous, oxygen and fluorine. Qualitative ratios of elements in composites depend on share of hydroxyapatite added to polymer. Mass ratio Ca/P = 2.27 does not depend on quality of hydroxyapatite in composite but is determined by chemical composition of initial HA.

Method of radio frequency magnetron sputtering of hydroxyapatite target allows modifying surface of composite scaffold by effective way. It is shown that modification of composite scaffold surface by the RFMS method increases surface roughness that is stimulating factor for attachment and proliferation of osteogenous cells.

It was shown by the Kelvin method that CaP coating formed by the RFMS of hydroxyapatite target changes surface potential of a scaffold moving it in the field of positive values in relation to ground.

Modification of polymer scaffold surface by RFMS would allow ranging its limiting wetting angle that must provide its ability to be impregnated with various drugs.

Proposed scaffolds after sterilization with ethylene oxide are nontoxic, apirogenous and sterile.

Tests *in vivo* have not revealed negative tissue reaction on implanted scaffold. Test of ectopic bone formation demonstrates positive result of implantation.

5. Acknowledgment

Authors expressed gratitude to professor I.A. Khlusov (SibSMU, Tomsk, Russia) for help in carrying out of investigations *in vivo*.
The work is performed with the support of Federal Target Program (state contract № 16.513.11.3075), RFBR (project № 11-08-98032-р_сибирь_а), and ADTP "Development of Scientific Potential of Higher Education, 2009-2011" (project № 2.1.1/14204).

6. References

American Academy of Orthopedic Surgeons. Facts on Orthopedic Surgeries. Available from: http://www.aaos.org/research/patientstats

Aronov A.M., Pichugin V.F., Eshenko E.V., Ryabtseva M.A., Surmenev R.A., Tverdokhlebov S.I., Shesterikov E.V. (2008). Thin calcium-phosphate coating produced by by rf-magnetron-sputtered and prospects for their use in biomedical engineering *Biomedical Engineering*, Vol. 42, No. 3, pp. 123-127

Aronov D., Rosenman G. (2007). Traps states spectroscopy studies and wettability modification of hydroxyapatite nano-bio-ceramics. *J. Appl. Phys*, Vol. 101

Banfi A., Muraglia A., Dozin B., Mastrogiacomo M., Cancedda R., Quarto R. (2000). Proliferation kinetics and differentiation potential of ex vivo expanded human bone marrow stromal cells: implications for their use in cell therapy. *Exp. Hematol.*, Vol. 28, pp. 707-715

Bruder S.P., Jaiswal N., Haynesworth S.E. (1997). Growth kinetics, selfrenewal, and the osteogenic potential of purified human mesenchymal stem cells during extensive subcultivation and following cryopreservation. *J. Cell Biochem.*, Vol. 64, pp. 278-294

Chen J., Wolke J.G.C. and de Groot K. (1994). Microstructure and crustallinity in hydroxyapatite coatings. *Biomaterials*, No. 15, pp. 396-399

Christenson E.M., Anseth K.S., van den Beucken J.J., Chan C.K., Ercan B., Jansen J.A., Laurencin C.T., Li W.J., Murugan R., Nair L.S., Ramakrishna S., Tuan R.S., Webster T.J., Mikos A.G. (2007). Nanobiomaterial applications in orthopedics. *J. Orthop. Res.*, Vol. 25, pp.11-22

Daculsi G., Legeros R., Heugheaert M., Barbieux I. (1990). Formation of carbonate apatite crystals after implantation of calcium phosphate ceramics. *Calcif. Tis. Int.*, Vol. 46, pp. 20-27

Desai T.A. (2000). Micro- and nanoscale structures for tissue engineering constructs. *Med. Eng. Phy.*, Vol. 22, pp. 595-606

Dutton J.J. (1991). Coralline hydroxyapatite as an ocular implant. *Ophthalmology*, Vol. 98, No. 3, pp. 370-377

Fernández-Parada J.M., Sardin G., Clèries L., Serra P., Ferrater C., Morenza J.L. (1998). Depostion of hydroxyapatite thin films by excimer laser ablation. *Thin Solid Films*, No. 317, pp. 393-396

Gauthier O., Bouler J.M., Weiss P., Bosco J., Daculsi G., Aguado E. (1999). Kinetic study of bone ingrowth and ceramic resorption associated with the implantation of calcium-phosphate bone substitutes. *J Biomed Mater Res.*, No. 47, pp. 28-35

Goldberg R.A., Holds J.B., Ebrahimpour J. (1992). Exposed hydroxyapatite orbital implants: report of six cases. *Ophthalmology*, Vol. 99, No. 5, pp. 831-836

Habibovic P., Barrere F., van Blitterswijk C. A., de Groot K, and Layrolle P. (2002). Biomimetic hydroxyapatite coating on metal implants. *J. Am. Ceram. Soc.*, No. 85, pp. 517-522

Hanusiac W. M. Polymeric Replamineform Biomaterials and A New Membrane Structure. PhD Thesis, Pennsylvania

Harris L.D., Kim B., Mooney D.J. (1998). Open pore biodegradable matrices formed with gas foaming. *J. Biomed. Mater. Res.*, Vol. 42, pp. 396-402

Holmes R.E. (1979). Bone regeneration within a coralline hydroxyapatite implant. *Plast. Reconstr. Surg.*, Vol. 63, No. 5, pp. 626-633

Holmes R., Mooney V., Bucholz R. and Tencer A. (1984). Coralline Hydroxyapatite Bone Graft Substitute. *Clin Orthop.*, Vol. 188, pp. 252 - 262

Horbett TA. (1994). The role of adsorbed proteins in animal cell adhesion. *Surf. Coll. B.*, Vol. 2, pp. 225-240

Hubbard W. (1974). Physiological Calcium Phosphate as Orthopedic Implant Material. PhD Thesis, Marquette University, Milwaukee, WI

Jones J.R. & Hench L. L. (2003). Regeneration of trabecular bone using porous ceramics. *Curr. Opin. Solid State Mater. Sci.*, Vol. 7, No. (4-5). pp. 301-307

Kanczler J.M. & Oreffo R.O. (2008). Osteogenesis and angiogenesis: the potential for engineering bone. *Eur. Cell Mater.*, Vol. 15, pp. 100-114

Ki C.S., Park S.Y., Kim H.J., Jung H.M., Woo K.M., Lee J.W., Park Y.H. (2008). Development of 3D nanofibrous fibroin scaffold with high porosity by electrospinning: implications for bone regeneration. *Biotechnol. Lett.*, Vol. 30, pp. 405-410

Kim B., Mooney D.J. (1998). Engineering smooth muscle tissue with a predefined structure. *J. Biomed. Mater. Res.*, Vol. 41, pp. 322-332

Kim T.G., Yoon J.J., Lee D.S., Park T.G. (2006). Gas foamed open porous biodegradable polymeric microspheres. *Biomaterials,* Vol. 27, pp. 152-159

Kim Y.D., Goldberg R.A., Shorr N., Steinsapir K.D. (1994). Management of exposed hydroxyapatite orbital implants. *Ophthalmology*, Vol. 101, No. 10, pp. 1709-1715

Kurtz S.M., Ong , K.L. Schmier J., Mowat F., Saleh K., Dybvik E., Karrholm J., Garellick G., Havelin L.I., Furnes O., Malchau H., Lau E. (2007). Future clinical and economic impact of revision total hip and knee arthroplasty. *J. Bone Joint Surg. Am.*, Vol. 89, No. 3, pp. 144-151

Kumar R., Cheang P., Khor K.A. (2003). Radio frequency (RF) suspension plasma sprayed ultra-fine hydroxyapatite (HA)/zirconia composite powders. *Biomaterials,* Vol. 24, pp. 2611-2621

Langer R. & Vacanti J.P. (1993). Tissue engineering. *Science*, Vol. 260, pp. 920-926

Mistry A.S., Mikos A.G. (2005). Tissue engineering strategies for bone regeneration. *Adv. Biochem. Eng. Biotechnol.*, Vol. 94, pp. 1-22

Lanza R.P., Butler D.H., Borland K.M., Staruk J.E., Faustman D.L., Solomon B.A., Muller T.E., Rupp R.G., Maki T., Monaco A.P. (1991). Xenotransplantation of canine, bovine, and porcine islets in diabetic rats without immunosuppression. *Proc. Nat. Acad. Sci. USA*, Vol. 88, pp. 11100-11104

Laurencin C.T., El-Amin S.F. (2008). Xenotransplantation in orthopedic surgery. *J. Am. Acad. Orthop. Surg.*, Vol. 16, pp. 4-8

Lee S.H. & Shin H. (2007). Matrices and scaffolds for delivery of bioactive molecules in bone and cartilage tissue engineering. *Adv. Drug Deliv. Rev.*, Vol. 59, pp. 339-359

Leeuwenburgh S.C., Wolke J.G., Siebers M.C., Schoonman J., Jansen J.A. (2006). In vitro and in vivo reactivity of porous, electrosprayed calcium phosphate coatings. *Biomaterials*, Vol. 27, pp. 3368-3378

Le Geros R.Z., Le Geros J.P., Daculsi G., Kijkowska R. (1995). Calcium phosphate biomaterials: preparation, properties, and biodegradation. (1995). In: *Encyclopedic Handbook of Biomaterials and Bioengineering*. New York. - Part A. - Materials. - Vol. 2

Le Geros R.Z., Orly I., Gregoire M., Daculsi D. (1991). Substrate surface dissolution and interfacial biological mineralization. The Bone-Biomaterial Interface Davies JE (ed). *University of Toronto Press*, Vol. 8, pp. 76-88

Li W., Laurencin C.T., Caterson E.J., Tuan R.S., Ko F.K. (2002). Electrospun nanofibrous structure: a novel scaffold for tissue engineering. *J. Biomed. Mater. Res.*, Vol. 60, pp. 613-621

McCaig C.D., Rajnicek A.M., Song B., Zhao M. (2005). Controlling cell behavior electrically: Current views and future potential. *Physiological Reviews*, Vol. 85, pp. 943-978

Malluche H. H., Meyer W., Sherman D., Massry S. G. (1982). Quantative Bone Histology In 84 Normal American Subjects: Morphometric Analysis and Evaluation of Variance in Illiac Bone. *Calcif Tissue Internat.*, Vol. 34, pp. 449-455

Mankin H.J., Hornicek F.J., Raskin K.A. Infection in massive bone allografts. (2005). *Clin. Orthop. Relat. Res.*, Vol. 432, pp. 210-216

Massry G.G. & Holds J.B. (1995). Coralline hydroxyapatite spheres as secondary orbital implants in anophthalmos. *Ophthalmology*, Vol. 102. No. 1. pp. 161-166

Melican M.C., Zimmerman M.C., Kocaj S.M., Parsons J.R. (1998). Osteoblast Behaviour on Different Hydroxyapatite Coatings With Adsorbed Osteoinductive Protein. *24lh Annual Meeting of the Society for Biomaterials*. - San Diego, California, U.S.A., p. 222

Merkx M., Maltha J, Freihofer H, Kuijpers, Jagtman A. (1999). Incorporation of particulated bone implants in the facial skeleton, *Biomaterials*, No. 20, pp. 2029-2035

Mikos A.G., Sarakinos G., Leite S.M., Vacanti J.P., Langer R. (1993). Laminated three-dimensional biodegradable foams for use in tissue engineering. *Biomaterials*, Vol. 14, pp. 323-330

Mooney D.J., Baldwin D.F., Suh N.P., Vacanti J.P., Langer R. (1996). Novel approach to fabricate porous sponges of poly(D,L-lactic-co-glycolic acid) without the use of organic solvents. *Biomaterials*, Vol. 17, pp. 1417-1422

Mo X.M., Xu C.Y., Kotaki M., Ramakrishna S. (2004). Electrospun P(LLA-CL) nanofiber: a biomimetic extracellular matrix for smooth muscle cell and endothelial cell proliferation. *Biomaterials*, Vol. 25, pp. 1883-1890

Nair L.S. & Laurencin C.T. (2006). Polymers as Biomaterials for Tissue Engineering and Controlled Drug Delivery. *Adv. Biochem. Engin. Biotechnol.*, Vol. 102, pp. 47-90

Nam Y.S. & Park T.G. (1999). Biodegradable polymeric microcellular foams by modified thermally induced phase separation method. *Biomaterials*, Vol. 20, pp. 1783-1790

Nam Y.S. & Park T.G. (1999). Porous biodegradable polymeric scaffolds prepared by thermally induced phase separation. *J. Biomed. Mater. Res.*, Vol. 47, pp. 8-17

Nam Y.S., Yoon J.J., Park T.G., (2000). A novel fabrication method for macroporous scaffolds using gas foaming salt as porogen additive. *J. Biomed. Mater. Res. (Appl. Biomater.)*, Vol. 53, pp. 1-7

Nishida J., Shimamura T. (2008). Methods of reconstruction for bone defect after tumor excision: a review of alternatives. *Med. Sci. Monit.*, Vol. 14, pp. RA107-RA113

Piatelli M., Favero G., Scarano A., Orsini G., Piatelli A. (1999). Bone reactions to anorganic bovine bone (Bio-Oss) used in sinus augmentation procedures: a histologic longterm report of 20 cases in humans. *Int. J. Oral. Maxillofac.*, V. 14, No. 6, pp. 835-840

Pichugin V.F., Surmenev R.A., Shesterikov E.V., Ryabtseva M.A., Eshenko E.V., Tverdokhlebov S.I., Prymak O., Epple M. (2008). The preparation of calcium-phosphate coating on titanium and nickel-titanium by rf-magnetron-sputtered deposition: composition, structure and micromechanical properties. *Surface and Coatings Technology,* Vol. 202, No. 16, pp. 3913-3920

Porter J.R., Ruckh T.T. and Popat K.C. (2009). Bone Tissue Engineering: *A Review in Bone Biomimetics and Drug Delivery Strategies. Biotechnol. Prog.*, Vol. 25, pp. 1539-1560

Rosenman G., Aronov D. (2006). Wettability engineering and bioactivation of hydroxyapatite nanoceramics. *Intern. Tech. Proc. Nanotech. Conf., Boston,* Vol. 2, pp. 91-94

Saltymakov M.S., Tverdokhlebov S.I., Pushkarev A.I., Volokitina T.L. (2010). Obtaining bioactive coatings on steel and Ti Substrates from ablation plasma. 3-rd Euro-Asian Pulsed Power Conference, *Proceedings of 18th International Conference on High-Power Particle Beams. Abstract Book,* October 10-14, 2010, Jeju, Korea, Korea Electrotrchnology Reseach Institute, Korea, p. 236

Santini J. T., Cima M. J., Langer R. (1999) A Controlled-Release Microchip. *Nature 397*, January 28, 1999, Available from http://www.nature.com/nature/journal/v397/n6717/abs/397335a0.html

Santini J.T., Richards A.C., Scheidt R., Cima J.M. and Langer R. (2000). Microchips as controlled drug delivery devices. *Angew. Chem, Int. Ed.*, Vol. 39, pp. 2396-2407

Schneider G. & Decher G. (2008). Functional core/shell nanoparticles via layer-by-layer assembly. Investigation of the experimental parameters for controlling particle aggregation and for enhancing dispersion stability. *Langmuir*, Vol. 24, pp. 1778-1789

Service R. F. (2000). Tissue engineers build new bone. *Science*, Vol. 289, pp. 1498-1500

Silber J.S., Anderson D.G., Daffner S.D., Brislin B.T., Leland J.M., Hilibrand A.S., Vaccaro A.R., Albert T.J. (2003). Donor site morbidity after anterior iliac crest bone harvest for single-level anterior cervical discectomy and fusion. *Spine*, Vol. 28, pp. 134-139

Thaller S. (1993). Reconstruction of cranial defects with anorganic bone mineral (Bio-Oss®) in a rabbit model. /Thaller S., Hoyt J, Borjeson K, Dart A, Tesluk H. *J. Craniofac. Surg.*, No. 4, pp. 79-84

Tofe A.J., Watson B.A., Cheung H.S. (1993). Characterization and performance of calcium phosphate coatings for implants. Eds. Horowitz E., Parr J.E. Philadelphia: *Amer. Soc. test, and materials*, p. 10

US Department of Health and Human Services. Healthcare Cost and Utilization Project. Available from http://www.hcup-us.ahrq.gov/reports/statbriefs

Vagaska B., Bacakova L., Filova E., Balik K. (2010). Osteogenic Cells on Bio-Inspired Materials for Bone Tissue Engineering. *Physiol. Res.*, Vol. 59, pp. 309-322

Valentini P., Abensur D., Densari D., Graziani J., Hammerle C. (1998). Histological evaluation of Bio-Oss® in a 2 stage sinus floor elevation and implantation procedure. *Clin. Oral. Impl. Res.*, No. 9, pp. 59-64

Vallet-Regır, M., Ruiz-Gonzarlez, L., Izquierdo-Barba, I. & Gonzarlez-Calbet, J. (2006). Revisiting silica based ordered mesoporous materials: medical applications. *J. Mater. Chem.*, Vol. 16, pp. 26-31

Walsh W.R., Chapman-Sheath P.J., Cain S., Debes J., Bruce W.J., Svehla M.J., Gillies R.M. (2003). A resorbable porous ceramic composite bone graft substitute in a rabbit metaphyseal defect model. *J. Orthop. Res.*,Vol. 21, pp. 655-661

Whang K., Thomas C.H., Healy K.E. (1995). A novel method to fabricate bioabsorbable scaffolds. *Polymer.*, Vol. 36, pp. 837-842

White E. & Shors E. C. (1986). Biomaterials Aspects of Interpore - 200 Porous Hydroxyapatite. *Dent. Clin. North. Am.* Vol. 30, pp. 49-67

Wolke J.G.C., de Blieck-Horgervorst, Dhert W.J.A., Klein C.P.A.T. and de Groot K. (1992). Studies on the thermal spraying of apatite bioceramics. *J. Thermal Spray Technol.*, No. 1, pp. 75-82

Woodard J.R., Hilldore A.J., Lan S.K., Park C.J., Morgan A.W., Eurell J.A., Clark S.G., Wheeler M.B., Jamison R.D., Wagoner Johnson A.J. (2007). The mechanical properties and osteoconductivity of hydroxyapatite bone scaffolds with multi-scale porosity. *Biomaterials*, Vol. 28, pp. 45-54

Yoon J.J. & Park T.G. (2001). Degradation behaviors of biodegradable macroporous scaffolds prepared by gas foaming of effervescent salts. *J. Biomed. Mater. Res.*, Vol. 55, pp. 401-408

Russian references

Barinov S.M. & Komlev V.S. (2005). *Bioceramics on the basis of calcium phosphates*, Nauka, Moscow, Russia

Cataeva V.M., Popova V.A., Sazhina B.I. (1975). *Handbook for plastics*, Vol. 1, Himia, Moscow, Russia

Guidance. (2003).*Vascular and inner organ stenting,* Publishing House "GRAAL", Moscow, Russia

Grafskaya N.D. (1967). Comparative estimation of reticulate polymer materials as allografts of abdominal walls at hernias: these of cand. Med. Science, Moscow

Karlov A.V. & Shakhov V.P. (2001). *The external fixation systems and mechanisms of optinal biomechanics*, STT, Tomsk, Russia

Karlov A.V. & Khlusov I.A. (2003). Dependence of reparative osteogenesis processes on surface properties of osteosynthesis implants. *Genius orthopedics,* No. 3, pp. 46-51

Khlusov I.A., Pichuguin V.F., Gostishchev E.A., Sharkeev Yu.P., et al. (2011). Influence of physical, chemical and biological manipulations on surface potential of calcium phosphate coatings on metallic substrates. *Bulletin of Siberian medicine*, No. 3, pp. 72-81

Mironov V.L. (2004). *Basics of Scanning Probe Microscopy*, Nizhny Novgorod, Russia

Panshin Yu.A., Malkevich S.G., Dunayevskaya Ts.S. (1978). *Fluoropolymer,* Himia, Leningrad, USSR

Struts V.K., Petrov A.V., Matvienko V.M., Pichuguin V.F., Tverdokhlebov S.I. (2011). Properties of calcium-phosphate coatings deposited from ablation plasma, produced by power ion beams. *Surface. X-ray, synchrotron and neutron investigations*, No. 5, pp. 97-100

Tverdokhlebov S.I., Shesterikov E.V., Malchikhina A.I. (2010). Using of method of explosive evaporation to obtaini calcium phosphate coatings on ceramic materials. *Modern ceramic materials and their use: Transaction of scientific – practical conference,* Novosibirsk, Russia, Sibprint, pp. 109-110

5

Doped Calcium Carbonate-Phosphate-Based Biomaterial for Active Osteogenesis

L. F. Koroleva[1], L. P. Larionov[2] and N.P. Gorbunova[3]
[1]*Institute of Engineering Science of the Russian Academy of Sciences, Ural Branch, Ekaterinburg,*
[2]*Ural State Medical Academy, Ekaterinburg,*
[3]*Institute of Geology and Geochemistry of the Russian Academy of Sciences, Ural Branch, Ekaterinburg,*
Russia

1. Introduction

The problems of modern medicine and biotechnology involve not only creation of implants replacing bone tissues and organs, but also synthesis of biologically active materials promoting the fullest restoration of tissues and maintenance of necessary functions of an organism. It is well known that calcium is one of the elements important for a living organism, for its cations control the transportation of inorganic ions and organic substances through cell membranes in the metabolic process involving the delivery and removal of reaction products from a cell. Interacting with regulatory proteins, calcium participates in nerve impulse transmission to muscles. Calcium is necessary for blood coagulation and participation in the synthesis of hormones, neuromediators and other controlling substances (1). Calcium is a building material for the bone tissue, its inorganic part. The solid residual of the bone tissue contains 70 % of calcium hydroxide phosphate (calcium hydroxyapatite) $Ca_{10}(PO_4)_6(OH)_2$ and 30 % of an organic component, namely, collagen fiber. The bone tissue should be characterized as an organic matrix impregnated by amorphous $Ca_3(PO_4)_2$ and crystals of calcium hydroxide phosphate synthesized in bone tissue osteoblast cells (2).

Ions Na^+, K^+, Mg^{2+}, Fe^{2+}, Cl^- and CO_3^{2-} are contained in the structure of calcium hydroxide phosphate of the bone tissue besides Ca^{2+} and PO_4^{3-}. The content of anions CO_3^{2-} in calcium hydroxide phosphate of the bone material can make up to 8 wt. %, and they substitute hydroxyl or phosphate groups. Therefore, in view of the carbonate groups introduced into the structure of calcium hydroxide phosphate, its probable formula will be as follows (3 - 5): $Ca_{10}(PO_4)_6(CO_3)_x(OH)_{2-x}$.

Actually, the crystal structure, as well as the structure of chemical bonds, of calcium hydroxide phosphate is much more complex because of vacancies in the crystal structure of both anion and cation nature. The vacancies can be filled with bivalent cations of trace elements received by a living organism and with anions $SiO_{2x}{}^{2-}$, SO_4^{2-} and Cl^-, F^-. The crystal structure of calcium hydroxyapatite is considered in (4, 5) where there is a simplified form of an elementary cell. However, practically in all scientific works accessible for viewing it is not mentioned that the structure of chemical bonds in calcium hydroxyapatites and apatites of the kind is more complex than their empirical formula and that it is not completely representative. Taking into consideration that phosphoric acids and their salts have basically polymeric structure with the formation of inorganic polymers due to hydrogen bonds and oxygen bridges, one can assume that calcium hydroxide phosphates are also characterized by the formation of inorganic polymers.

It is well known that in an organism there is a complex system of storage and release of calcium, which involves the hormone of the parathyroid gland, calcitonin and vitamin D_3. If an organism is unable to assimilate calcium because of age-related and hormonal changes, the lack of calcium begins to be filled with the dissolution of calcium hydroxide phosphate of the bone tissue. As a result, the bone tissue becomes less strong. Besides, deposition of phosphate salts in the cartilaginous connective tissue and on vessel walls is observed. A prominent feature of the growth of bones, teeth and other structures is the accumulation of calcium. On the other hand, the accumulation of calcium in atypical sites leads to the formation of stones, osteoarthritis, cataracts and arterial abnormalities (1). The entrance of calcium into an organism can proceed in the form of easily assimilated phosphates, which are also necessary for the synthesis of adenosine triphosphoric acid accumulating energy and participating in active transportation of ions through cell membranes. As after 55 the majority mankind suffers from various diseases of joints, lower strength of the bone tissue, osteochondrosis, osteoporosis and frequent fractures, it is necessary to create a material based on inorganic calcium phosphates easily assimilated by a living organism, and not only through the gastrointestinal tract. It is well known that, when calcium phosphate (hydroxyapatite) is introduced into the bone tissue, as a result of slow resorption in an organism and involving in metabolism, osteogenesis improves, but calcium phosphates fail to get into an organism through the skin. The solution to this problem is biomaterial developed on the basis of nanocrystalline doped microelements of calcium carbonate phosphates with a rapid impact on the process of osteogenesis and with the ability to penetrate into the organism through the skin, i.e., through the membranes of living cells (6 -8).

Calcium phosphates are studied all over the world. Methods of synthesizing calcium hydroxide phosphates are known. They consist in the following: precipitation from salts of calcium (or hydroxide, or oxide, or carbonate) with addition of *o*-phosphoric acid or mono- or double-substituted phosphate salts with the subsequent hydrolysis in the solution, under hydrothermal conditions, or as a result of pyrolysis (9 – 23). Methods for synthesizing calcium hydroxide phosphates are most exhaustively discussed in (4). It is hardly possible to adduce all the references. The issues concerning methods of production of calcium phosphates, their structure and properties are most fully elucidated in (14).

These are problem of a resorption of calcium hydroxyapatite and osteogenesis in vivo organisms important (24 - 27). However, the patent and scientific literature does not offer any preparations based on inorganic calcium phosphates influencing the metabolism of calcium in a living organism through the skin.

The aim of this work is to synthesize calcium carbonate-phosphates doped with cations, which are easily assimilated by a living organism, including through the skin. It presents a study of their crystal phases, chemical composition and particle size analysis, as well as their biological activity in the processes of osteogenesis.

2. Materials and methods

For synthesizing samples of doped calcium carbonate-phosphate, calcium carbonate of three crystal structures was used. They are calcite (rhombohedral), vaterite (hexagonal) and aragonite (orthorhombic). Precipitation of calcium carbonate-phosphate was performed by *o*-phosphoric acid (2 mol/l), which was added dropwise into a calcium carbonate suspension in an ammonium chloride solution (2 mol/l) at 45 to 55°C. The size of the pH environment varied between 5.2 and 6.5 depending on the molar ratio Ca/P (1.55 to 1.67). Doping cations were added during calcium carbonate precipitation: Fe^{2+} and Mg^{2+} 0.0004–0.06; Zn^{2+} 0.0015–0.002; K^{+} 0.001– 0.01; SiO_2 0.0002– 0.006; and Mn^{2+} 0.00002 - 0.001 mol %. The choice of the calcium-phosphorus - cations-doped molar ratio was caused by the known concentrations of these elements in the bone tissue (1). The precipitate of synthesized calcium carbonate-phosphates was separated by filtering, washed by water and dried at temperatures not higher than 75°C.

The samples thus obtained were characterized by X-ray diffraction (XRD) (DRON-2 diffractometer, Cu*K*α radiation; STADI-P diffractometer, software for diffraction peak identification using JCPDS–ICDD PDF2 data); IR spectroscopy (Shimadzu JR-475 spectrophotometer, KBr disk method) and differential thermal analysis (DTG) (MOM thermoanalytical system) at a heating rate of 10 to 11deg/min within the range of temperatures from 20 to 1000°C, with a weight of 500 mg. The particle size analysis of the samples was performed by gravitational centrifugal sedimentation with the use of the SA-CP2 analyzer produced by Shimadzu, Japan (dispersion medium viscosity 0.0093 P, density 1.0 g/cm^3).

The chemical composition (Ca, P, Fe, Mg, Zn, Mn, K, Si) was determined by standard techniques of complexometric method (28) and X-ray fluorescent analyses with the use of the EDX-900HS energy dispersion spectrometer (Shimadzu, Japan). The mechanical strength of the bone and dental tissues was studied with the application of the method of stress determination in the bone tissue transverse section (29, 30). The calculation was made by the formula $\boldsymbol{P=a\ F/S}$, where P is mechanical strength (shearing stress), MPa; S is the cross-sectional area of the specimen to produce the stress, mm^2; F is the load applied to cut the bone and dental tissues, kg-wt. The relative error of the method was 2.5 %. *Figure* 1 is presented apparatus for research transverse mechanical strength of the bone and dental tissues.

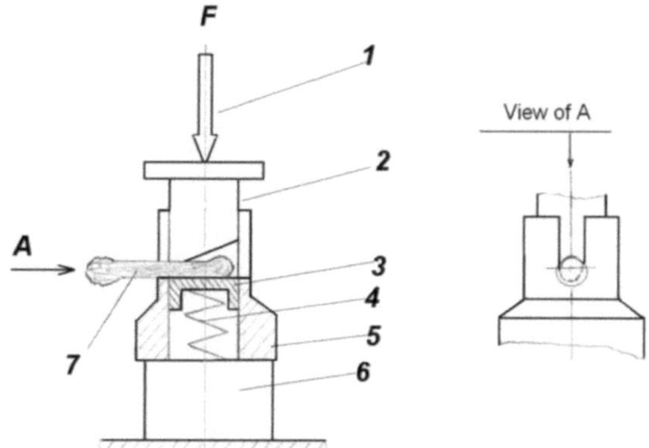

Fig. 1. Instrument for research transverse mechanical strength of the bone and dental tissues: 1-screw press; 2- poise; 3- pillar; 4- spring; 5 – spigot-matrix; 6 – force sensor; 7- sample of bone and dental tissue

3. Results and discussion

3.1 The synthesis of doped calcium carbonate- phosphate

The mechanism of obtaining this biomaterial is quite difficult, and this process can be considered oscillating reactions of calcium in a living organism. Reaction of the synthesis of doped calcium carbonate phosphates, which were described in (6-8), include several initial compounds as a calcium carbonate of three polymorphic crystal forms (calcite, aragonite, and vaterite), ortho–phosphoric acid, ammonium chloride, ammonium hydroxide, and microelements of the living organism (K^+, Mg^{2+}, Fe^{2+}, Zn^{2+}, Mn^{2+}, SiO_2). The formation of complex of $M_{g-x}M_x(OH)_2[(CO_3)_{x-2}\cdot H_2O]$ were described in (7, 8).
For example, in the medium of ammonium hydroxide, three polymorphic forms of $CaCO_3$ can form ammonium met stable Hydroxycarbonates complexes on the following scheme:

$$CaCO_3 + NH_4OH \rightleftarrows NH_4CaCO_3OH \tag{1}$$

Or in general terms:

$$A \rightleftarrows X \tag{2}$$

The formation of three types of crystal structures of calcium carbonate (in the medium of ammonium hydroxide and ammonium chloride) is typical for the reaction (1): calcite, vaterite, and aragonite, which was proven by the data of XRD (*Figure 2). SEM micrographs of synthetic calcium carbonate: calcite, vaterite, and aragonite shown in *Figure* 3.

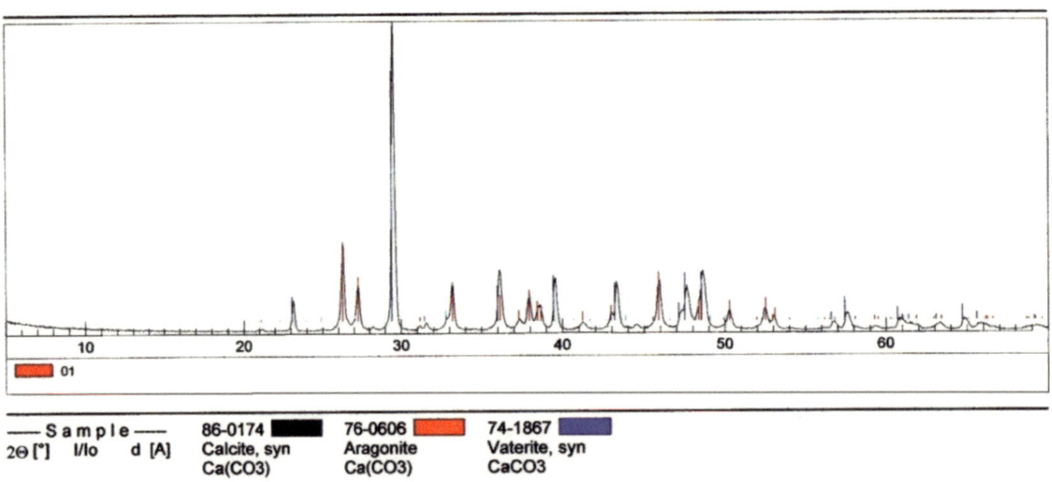

Fig. 2. XRD patterns of calcium carbonate: calcite (53 wt.%), vaterite (6 wt.%) and aragonite (41 wt.%)

Under the action of *ortho*-phosphate acid in the presence of magnesium cations and silicon dioxide, carbonate is replaced in the phosphate acid with the formation of $CaHPO_4$ (brushite) or $Ca_8H_2(PO_4)_6\cdot$ according to the reaction:

$$NH_4CaCO_3OH + H_3PO_4 = NH_4OH + CaHPO_4 \tag{3}$$

$$10NH_4CaCO_3OH + 6H_3PO_4 = Ca_8H_2(PO_4)_6 + 2CaCO_3 + 8CO_2 + 10NH_4OH + 8H_2O \tag{4}$$

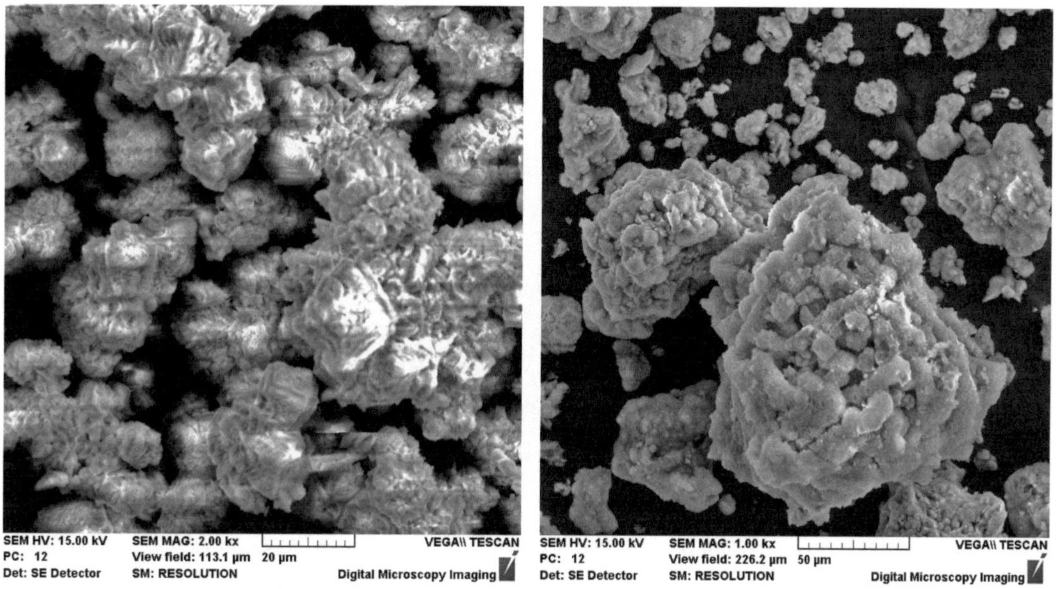

a) b)

Fig. 3. Scannig electron micrographs of calcium carbonate (a): calcite, vaterite, and aragonite; of doped Fe 0.004; Mg 0.007; Zn 0.002; Mn 0.00002 mol.% calcium carbonate-phosphate (b)

Or in general terms:

$$B + X \rightarrow Y + C \qquad (5)$$

In the environment of ammonium chloride with the addition of *o*-phosphoric acid, with the pH environment from 5.2 to 6.5, calcium phosphate chloride may form from precipitated calcium carbonate, for example, by the following equation (for convenience of writing equations by integers in a formula, while XRD analysis the number of atoms shows fractional):

$$5CaCO_3 + 2H_3PO_4 + 2NH_4Cl + 2\,NH_4OH = 2Ca_5(PO_4)_2(OH)_2Cl_2 + 5CO_2 + \\ + 5H_2O + 4NH_3 \qquad (6)$$

$$Ca_8H_2(PO_4)_6 + 2CaCO_3 + NH_4Cl + NH_3 \rightleftarrows Ca_{10}(PO_4)_6OHCl + 2NH_4HCO_3 \qquad (7,8)$$

Or in general terms:

$$C \rightleftarrows R$$

According to the law of mass action speed of responce (7, 8) characterize by the equation:

$$\frac{dx_4}{dt} = k_4[NH_4^+][Cl^-][NH_3];$$

$$\frac{dx_5}{dt} = k_5[NH_4^+]^2[HCO_3^-]^2$$

$$3CaHPO_4 + 2\,CaCO_3 + 2\,NH_4Cl + 2\,NH_3 + 3\,H_2O + CO_2 \rightleftarrows$$
$$\rightleftarrows Ca_5(PO_4)_2(OH)_2Cl_2 + 3\,NH_4HCO_3 + NH_4H_2PO_4 \qquad (9,10)$$

Or in general terms:

$$C \rightleftarrows R \qquad (11)$$

Reaction rate (9, 10) characterize by the equation:

$$\frac{dx_6}{dt} = k_6\left[NH_4^+\right]^2\left[Cl^-\right]^2\left[NH_3\right]^2\left[CO_2\right]$$

$$\frac{dx_7}{dt} = k_7[NH_4^+]^4[HCO_3^-]^3[H_2PO_4^-].$$

In addition is transfomation cycle with response:

$$CaHPO_4 \rightleftarrows CaCO_3$$

Or in general terms:

$$C \rightleftarrows A \qquad (12)$$

Doping of calcium carbonate-phosphate with Mg^{2+} - cations leads to the formation of the following phases in them: octacalcium phosphate hydrogen, brushite, besides, the phases of calcite and aragonite partially remain there. Simultaneous doping with Fe^{2+} and Mg^{2+} cations causes the formation of the same phases as in case of introduction of Fe^{2+} cations alone, however, the calcium hydrogen phosphate $Ca_8H_2(PO_4)_6 \cdot 5H_2O$ and calcium phosphate chloride hydroxide $Ca_{9.70}P_{6.04}O_{23.86}(OH)_{2.01}Cl_{2.35}$. The insertion of cations Fe^{2+}, Mg^2 leads to the basic crystal phase of octacalcium phosphate hydrogen $Ca_8H_2(PO_4)_6\ 5H_2O$.
The next stage in the presence of such doping microelements as Fe^{2+}, Mg^2, Zn^{2+} K^+, Si^{4+}, Mn^{2+} is the formation of calcium phosphate chloride hydroxide according to the following scheme:

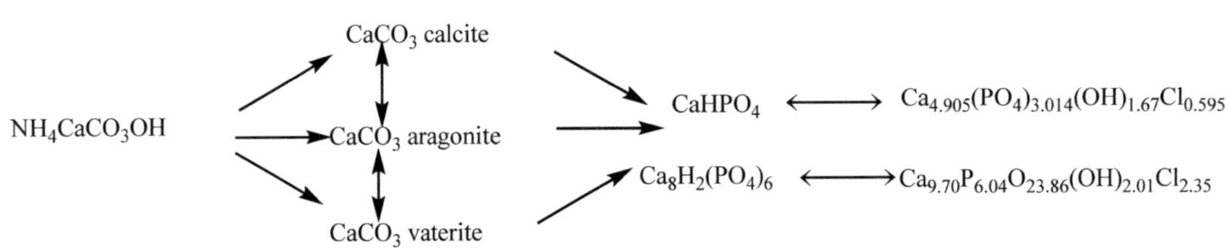

The simplest classic example of the existence of autooscillations in the system of chemical reactions is the trimolecular model ("brusselator") offered by I.R. Prigozhine and R. Lefebre (31). The main purpose for the study of this model was to determine the qualitative types of behavior, which are compatible with the fundamental laws of chemical and biological kinetics. In this context, the brusselator plays the role of a basic model, like a harmonic oscillator in physics. A classic brusselator model describes the hypothetical scheme of chemical reactions:

$$A \rightarrow X$$

$$B+X \rightarrow Y+C$$

$$2X+Y \rightarrow 3X$$

$$X \rightarrow R$$

$$A+B \rightarrow R+C. \quad (13)$$

The key is the stage of transformation of two *X* molecules and one *Y* molecule into *X* (the so-called trimolecular reaction). Such a reaction is possible in processes with the participation of ferments with two catalytic centers. The nonlinearity of this reaction, coupled with processes of diffusion of the substance, well as the formation spatial structures in an initially homogeneous system of morphogenesis. Although the trimolecular stage in chemical kinetics is not as common as in biomolecular processes, expressions for the speed of some chemical reactions in some definite cases can be called cubic - type. Such equations are called "reaction diffusion"equations. The whole system has an oscillating character and can be presented as a brusselator of the simplest implementation of cubic nonlinearity by the following chemical reaction:

$$2X + Y \rightarrow 3X \quad (14)$$

If the final products *C* and *R* are immediately removed from the reaction, then the scheme of the reactions (in the case of a point system) can be given by the following system of equations:

$$\frac{dx}{dt} = A + X^2Y - (B+1)X$$

$$\frac{dy}{dt} = BX - X^2Y.$$

Inserting doping cations Mg^{2+} and K^+ leads to the synthesis of the basic phase of calcium phosphate hydrogen $Ca_8H_2(PO_4)_6$ as the additional phase of calcium phosphate chloride hydroxide $Ca_{9.70}P_{6.04}O_{23.86}(OH)_{2.01}$ $Cl_{2.35}$ (up to 7 wt %) and calcium carbonate phosphate and potassium hydrate phosphate hydrogen $Ca_8H_2(PO_4)_6 \cdot H_2O\text{-}KHCO_3\text{-}H_2O$ (up to 6 wt %, *Table 1*). The regularities of the concentration change of hydroxychlorapatite, chloride, and magnesium in the products of reaction in the synthesis of calcium carbonate phosphate for the reaction with visible cations Mg^{2+}, Fe^{2+}, Zn^{2+}, and Mn^{2+} are shown in *Figure 4.*

The kinetic curves of concentration changes in the synthesis of doped calcium carbonate-phosphate are similar to the kinetics of concentration changes and the phase picture of the fructose-6-phosphate and fructose - diphosphate system.

Therefore, the oscillating dynamics of the brusselator model and modeling with waves, which are proposed for the fructose-6-phosphate and fructose-diphosphate system in (31, 32). For comparison, see model of intracellular calcium oscillations, as described in (33-37), *Figure 5.*

Oscillating character synthesis of the doped calcium carbonate-phosphate reply in the filtering and washing process doped calcium carbonate-phosphate precipitation what shown in *Figure 6.*

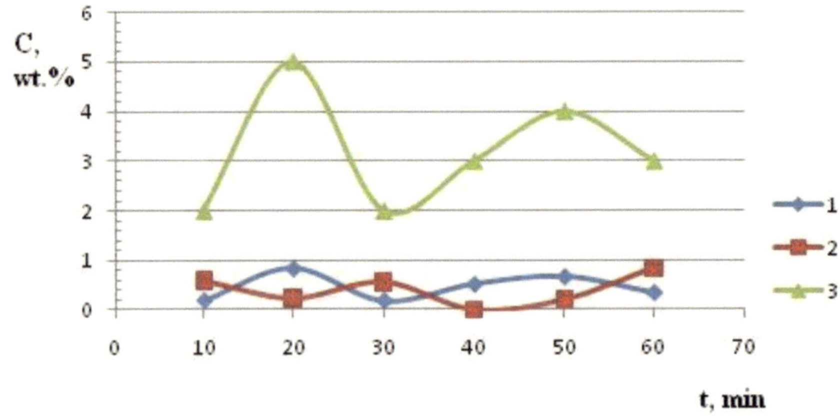

Fig. 4. The kinetics of concentration dependencies of the chloride-ions (1), Mg^{2+} (2) and calcium chloride-hydroxide phosphate (3) precipitation on a time reaction

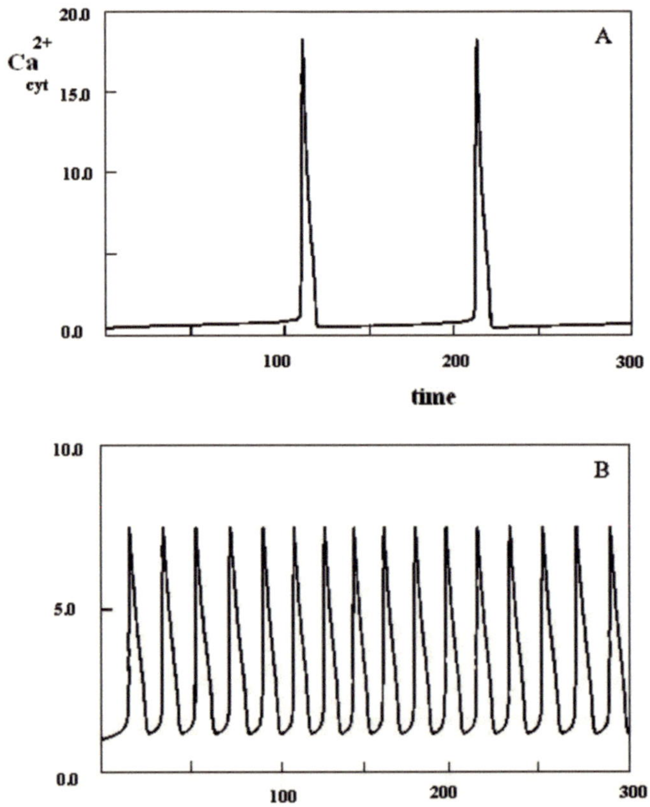

Fig. 5. Model fluctuations in intracellular calcium. Kinetics of Ca concentration in different settings (33)

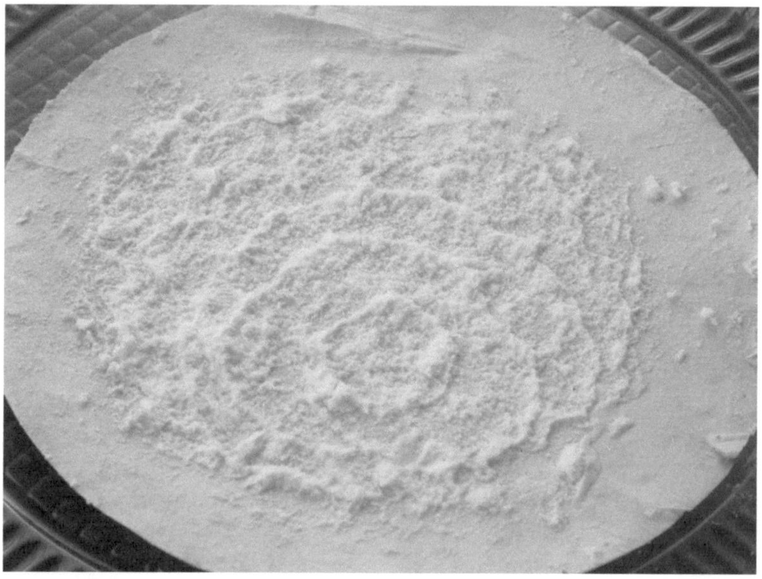

Fig. 6. Oscillating character in the filtering and washing process of the doped calcium carbonate-phosphate precipitation

The results of X-ray diffraction and chemical analysis confirm this. Typical X-ray diffraction pattern of doped calcium carbonate-phosphate samples are presented in *Figure* 7. SEM-micrographs of synthetic doped calcium carbonate-phosphate shown in *Figure 3.*

The composition is also confirmed by the chemical analysis data and the obtained IR-spectra of calcium carbonate-phosphate samples. *Figure* 8 presents typical IR-spectra of calcium carbonate-phosphate samples doped with iron, magnesium, zinc, manganese where there are bands of absorption of valence vibration δ_v of the PO_4^{3+} group 525, 560, 600 cm^{-1}, bands of absorption of symmetric vibrations ν_1 865-870 and 960-980 cm^{-1} and asymmetric vibrations ν_3 1040 - 1050 and 1100 -1130cm^{-1}, and also bands of absorption of the deformation vibration ν_3 of the CO_3^{2-} group 1400 cm^{-1}. The band of absorption of 1630 -1650 cm^{-1} corresponds to the deformation vibrations of OH^- water groups. The band of absorption 3150, 3480 cm^{-1} corresponds to the valence vibration of water and characterizes the presence crystallization water. The values for the triplet of the valence vibration of the phosphate group δ_v are close to those presented in (9 – 11). A comparison between the IR-spectra of the calcium carbonate-phosphate samples and brushite $CaHPO_4 \cdot 2H_2O$ formed from calcium oxide revealed a difference. It has been found that brushite is characterized by bands of absorption of valence vibration δ_v of group PO_4^{3+} 530, 575, 600 cm^{-1}, bands of absorption of symmetric vibrations ν_1 790, 870 and 985 cm^{-1} and asymmetric vibrations ν_3 1060, 1135 and 1210 cm^{-1}, as well as bands of absorption of deformation vibration of the OH^- group 1645 cm^{-1}.

DTG-analysis establishes that the calcium hydroxyapatite crystallization temperature is 840°C, which proves to be true judging by the endothermic effect on the thermograph. At temperatures 130, 190 and 240°C, endothermic effects are caused by the dehydration of crystallization waters and the removal of hydrogen ions. The general loss of the weight of the samples dried up at a temperature of 75°C makes 17.5 to 18.5 wt. %, and this agrees well with the chemical and phase analysis *(Figure* 9*).*

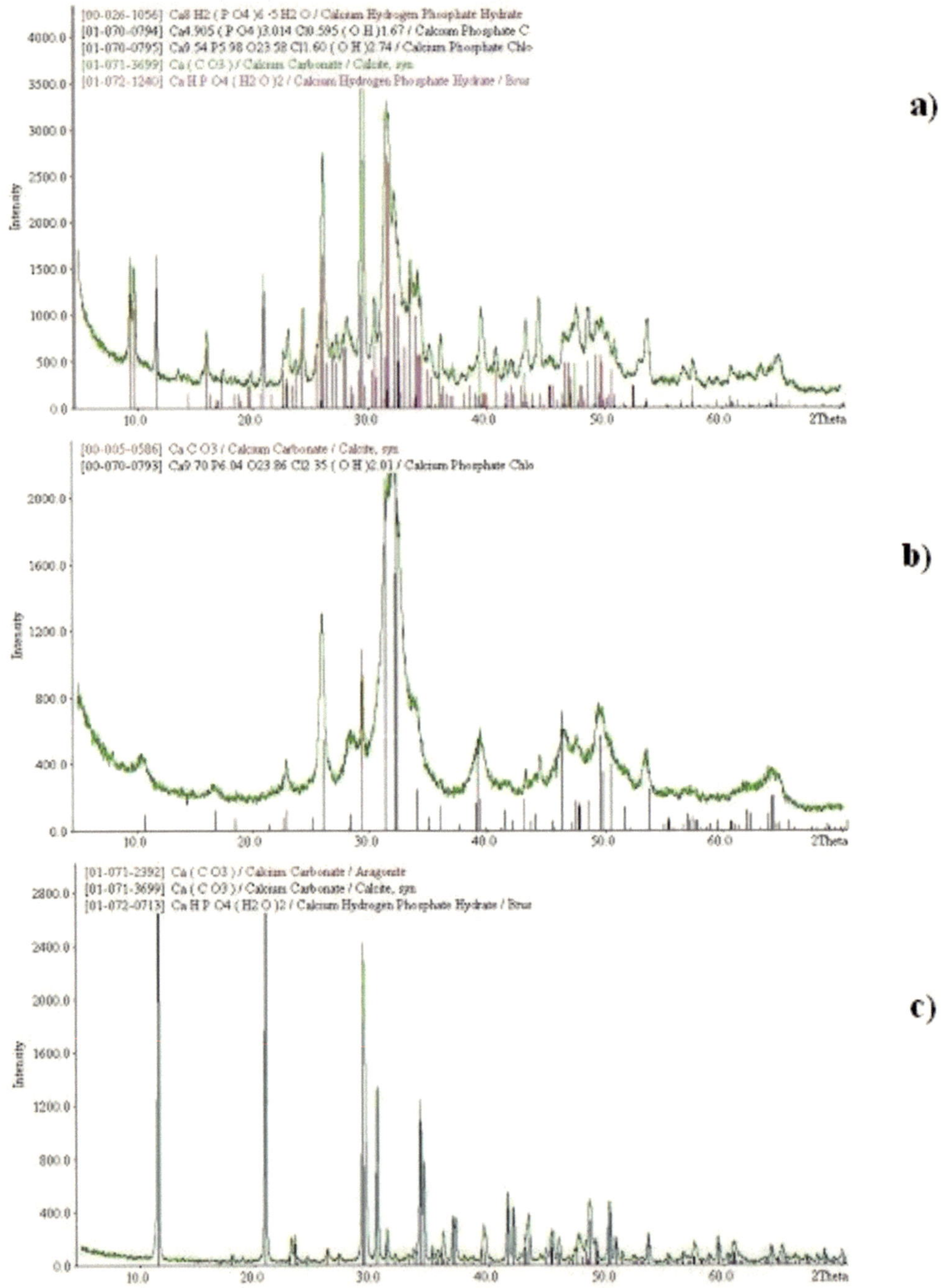

Fig. 7. XRD patterns of (a) iron, magnesium, zinc doped; (b) iron, magnesium, zinc, manganese doped; (c) iron, magnesium, silica doped calcium carbonate phosphate

Found, mol. %						Solid phase concentration, wt.%
Fe	Mg	Zn	K	Mn	SiO_2	
0.001	0.02	-	-	-	-	$Ca_8H_2(PO_4)_6*5H_2O$ 76% $Ca_{9.70}P_{6.04}O_{23.86}Cl_{2.35}(OH)_{2.01}$ 18%
0.001	0.005	0.002	-	0.001	-	$CaHPO_4*2H_2O$ 72% $Ca_{9.70}P_{6.04}O_{23.86}Cl_{2.35}(OH)_{2.01}$ 13%
0.001	0.004	0.002				$CaHPO_4*2H_2O$ 72% $Ca_{9.70}P_{6.04}O_{23.86}Cl_{2.35}(OH)_{2.01}$ 13%
0.002	0.06	0.002				$CaHPO_4*2H_2O$ 70% $Ca_{9.70}P_{6.04}O_{23.86}Cl_{2.35}(OH)_{2.01}$ 18%
0.002	0.01	0.002				$CaHPO_4*2H_2O$ 70% $Ca_{9.70}P_{6.04}O_{23.86}Cl_{2.35}(OH)_{2.01}$ 18%
0.003	0.02	-	0.001	-	-	$CaHPO_4*2H_2O$ 80%
-	0.06	-	0.001	-	-	$Ca_8H_2(PO_4)_6*5H_2O$ 85% $Ca_{9.70}P_{6.04}O_{23.86}Cl_{2.35}(OH)_{2.01}$ 7 % $Ca_8H_2(PO_4)_6*H_2O$-$KHCO_3$-H_2O 6%
-	0.003	-	-	-	0.002	$CaHPO_4*2H_2O$ 60% $Ca_8H_2(PO_4)_6*5H_2O$ 16%
-	0.01	-	0.001	-	-	$CaHPO_4*2H_2O$ 80%
0.0004	0.035	0.002	-	-	-	$Ca_8H_2(PO_4)_6*5H_2O$ 86% $Ca_{9.70}P_{6.04}O_{23.86}Cl_{2.35}(OH)_{2.01}$ 2% $CaHPO_4*2H_2O$ 6% $Ca_{4.905}(PO_4)_{3.014}Cl_{0.595}(OH)_{1.67}$ 1%
-	0.02	-	-	-	-	$CaHPO_4*2H_2O$ 10% $Ca_8H_2(PO_4)_6*5H_2O$ 50%
0.0004	0.02				0.0006	$CaHPO_4*2H_2O$ 84%
0.004	0.007	0.002	-	0.00002	-	$Ca_{9.70}P_{6.04}O_{23.86}Cl_{2.35}(OH)_{2.01}$ 75% $CaCO_3$ 25%

Table 1. The phase and chemical composition of calcium carbonate-phosphate samples

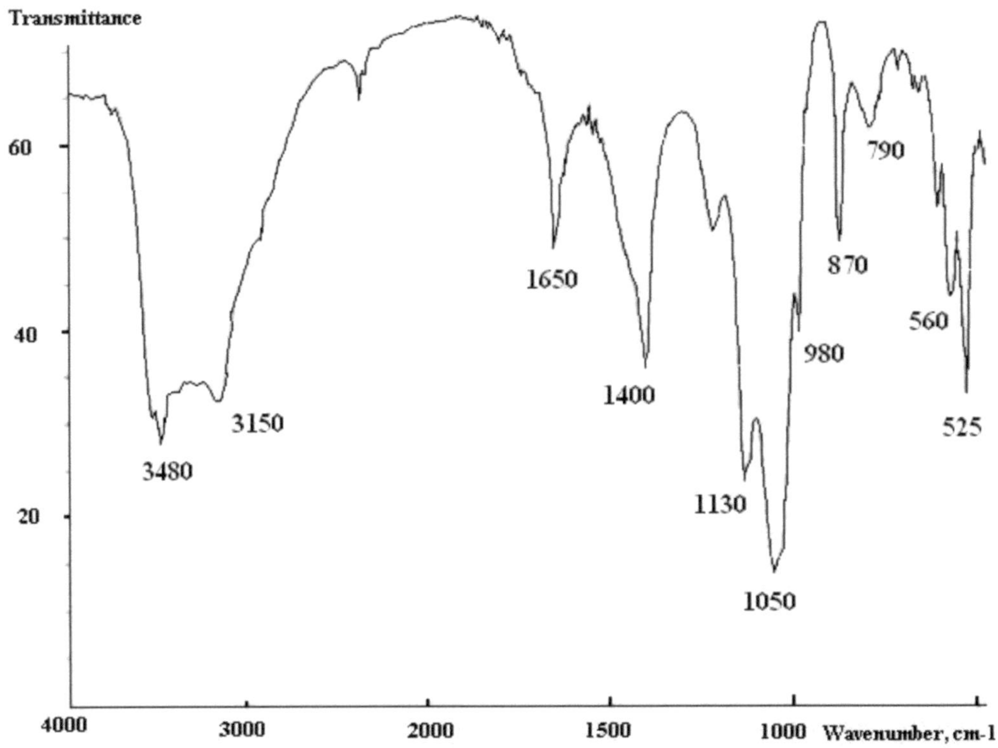

Fig. 8. Typical IR-spectra of calcium carbonate-phosphate samples doped with iron, magnesium, zinc, manganese.

Thus, doping cations of Fe^{2+}, Mg^{2}, Zn^{2+} K^{+}, Mn^{2+} and Si^{4+} have an effect on the phase equilibrium in the system $CaCO_3$ - H_3PO_4 - NH_4Cl, as well as on the end products of the process of sedimentation and their properties. It is calcium phosphate chloride and calcium hydrogen phosphate that are general crystal phases for iron- and magnesium-doped samples. The particle-size analysis has shown that the composition of calcium carbonate-phosphate samples is polydisperse.

The basic fraction of particles ranges from 5 to 20 microns for samples doped with cations simultaneously. In addition the ultradispersed fraction with the size of particles up to 10 nm in amounts of 1.5 % is observed, and this allows the material to be especially active in all the samples. It is noted that material dispersiveness enables the material to get through the skin of an organism. The characteristic curves of the particle-size analysis of the samples are adduced in *Figure 10*.

3.2 Studying biological activity

The influence of the doped calcium carbonate-phosphate on the bone and dental tissues of a living organism was investigated experimentally in white rats. A 1 % water suspension of calcium carbonate-phosphates was introduced inside animals through an enteric tube in amounts of 5 ml within 40 days, 30 mg per 1 kg of live weight (there were five groups of 10 animals, namely, I – placebo, II – within 10 days, III – within 20 days, IV – within 30 days, V

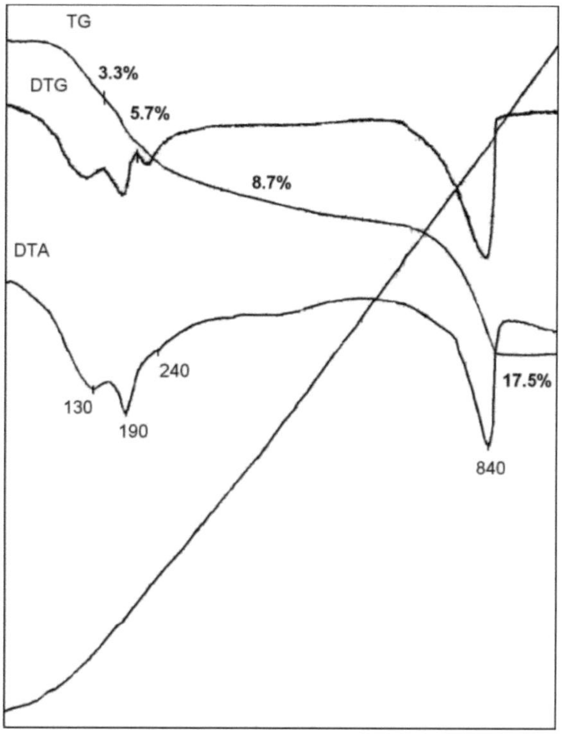

Fig. 9. A characteristic DTA-curve of calcium carbonate-phosphate samples doped with cations of iron and magnesium

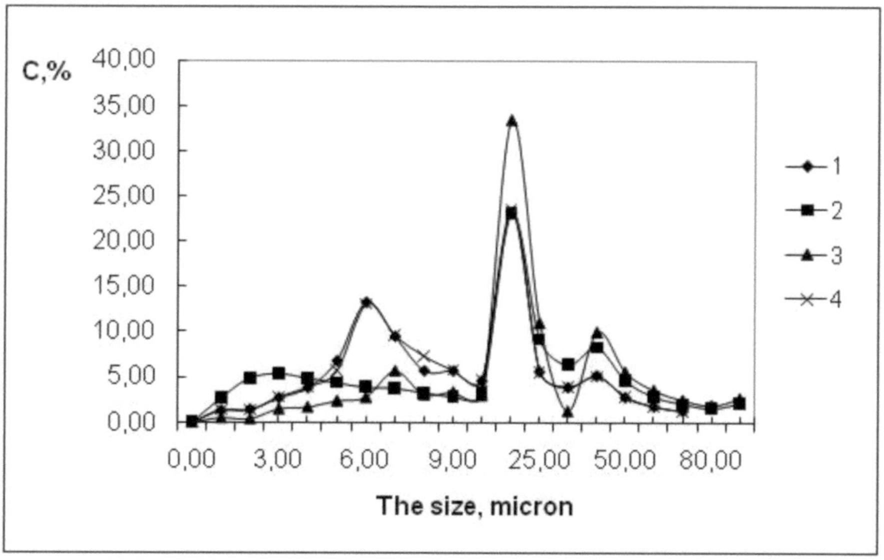

Fig. 10. Differential particle size distributions of calcium carbonate phosphates prepared from them: (*1*) doped with 0.02 mol % Fe, (*2*) doped with 0.02 mol % Mg, (*3*) doped with 0.02 mol % Fe and 0.02 mol% Mg, (*4*) undoped

– within 40 days). The results are illustrated in *Table* 2 showing the transverse mechanical strength (shear stress) of the bone tissue (femur) and the dental enamel as a function of the duration suspension introduction into animals. As a result, it has been found that there is a 13% increase in the mechanical strength (shear stress) of the bone tissue and a 7 % increase in the strength of the dental tissue (enamel), and this enables us to make an assumption of strengthened osteogenesis in a living organism.

Groups on 10 animals	Shear strength of the bone tissue, MPa	Standard deviation, S^2	Content of Ca of the bone tissue, wt. %	Standard deviation, S^2	Shear strength of dental enamel, MPa	Standard deviation S^2	Content of Fe, wt. %	Standard deviation, S^2	Content of Mg, wt. %	Standard deviation, S^2
I	24.1	0.23	40.25	0.14	63.8	1.95	0.78	0.07	0.06	0.01
II	17.2	0.98	41.72	0.45	50.0	1.20	0.40	0.09	0.24	0.04
III	23.0	0.15	40.06	0.69	68.1	1.83	0.63	0.03	0.26	0.01
IV	26.5	0.46	41.53	0.12	56.1	1.75	0.92	0.05	0.16	0.01
V	27.3	0.59	41.78	0.10	57.9	1.90	0.70	0.05	0.22	0.03

Table 2. Processed experimental data on the effect of doped calcium carbonate-phosphate on the mechanical strength of the bone tissue and the concentration of iron and magnesium in dental enamel

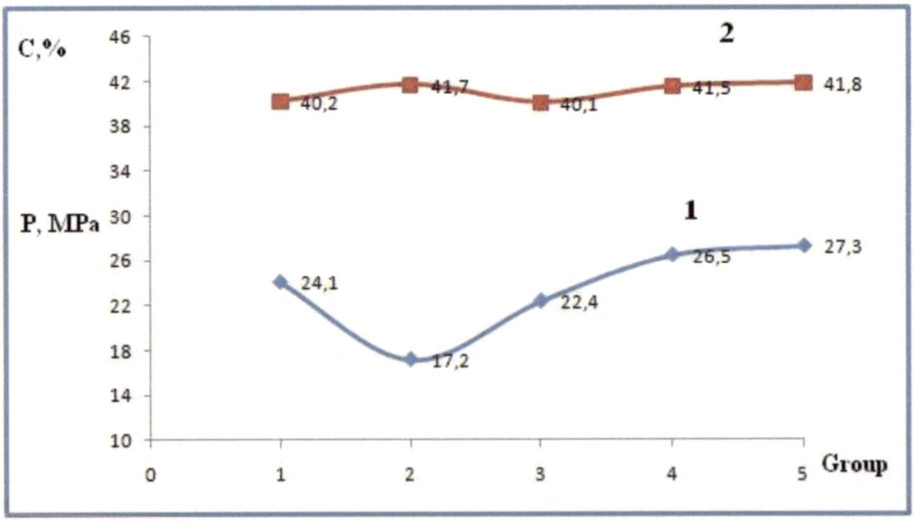

a)

Fig. 11. (Continued)

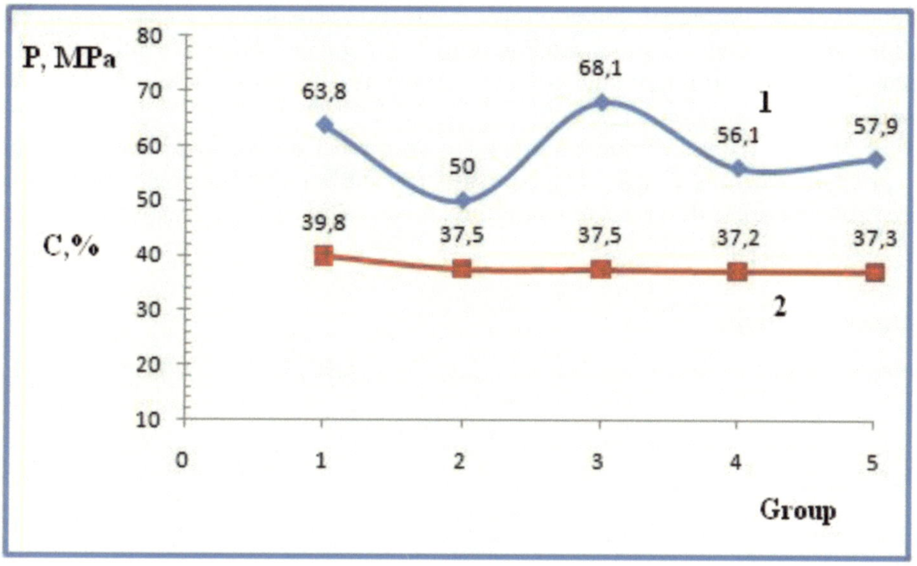

b)

Fig. 11. Impact doped calcium carbonate-phosphate an bone tissue strength (curve 1, fig. a) and bone tissue calcium concentration (curve 2, fig. a) and impact an tooth tissue strength (curve 1, fig. 11b) and tooth tissue calcium concentration (curve 2, fig. 11 b)

It is necessary to note that the first 10 days see a decrease in mechanical strength for the bone and dental tissues, and this is attributed to the insufficient number of receptors generated to assimilate calcium and phosphorus at the first stage. The results obtained have been processed by means of methods of mathematical statistics and the sampling has been verified for the normal distribution of the results. The comparison of the results with known ones (29) demonstrates a good agreement.

The content of calcium in the bone tissue, iron and magnesium in the dental enamel of animals as dependent on the introduction of calcium phosphates doped with magnesium and iron is presented in *Table 2* and in *Figure 11.* The changes in the mechanical strength of dental enamel and the content of iron and magnesium prove the activity of calcium phosphates and their influence on osteogenesis.

4. Conclusion

Thus, synthesized and investigated doped calcium carbonate-phosphate doped with cations represent a complex phase composition and constitute a biologically active material. The introduction of cations Fe^{2+}, Mg^{2+}, Zn^{2+}, K^{+}, Mn^{2+} and Si^{4+} changes the phase equilibrium in the $CaCO_3$ - NH_4Cl - H_3PO_4 system and leads to the formation of calcium phosphate chloride hydroxide, octacalcium hydrogen phosphate, brushite as the most active components participating in osteogenesis and the strengthening of the bone and dental tissues. By virtue of the kinetic data of the reaction of the interaction between orthophosphate acid and calcium hydroxycarbonate complexes in the synthesis process of nanocrystalline doped calcium carbonate phosphate, this system can be submitted as being chemically oscillating, i.e., oscillating in time. To describe this oscillating system, one can use a brusselator of the simplest cubic nonlinear realization. The kinetic curves of concentrated changes in the synthesis of nanocrystalline doped calcium carbonate phosphates are similar to the kinetics of concentration changes and phase pattern of the fructose-6-phosphate and fructose di-phosphate systems, respectively. The final reaction product output is determined as a result of oscillations. Doping cations have an impact on the formation of biologically active phosphate compounds. Doped calcium carbonate-phosphate are promising biocompatible materials designed to strengthen the bone and dental tissues and to replenish calcium in a living organism.

5. Acknowledgment

This research was funded by the Russian Basic Research Fund - Urals, project No 07-03-96076-[r].

6. References

[1] Hughes M.N. The Inorganic Chemistry of Biological Processes. Moscow: Mir, 1983. p. 348-358.
[2] Sapin M.R, Bilich G.L. Human anatomy. Moscow, 2000; v. 1. p. 96-111.
[3] Bibikov V.Yu., Smirnov V.V., Fadeeva, I.V. Ray G.V., Ferro D., Barinov S.M., Shvorneva. L.I. Intensification of sintering carbonate-hydroxyapatite of ceramics for bone implants. Perspectivniye materialy, 2005; 6, p. 43-48. ISSN1028-978X
[4] Tretyakov Yu.D. Development of inorganic chemistry as a fundamental base for the design of new generations of functional materials. Uspekhi khimii, 2004; 73(9), p. 899- 916. ISSN: 0042-1308; ISSN: 1817-5651
[5] Veresov A.G. Putlyaev V.I., Tretyakov Yu.D. Chemistry of inorganic biomaterials on the basis of calcium phosphates. The Russian chemical journal of the society named after D.I. Mendeleev. 2004; 48 (4), p. 52-64.
[6] Koroleva L.F. Doped calcium phosphates—a promising biomaterial, Perspekt. Mater. 2007; 4, p. 30–36. ISSN 1028-978X
[7] Koroleva L.F. Doped Nanocrystalline Calcium Carbonate Phosphates, Inorganic Mater. 2010; 46 (4), p. 405–411. ISSN 0020-1685.
[8] Koroleva L.F. An Oscillating Mechanism in the Synthesis of Doped Nanocrystalline Calcium Carbonate Phosphates. Nanotechnologies in Russia, 2010; 5 (9–10), p. 635–640. ISSN 1995-0780.
[9] Bouyer E, Gitzhofer F, Boulos M.I. Morphological study of hydroxyapatite nanocrystal suspension. J. Mater Sci: Mater Med 2000; 11, p. 523-531. ISSN 0957-4530.
[10] Changsheng Liu, Yue Huang, Wei Shen, Jinghua Cui. Kinetics of hydroxyapatite precipitation at pH 10 to 11. Biomaterials. 2001; 22, p. 301-306. ISSN: 0142-9612
[11] Rodicheva G.V., Orlovsky V.P, Privalov V.P, Barinov S.M., Pustikelli F. S., Oskarson S. Synthesis and physical chemical research of calcium carbonate-hydroxyapatite of type A. J. Inorganic chemistry. 2001; 46, 11, p.1798-1802. ISSN 0036-0236: ISSN 1531-8613
[12] Jaroslav Cihlar and Klara Castkova. Direct Synthesis of Nanocrystalline Hydroxyapatite by Hydrothermal Hydrolysis of Alkylphosphates. Monatshefte für Chemie / Chemical Monthly. 2002; 133 (6), p. 761-771. ISSN: 0026-9247; ISSN: 1434-4475.

[13] Tasi C., Aldinger F. Formation of apatitic calcium phosphates in a Na-K-phosphate solution of pH 7.4. J. Mater Sci: Mater Med. 2005; 16, p.167– 174. ISSN 0957-4530
[14] Barinov S.M, Komlev V.S. Calcium phosphate based bioceramics. Moscow, Nauka, 2005. 204 p. ISBN 5-02-033724-2
[15] Rui-Xue Sunl, Yu-Peng Lu. Fabrication and characterization of porous hydroxyapatite microspheres by spray-drying method. Frontiers of Materials Science in China. 2008; 2, p. 95-98. ISSN 2095-025X; ISSN 2095-0268.
[16] Hong L., Min Ying Zhu, Li Hua Li, Chang Ren Zhou. Processing of nanocrystalline hydroxyapatite particles via reverse microemulsions. J. Mater Science. 2008; 43, p.384–389. ISSN 0022-2461; ISSN 1573-4803
[17] Sherina Peroos, Zhimei Du, Nora henriette de Leeuw. A computer modeling study of uptake, structure and distribution of carbonate defects in hydroxyl-apatite. Biomaterials. 2006; 27 (9), p.2156-2161. ISSN 0142-9612.
[18] Kitikova N.V., Shashkova I.L., Zonov Yu. G., Sycheva O.A., Rat'ko A.I. Effect of phase transformations during synthesis on the chemical composition and structure of calcium-deficient hydroxyapatite. Inorganic Materials. 2007, V. 43, p. 319-324. . ISSN 0020-1685.
[19] Fomin A. S., Barinov S.M., V. M. Ievlev,V. V. Smirnov, B. P. Mikhailov, Belonogov E. K., Drozdova N. A. Nanocrystalline Hydroxyapatite Ceramics Produced by Low-Temperature Sintering after High-Pressure Treatment. Doklady Chemistry. 2008; 418 (1), p. 22–25. ISSN 0012-5008.
[20] Rui-xue Suni, Yu-peng Lu. Fabrication and characterization of porous hydroxyapatite microspheres by spray-drying method. Frontiers of Materials Science in China. 2008; 2, p.95-98.
[21] YuLing Jamie Han,. Say Chye Joachim Loo, Ngoc Thao Phung , Freddy Boey,. Jan Ma. Controlled size and morphology of EDTMP-doped hydroxyapatite nanoparticles as model for 153Samarium-EDTMP doping. J. Mater Sci: Mater Med. 2008; 19; p. 2993–3003. ISSN 0957-4530
[22] Ines S. Neira, Yury V. Kolen'ko, Oleg I. Lebedev, Gustaaf Van Tendeloo, Himadri S. Gupta, Nobuhiro Matsushita, Masahiro Yoshimura, Francisco Guitian. Rational synthesis of a nanocrystalline calcium phosphate cement exhibiting rapid conversion to hydroxyapatite. Materials Science and Engineering C 2009; 29, p. 2124–2132. ISSN 0928-4931
[23] A. Generosi, J. V. Rau, V. Rossi Albertini, B. Paci. Crystallization process of carbonate substituted hydroxyapatite nanoparticles in toothpastes upon hysiological conditions: an in situ time-resolved X-ray diffraction study. J. Mater Sci: Mater Med. 2010; 21, p. 445–450. ISSN 0957-4530
[24] Hazegawa M, Doi Y. and Uchida A. Cell-mediated bioresorption of sintered carbonate apatite in rabbits. J. Bone Joint Surg. 2003; 85 (B), p.142-147.
[25] M. Mullender, A.J. El Haj, Y. Yang, M.A. van Duin, E. H. Burger I J. Klein-Nulend. Mechanotransduction of bone cells in vitro: mechanobiology of bone tissue. Med. Biol. Eng. Comput. 2004; 42, p. 14–21. ISSN: 0140-0118; ISSN: 1741-0444.
[26] Chen Lai, Ying Jun Wang and Kun Wei. Nucleation kinetics of calcium phosphate nanoparticles in reverse micelle solution. Colloids and Surfaces A. 2007; 299 (1-3), p.203-208. ISSN: 0927-7757.

[27] J. Brandt, S. Henning, G. Michler, W. Hein, A. Bernstein, M. Schulz. Nanocrystalline hydroxyapatite for bone repair: an animal study. J Mater Sci: Mater Med (2010) 21, p. 283–294. ISSN 0957-4530

[28] Peters Dennis G, Hayes John M., Hieftje Gary M. Chemical Separations and Measurements. Theory and Practice of Analytical Chemistry. Moscow, 1978, Part 1.

[29] German J, Liebowitz H. Mechanics of destruction of the bone tissue. In the book: Fracture of nonmetals and composites. Editor Liebowitz H. Moscow, Mir, 1976; vol. 7, Part 2: p.391-463.

[30] Koroleva L.F., Larionov L.P., and Gorbunova N.P., Doped calcium carbonate phosphates—an effective ultradispersed biomaterial for substitution and strengthening of bony tooth tissues, in Proceedings of the International Forum on Nanotechnologies "Rusnanotech 08," Moscow, Russia, 3-5 December, 2008; 1, p. 505–507.

[31] Prigozhine I. R., Lefebre R., Symmetry breaking instabilities indissipative Systems. J. Chem. Phys.1968; 48:1665–1700. ISSN 0021-9606; ISSN 1089-7690.

[32] Oscillations and Traveling Waves in Chemical Systems, Ed. by R. J. Field and M. Burger (Wiley, New York, 1985; Mir, Moscow, 1988).

[33] Higgins J.A. A chemical mechanism for oscillations in glicolitic intermediates in yeast cells. Proc. Nat. Acad. Sci. USA, 1954; v. 51. ISSN 0027-8424.

[34] Higgins J.A. The theory of oscillating reactions. Ing. Chem. 1967;.59, (5).

[35] Dupont G., Goldbetter A. Theoretical insights into the origin of signal-induced calcium oscillations: From experiments to theoretical models. Acad. Press. London. 1989; p. 461-474.

[36] Dupont G, Goldbetter A. Protein phosphorylation driven by intracellular calcium oscillations: a kinetic analysis. Biophys. Chem. 1992; 42, p. 257–270. ISSN: 0301-4622.

[37] Dupont G. and Goldbetter A. Oscillations and waves of citosolic calsium: insights from theoretical models. Bioessays. 1992; 14: 485-493.

6

Osteogenesis of Adipose-Derived Stem Cells

Xiaoxiao Cai, Xiaoxia Su, Guo Li, Jing Wang and Yunfeng Lin*
State Key Laboratory of Oral Diseases,
West China School of Stomatology, Sichuan University,
P. R. China

1. Introduction

Mesenchymal stem cells (MSCs) are a group of multipotent adult-derived stem cells that can be isolated from the organs and tissues, including the bone marrow, ligaments, muscle and adipose tissue [1, 2]. MSCs may undergo self-renewal for several generations while maintaining their capacity to differentiate into multi-lineage tissues such as bone, cartilage, muscle and fat [3]. Bone marrow stem cells (BMSCs), one of the earliest multipotent stem cells to attract researchers' attention, have been studied for years and have gained some achievements. However, the stem cell population in bone marrow is estimated to be approximately 1 per 10^5 cells, and other tissues contain even fewer stem cells. Recently, research interest in the therapeutic potential of adipose derived stem cells (ASCs) has grown rapidly. Compared with BMSCs, ASCs are easier to obtain, have lower donor site morbidity, grow quickly, and are harvested in large numbers from small volumes of adipose tissue [4]. During culture in vitro, ASCs can be expanded for more passages because of their proliferative capacity, and they maintain their function after expansion or cryopreservation like BMSCs. ASCs demonstrate substantial in vitro and in vivo bone formation capacity that is similar to or greater than that of BMSCs [5]. Moreover, ASCs secrete potent growth factors, such as fibroblast growth factor-2 (FGF-2) and vascular endothelial growth factor (VEGF), to stimulate angiogenesis, which is of vital importance for osteogenesis [6]. Bone tissue engineering offers a promising method for the repair of bone deficiencies caused by fractures, bone loss, and tumors. In bone regeneration, the use of ASCs has received attention because of the self-renewal ability and high proliferative capacity of these cells and because of their potential for osteogenic differentiation. Therefore, it is of significance to study the osteogenesis mechanism of ASCs for future clinical applications.

2. The isolation and culture of ASCs

Adipose tissue is composed of adipocytes and a heterogeneous set of cell populations, which, upon isolation, are termed the stromal vascular fraction (SVF), that surround and support the adipocytes [7]. The SVF includes ASCs, cells from the microvasculature such as vascular endothelial cells and their progenitors, vascular smooth muscle cells, cells with hematopoietic progenitor activity and leukocytes. Despite the fact that the SVF is a heterogeneous cell population, the subsequent expansion of ASCs selects for a relatively

* Corresponding Author

homogeneous cell population that is enriched for cells expressing a stromal immunophenotype, when compared with the heterogeneity of the crude SVF.

The ASCs that were isolated from the inguinal fat pads of mice were harvested as follows. Eight-week-old BALB/c mice were used in the study, in accordance with the International Guiding Principles for Animal Research (1985). All of the surgical procedures were performed under approved anesthetic methods using Nembutal at 35 mg/kg. Inguinal fat pads were harvested from the mice and extensively washed with sterile phosphate-buffered saline (PBS) to remove contaminating debris. Then, the fat pads were incubated with 0.075% type I collagenase in PBS for 60 min at 37°C with agitation. After removing the collagenase by dilution with PBS, the cells that were released from the adipose specimens were filtered through a 100 µm mesh to remove the tissue debris and were collected by centrifugation at 1,200 g for 10 min. This treatment resulted in the separation of harvested fat into three layers: the infranatant (the lowest layer, which is composed of blood, tissue fluid and local anesthetic), the middle portion (primarily fatty tissue), and the supranatant (the upper layer, which is the least dense and consists of lipids). The pellet from the infranatant was resuspended and incubated to remove contaminating red blood cells. Then, the pellet was washed three times with PBS and seeded on plastic tissue culture dishes in growth medium containing α-MEM, 10% fetal bovine serum (FBS), 100 U/mL penicillin, and 100 mg/mL streptomycin. The ASCs were maintained in a humidified atmosphere of 5% CO2 at 37 °C. The cells were passaged three times prior to osteogenic differentiation. After their transfer into specific medium containing dexamethasone (10^{-8} mol/L), ascorbic acid (50 mg/L), and β-glycerophosphate (10 mmol/L), the ASCs exhibited an obvious phenotype alteration and became osteogenic. The medium was replaced every 3–4 days for 14 days until the differentiated cells were confluent.

ASCs are adherent cells, which display a fibroblast-like morphology and align with a spindle-like or eddy-like shape. ASCs have proven to be difficult to identify in culture. Some studies have focused on particular cell markers to more easily recognize ASCs. Dominici et al. demonstrated that ASCs must express CD105, CD73 and CD90, and lack expression of the CD45, CD34, CD133, CD14 or CD11b, CD79α or CD19 and HLA-DR surface molecules [6]. Mitchell et al. found that stromal cell–associated markers (CD13, CD29, CD44, CD63, CD73, CD90, and CD166) were initially low on SVF cells and increased significantly with successive passages [7]. Lin et al. observed the behavior of ASCs in culture, likened them to vascular and endothelial cells, and pinpointed markers CD34+/CD31-/CD104b- /SMA- in this differentiation [8]. The markers that are uniformly reported to be highly expressed are CD13, CD29, CD44, CD73, CD90, CD105, CD166 and MHC-I, while markers of the hematopoietic and angiogenic lineages, such as CD31, CD45 and CD133, have been reported to be lowly expressed or unexpressed on ASCs. MHC-II has also been found to be absent on ASCs. Moderate expression, in which the surface marker expression level is lower than 50%, has been reported for markers CD9, CD34, CD49d, CD106, CD146 and STRO-1.

ASCs have the ability to differentiate into cells of several lineages such as adipocytes, osteoblasts, chondrocytes, myocytes, endothelial cells, hematopoietic cells, hepatocytes and neuronal cells.

3. The mechanisms of osteogenesis – Growth factors and cytokines

The bone regeneration and repair process is not completely understood, and its molecular mechanisms have recently been paid an increasing amount of attention. Traditionally, the process of bone healing has been defined by four stages: inflammation and clot formation, cellular infiltration and soft-callus formation, hard-callus formation, and remodeling. The mechanisms that drive the ASCs into the osteoblast lineage are still not clear, but research on growth factors and cytokines have provided much information about the effect of signaling molecules on cell proliferation, differentiation, adhesion, migration, and ultimate bone formation. Engineered tissues can be formed more efficiently by delivering genes that encode growth factors into ASCs through the use of electroporation, calcium phosphate precipitation transfection or lipofection of plasmids or viral vectors [9]. It is possible to accelerate the bone healing and regeneration process by gene transfection [10]. Therefore, the incorporation of the appropriate growth factors or cytokines within a progenitor population will allow for their use in bone regeneration.

A host of growth factors and cytokines are involved in the process of bone formation in developmental biology and distraction osteogenesis. BMPs, which are already used in the clinic, seem to be the most promising candidate cytokines in osteogensis and ectopic bone formation. With the exception of BMP-1, BMPs are members of the TGF-β superfamily that were originally isolated from bovine bone extracts and were found to induce ectopic bone formation subcutaneously in rats [11]. This group of proteins includes sixteen BMPs and comprises nearly one-third of the TGF-β superfamily. BMPs are also involved in mesoderm induction, skeletal patterning and limb development [12]. BMPs transmit their signals via ligand binding to the heteromeric complex of types I and II serine/threonine kinase receptors on the cell surface[13]. The ligand signal is then transduced intracellularly via activation of the SMAD (signaling mothers against decapentaplegic) proteins, and then phosphorylated R-Smads and Smad4 subsequently migrate to the nucleus to effect the expression of the target gene and promote the osteogenic differentiation. BMP signaling also has been known to be transmitted via the MAPK (mitogen-activated protein kinase) pathway. Various subtypes of BMPs are observed to be expressed in obviously relevant tissues; for example, BMP-2 is expressed in the cartilage, periosteum and compact bone tissues. BMP-2, BMP-4, and BMP-7 exhibit good bone-forming activity when combined with collagen, hydroxyapatite (HA) and degradable high molecular polymer (HMP) in different animal bone defects experiments[14]. BMPs control both intramembranous and endochondral ossification through the chemotaxis and mitosis of mesenchymal cells, the induction of a mesenchymal commitment to osteogenic or chondrogenic differentiation, and programmed cell death. BMPs stimulate osteogenic differentiation in multiple cell lines, including fibroblasts, chondrocytes, BMSCs and ASCs. The effect of BMPs has also been noted to be concentration dependent. At low concentrations, BMPs foster chemotaxis and cellular proliferation, while at high concentrations, BMPs induce bone formation [15]. BMPs are more potent at inducing bone formation as heterodimers than as homodimers. In culture, BMP-2/6, BMP-2/7, and BMP-4/7 heterodimers have been shown to promote higher alkaline phosphatase levels than homodimer combinations [16, 17, 18]; these data have also been corroborated in vivo [19]. BMP-2, BMP-4, BMP-6, BMP-7, and BMP-9 are considered to be the most osteoinductive of the BMP proteins [20]. It is believed that BMPs regulate osteoblast differentiation via the increased transcription of core-binding factor-1/Runt–related family 2 (Cbfa1/Runx2), a molecule that is known to be necessary for commitment along an osteoblastic lineage [14]. The BMP and Wnt singling pathways regulate the osteoblastic differentiation of mesenchymal stem cells (MSCs). The Wnt pathway plays an essential role in bone regeneration, and it has been observed that Notch-1 overexpression inhibits osteoblastogenesis by suppressing Wnt/beta-catenin but not BMP signaling [21].Notch enhances the BMP-2-induced osteoblastic differentiation by overexpression of Delta1/Jagged1-activated Notch1 signaling in MC3T3-E1 cells [22]. Hence, there are many singling pathways play role in osteogensis. Here, our group has focused on BMP-2 and Notch.

BMP-2 is a pleiotropic regulator that governs the key steps in the bone induction cascade such as the chemotaxis, mitosis and differentiation of mesenchymal stem cells in the process of bone healing [23, 24]. There have been some reports describing the effectiveness of BMP-2 in the osteogenesis of BMSCs and ASCs, but it is unclear whether BMP-2-enhanced ASCs can heal large bone defects [10, 25]. Our group harvested ASCs from normal SD rats and transfected them with the BMP-2 gene before they were loaded onto alginate gel. The ability for bone regeneration was determined in critical-size rat cranial defects. An 8-mm diameter defect was created in the calvarias of 36 rats, and then these rats were divided into three groups. In the experimental group, the defects were filled with alginate gel combined with BMP-2-transfected ASCs; in the negative control group, the defects were filled with alginate gel mixed with normal ASCs; in the blank controls, the defects were filled with cell-free alginate gel. To identify the molecular events leading to the formation of new bone, we investigated the expression of biochemical markers by using RT-PCR and western blotting over the course of the BMP-2 enhanced ASCs differentiation. In the experimental group, weak osteogenesis was noted in the epidural region of the border of the defect at 8 weeks. After 16 weeks of treatment, the continued formations of new bone throughout the defects were observed. In the negative control group, bone islets formed by interstitial osteogenesis were observed in various connective tissues after 16 weeks. In the blank control group, the alginate gel was absorbed at 4 weeks. The RT-PCR analysis of OPN, OCN, RUNX2 and BMP-2 demonstrated that there was a significant difference in the expression of these genes between the experimental and control groups. Continued high expression of OPN, OCN, RUNX2 and BMP-2 was observed throughout the progression of the experimental group both in vitro and in vivo. In the negative control group, these genes were observed neither in vitro nor in vivo at 8 weeks; only at 16 weeks after surgery, a weak expression of these genes was observed. In the blank control group, these genes were not detected at 8 and 16 weeks post surgery. The western blot results were similar to the RT-PCR results, but the OPN, OCN, RUNX2, and BMP-2 proteins were not observed in the negative and blank control groups. The expression of OPN and OCN inside of the cranial defects made sure that osteogenesis and the maturation of BMP-2-enhanced ASCs occurred. Our research indicated that alginate gel with BMP-2-enhanced ASCs was necessary for critical-size defect repair, and load-bearing alginate with BMP-2-enhanced ASCs can be applied in engineering approaches for further clinical use.

Notch signaling plays a key role in the determination of cell fate and in the progenitor's maintenance in the normal development of many tissues and cell types. An evolutionarily conserved mechanism is to maintain a balance between the differentiation and proliferation of a diverse range of stem/progenitor cells and to enable them to adopt distinct cell fates [26]. Previous investigations have shown that Notch signaling positively regulates the osteoblastogenesis of several types of cells, such as murine bone marrow mesenchymal progenitors [27], ST-2 marrow stromal cells [21], Kusa mesenchymal progenitor cells [28], M3T3-E1 osteoblastic cells [29] and C2C12 myoblasts [30]. Other research has concluded that Notch is a positive regulator of osteogenesis in COS-7 cells [31] and MC3T3-E1 cells [32]. However, the enhancement of osteogenic gene expression was not observed in Tezuka's report.

In mammals, Notch signaling is mediated by the intracellular interactions of type I transmembrane ligands, such as Delta and Serrate, with Notch receptors (Notch-1, Notch-2, Notch-3 and Notch-4). Once it is bound to its ligand, the Notch receptor is cleaved by the metalloprotease TNF-a converting enzyme and the γ-secretase complex, at two sites, to generate the Notch intracellular domain (NICD) [33].This domain is transported to the nucleus and binds a CCAAT-binding protein (CBF-1), which is also called CSL. CSL acts as a transcriptional repressor in the absence of NICD, which recruits a co-repressor complex and inhibits the transcription of target genes that contain the CCAAT binding sites[34,35]. As a consequence of binding, NICD displaces the repressor complex of CSL and recruits nuclear co-activators, such as mastermind-like 1 (MAML1) and histone acetyltransferases[36], to convert CSL into a transcriptional activator. Notch activation through the CSL-NICD interactions can activate the transcription of various target genes, including Hes (Hairy /Enhancer of Split) [37], Hes-related repressor protein (HERP)[38,39], nuclear factor-κB (NF-κB) [40] and PPAR (peroxisome-proliferator-activated receptor) [41].

The Notch system is known to be an evolutionarily conserved mechanism that balances the differentiation and proliferation of stem/ progenitor cells [42], with NICD acting to keep the cells in an undifferentiated state during development [43]. N- [N- (3,5- Difluorophenacety l)-L-alanyl]-S-phenylglycine *t*- butyl ester (DAPT) is a γ- secretase inhibitor that can block Notch signaling by preventing the cleavage of Notch receptors, which has been widely used to evaluate the biological behaviors and Notch signaling pathway in various cells such as BMSCs, muscle stem cells, neural stem cells, and human tongue carcinoma cells [42]. It will be beneficial to consider the influence on the osteogenesis of ASCs by regulating Notch signaling with DAPT. We investigated, for the first time, the effects of DAPT on the proliferation and osteogenesis of ASCs by using an in vitro 1,25-Dihydroxyvitamin D_3(VD_3)-induced osteogenic differentiation system. The results showed that ASCs cultured in DAPT had significantly decreased CFU numbers in comparison with those cultured in control medium during a 2-week culture period. DAPT clearly inhibited the ASCs' proliferation at all doses, which indicated that ASCs responded with decreased growth when the Notch pathway was blocked. The alizarin red results indicate that the addition of DAPT to the VD_3 treatments increased osteogenesis in ASCs. Real-time PCR showed the expression levels of the Notch downstream target genes, Hes-1 and Hey-1, were decreased after DAPT treatment. Immunofluorescence staining revealed that Hey-1 was down-regulated when Notch signaling was inhibited by DAPT. However, Real-time PCR and Western blot analysis showed the up-regulation of Runx2 and OSX after DAPT treatment. Hey-1, which is expressed in the nucleus of ASCs and acts as a transcriptional repressor, was down-regulated when Notch signaling was inhibited by DAPT, whereas the expression of Runx2, an essential transcription factor that is required for osteogenesis, was increased in the nucleus of osteogenic ASCs after DAPT treatment. This finding indicates that the Runx2 dependent osteogenic differentiation of ASCs was enhanced when the interaction between Runx2 and the Notch target gene Hey-1 was suppressed in the presence of DAPT. In accordance with what has previously been reported, Notch repressed osteoblastic differentiation through its target genes and Runx2 [44]. Therefore, our study demonstrated that DAPT reduced the proliferation and enhanced the osteogenesis of ASCs via the regulation of Notch and Runx2 expression. We also found that the adipogenesis of mouse adipose-derived stem cells (mASCs) can be enhanced by the coordinated regulation of Notch and PPAR-γ. DAPT comprehensively inhibited the Notch signaling pathway and consequently influenced Hes-1 expression, which may directly or indirectly reduce DLK-1

/Pref-1, an inhibitor of the adipogenic transcription activator PPAR-γ. The continuous repression of DLK-1/Pref-1 with the activation of PPAR-γ dephosphorylation promotes the adipogenesis of mASCs. All of these findings imply that Notch signaling plays an important role in the fate determination of ASCs.

The FGFs (fibroblast growth factors) are a highly conserved family of twenty-four proteins that transmit their signals via a family of four transmembrane tyrosine kinases. The most abundant ligand of the family, FGF-2 may increase osteoblast proliferation and bone formation both in vitro and in vivo [45]. Exogenous FGF-2 was able to rescue the decreased bone nodule formation in osteoblast cultures from these transgenic mice.

TGF-β (transforming growth factor-β) enhances the osteogenic differentiation of MSCs by promoting mitosis, calcium phosphate deposition, Col I synthesis and adipogenesis suppression. The expression of IGF-1 mRNA, which is up-regulated by TGF-βs, may also promote the osteogenic differentiation of BMSCs.

IGF-2 (insulin-like growth factor) has been known to stimulate bone collagen synthesis, osteogenesis and chondrogenesis. In a transgenic mouse, where the IGF expression was up-regulated in osteoblasts, bone formation of the distal femur increased as compared with the control group [46]. Histology showed no increase in the number of osteoblasts, which suggests that IGF-1 up-regulated the activity of the existing bone-forming cells. The size and bone-formation rates of the IGF-1 knockout mice were significantly reduced as compared with their wild-type littermates [47].

PDGF (platelet-derived growth factor) has also been demonstrated to be a potent stimulus for osteoblast proliferation, chemotaxis, and collagen activity. PDGF is now being used clinically in periodontics; the application of recombinant human PDGF in a tricalcium phosphate matrix significantly increased periodontal bone formation. [48]

Hormones, including estrogen, glucocorticoid, and parathyroid hormone, are also considered to influence the bone metabolism directly or indirectly. Estrogen up-regulates the transcriptional expression of osteoblast-related genes such as ALP, Cbal, BMP-2 and TGF-1. Physiological concentrations of glucocorticoid can stimulate the osteoblastic differentiation of MSCs. However, an inhibition of osteoblast proliferation and apoptosis and a reduction of active osteoblast-composition, which may lead to osteoporosis, may be observed if large doses of glucocorticoid are applied for a long period of time. In mature bone tissue, parathyroid hormone either decomposes or synthesizes bone by promoting bone growth or filling up lacunas created by osteoclast[49].

Bone formation by the implantation of ASCs must be preceded by the in vitro osteogenic differentiation of these cells. The differentiation procedure has the disadvantage of requiring additional culture time and steps, including the use of large amounts of costly growth factors such as bone morphogenetic protein (BMP), and dexamethasone, which may be cytotoxic to cells, prior to implantation to achieve therapeutic efficacy. New methods aimed at reducing the culture period and the amount of required growth factors and enhancing the efficiency of osteogenesis and thus of bone regeneration should be developed. One approach is the delivery of cytokines by incorporating these molecules into scaffolds such as microspheres and liposome. This approach would allow the growth factors to be retained at the site of interest for an extended period of time while maintaining the proteins' biological activity. Moreover, engineered ASCs that are produced by gene transduction by various virus-vectors have evolved to be an attractive option to ameliorate bone repair, especially large bone defects. Transfecting ASCs with genes for BMP-2, BMP-4, BMP-7, Runx-2 or

Osterix is considered to promote bone formation in vivo following implantation of the ASCs [10, 24, 25].

4. Ectopic bone formation of ASCs and In situ repair of critical – Size cranial defects

Bone grafting and bone substitutes are required in many orthopedic and dental procedures such as spinal fusion, the revision of hip prostheses, the repair of non-healing fractures, or the reconstruction of large bone defects. Although autografts are the gold standard for the clinical repair of large defects, unsatisfactory results occur in as many as 30% of cases [50], and autografting can be restricted by donor tissue shortage and morbidity [51]. Allografts are limited in usage owing to immunological rejection, possible transmission of infectious diseases and premature resorption. Bone marrow-derived mesenchymal stem cells (BMSCs) are particularly promising as they can heal large segmental defects and can be genetically modified to augment in vivo bone formation [52,53]. ASCs and BMSCs are similar with respect to growth, morphology, immunoprivileged properties and the ability to differentiate into chondrocytes, osteoblasts and adipocytes [54].Furthermore, ASCs are reported to be slightly better than BMSCs with regard to osteogenic and chondrogenic differentiation potential; ASCs are also easy to isolate through liposuction and are available in large quantities, which has prompted the use of ASCs to repair cranial defects in animals and in clinical studies [55].

ASCs have osteogenic differentiation potential. Additionally, the biomaterial and the medium that were used enhanced the osteogenic differentiation of the cells. The ASCs showed an ability to adhere to and proliferate on scaffolds in vitro. In vivo, ASCs survive in low oxygen environments, which makes them good candidates for cell-based therapies in which the oxygen supply may be limited during the post implantation period when a blood supply is lacking[56]. However, ASCs secrete angiogenic cytokines such as vascular endothelial growth factor and hepatocyte growth factor, and these are considered to contribute to the angiogenic properties of ASCs[57]. It was considered that the transplanted ASCs produce cytokines and chemokines that act as homing signals to attract endogenous stem cells and progenitor cells to the site of injury. Thus, the presence of ASCs may enhance the osteogenic and angiogenic conditions of the construct in vivo, and the bone-forming capacity of ASCs in combination with various scaffold materials has been well reported [58]. Inorganic materials such as bioceramics, biodegradable polymer materials and composite materials have been commonly used in combination with ASCs to repair bone defects; for example, hydroxyapatite (HA)/tricalcium phosphate (TCP)[59], PLGA[60], chitooligosaccharide (COS)[61], fibrin/HA[62], and biphasic calcium phosphate nanocomposite (NanoBCP)[63] have all been used for these purposes. Heather L. et al. [64] examined the cell coverage and cell function of ASCs on different biomaterials, such as silicone rubber, fibronectin, dualligand , oxygen plasma plus fibronectin, polyimide and polyurethane. They found that cell attachment was very strong on both polyimide and polyurethane for all of the attachment methods; none of the attachment methods caused any differences in basic cell functions, including proliferation, metabolism, intracellular ATP concentration, and caspase-3 activity. However, ectopic bone formation inside of the porous ceramic blocks revealed that the material properties such as composition, geometry, porosity, size, and microstructure might be important but not sufficient parameters for evaluating appropriate bone formation [65].Moreover, β-TCP granules have been in clinical

use in Europe for over 20 years under the name CEROS 82, and investigations have been published concerning the clinical value of Chronos1 β-TCP in the bone environment [66].
Cytokines can induce healing in satisfactory biologic environments and are reported to improve the ability of ASCs to form bone when supplied in osteoinductive medium or coated onto biomaterials [62]; however, contradictory reports have been published with regards to this finding [67]. Engineered ASCs combined with gene modification have evolved to be an attractive option to ameliorate bone repair, especially large bone defects [68]. The co-delivery of BMP-2 and Runx-2 was a useful tool to enhance the osteogenesis of ASCs both in vitro and in vivo [69]. BMP-2/VEGF-[70], Runx2- or Osterix-transfected ASCs promoted bone formation in vivo following implantation [71].
Some researchers believed that ASCs should be induced into osteogenic lineages before they are seeded into scaffolds as more new bone tissues were observed when osteogenetic differentiation ASCs were seeded on PLGA in a rat critical-sized calvarial defect model [72,63]; this approach also had the advantage of avoiding the use of cytotoxic dexamethasone and had an additional culture period when it was used in a clinical application. Additionally, the physiological differences between individuals might influence the osteogenic and proliferative capacity of the expanded cells, as well as the microenvironment in the recipient site. The number and concentration of osteogenic cells in a scaffold are important for successful bone formation in vivo [73, 74].
Ectopic and in situ repair of cranial bone defects with ASCs and various scaffolds have been observed in mouse, rabbit and canine models [75, 76, 77]. Ectopic bone formation, inside of a muscle free flap, with autoASCs has been performed to reconstruct a large bony defect [56]. Ectopic bone formation was found when BMP-2- (BMP-2-ASC) or BMP-2/ Runx2- (BMP-2/ Runx2-ASC) transfected ASCs were seeded on PLGA biodegradable scaffolds and then implanted into the dorsal subcutaneous spaces of the mice [69]. ASCs are considered to be a suitable resource for cranial defects. The preferential expression of the HMWFGF-2 form is associated with a more osteogenic differentiated state of calvarial osteoblast. Murine ASCs undergoing osteogenesis recapitulate the in vivo osteogenic differentiation expression pattern of FGF ligands and receptors of calvarial mesenchymal cells during their own osteogenic differentiation[78]. Chin-Yu Lin et al. [70] confirmed the potential of the FLP/ Frt-mediated baculoviral vector recombination for sustained BMP-2 /VEGF expression in ASCs, and implantation of the engineered ASCs not only accelerated the weight-bearing segmental bone defect healing but also ameliorated the bone metabolism, bone volume, bone density, angiogenesis and mechanical properties so as to repair the massive bone defects. Additionally, 84% to 99% of the in situ new bone was derived from implanted cells when hASCs were transplanted onto PLGA to repair critical-size rat cranial defects successfully [72]. ASCs have been used clinically in a microvascular flap composed of autoASCs, and β-TCP and BMP-2 have been successfully used in a large bone defects reconstruction surgery [79]. Additionally, ASCs cultured in platelet- rich plasma have been successfully used to regenerate bone in rats' periodontal tissue defects [80].
Our group has performed research on the formation of ectopic and in situ new bone by osteogenic ASCs combined with biphasic calcium phosphate nanocomposite (NanoBCP), with high strength and porous structures. The NanoBCP constructs containing osteogenic ASCs were transplanted into nude mice subcutaneously for 8 weeks to acquire the physiological behavior of induced ASCs during ectopic differentiation in vivo. Critical-size rat cranial defects were used as the model to determine the efficiency of engineered constructs in the generation of new bone in situ. Histological analysis of the retrieved

specimens from nude mice in the experimental group showed obvious ectopic bone formation, and there was positive expression of osteopontin (OPN) and osteocalcin (OCN) at the RNA and protein levels. There was complete repair of the cranial defects in the experimental group, but only partial repair in the negative controls. Combining osteogenic ASCs with NanoBCP can lead to the formation of ectopic new bone. Furthermore, the approach can also stimulate bone regeneration and repair for large bone defects. Based on our results, we thought that load-bearing NanoBCP with ASCs could be applied in engineering approaches for further clinical usage. Patients' own ASCs would be an ideal cell source for bone tissue engineering, and autologous non-immunogenic bone tissues could be easily regenerated with this approach for the repair of large size bone defects.
Our goal is to develop a less invasive and more effective method for clinical use in bone regeneration. However, most of the animal models that are chosen for studies clearly belong to low-order phylogenetic species with a characteristically high potential for osteogenesis, and extending the experimental results relative to rate and amount of bone regeneration from animal models to humans is difficult. Additionally, the size of the defects that are likely to be treated in human subjects is usually much greater than those that were evaluated in this study. Consequently, a further investigation of large animal vertical augmentation models will be necessary before a similar protocol could be applied to bone reconstruction in the clinic.

5. New research in the field

The use of ASCs as an autologous and self-replenishing source for a variety of differentiated cell phenotypes provides much promise for reconstructive surgery. Therefore, research of ASCs and osteogenesis has been the focus of attention in recent years, both in basic research and clinical application.
The animal species for ASC cell sourcing have been expanded. ASCs can be recovered from wild Scandinavian brown bears and then grown in standard cell culture medium in monolayer cultures; ASCs from yearlings spontaneously formed bone-like nodules surrounded by cartilaginous deposits, which suggested the differentiation into osteogenic and chondrogenic lineages[81]. This is the first report of ASCs spontaneously forming extracellular matrix that is characteristic of bone and cartilage in the absence of specific inducers, and this ability appears to be lost gradually with age. Therefore, hibernating brown bears are considered as a model to study the osteogenesis mechanisms and disuse osteoporosis. ASCs were reported to be isolated based on a gradient solution and enzymatic digestion, and then several cell components were harvested. Rada T. et al. developed a method based on the use of immunomagnetic beads coated with specific antibodies, which could be used to study niches in ASC populations [82]. ASCs are further found to express stem cell markers (Oct4, Nanog, CD90 and CD105) and lineage-specific markers following induction; the expression of ALP, phosphoprotein (SPP1), Runx2 and OCN mRNA were positive in osteogenic lineages, and peroxisome proliferator activated receptor (PPARγ2) mRNA was positive in adipogenic lineages[837]. These cells are similar to but distinct from other adult stem cells. The expression of chemokine receptors such as CCR1/4/7 and CXCR6/4 in hASCs was higher than in BMSCs [84]. These receptors and their ligands and adhesion molecules play an important role in the tissue specific homing of leukocytes and have also been implicated in the trafficking of hematopoietic precursors into and through the tissues. Thus, ASCs may show a better migration and homing capacity, and they may be

a better candidate for bone regeneration. Meanwhile, a protocol for labeling ASCs with a readily available PET tracer, FDG, has been developed [85]. ASCs can be safely labeled with FDG concentrations up to 25 Bq/cell, without compromising their biological function. The initial biodistribution of the implanted FDG-labeled stem cells can be monitored using microPET imaging; this may provide a favorable method for long-term in vivo tracking for clinical usage.

Some new research on the osteoblast differentiation of ASCs and related factors should be noted. BMP-2 governs the key steps in the bone induction cascade such as chemotaxis, mitosis, and the differentiation of mesenchymal stem cells, which is applied in the clinical routine [86]. However, BMP-2 has a significant disadvantage; when it is used alone, it may induce a surplus of callus formation, and bone may develop in muscles (heterotopic ossification) [87]. However, Claudia K et al. just reported that the combination of ASCs and BMP-2 in a fibrin matrix significantly reduces callus formation when compared with BMP-2 alone [88]. Lin et al. reported that, compared with ASCs transiently expressing BMP-2, ASCs persistently expressing BMP-2 not only accelerated the healing of a weight-bearing segmental bone defect but also ameliorated the bone metabolism, bone volume, bone density, angiogenesis and mechanical properties [70]. BMP-6 also has been demonstrated to induce the osteogenic and chondrogenic differentiation of MSCs for tissue engineering and regenerative applications [89, 90]. HASCs were considered to express all components of the BMP/BMP receptor signaling pathway and respond to BMP-4 inducing up-regulated expression of its specific target genes Id1-Id4 [91]. BMP-4 effects on hASCs are dose-dependent. High doses significantly increased apoptosis and drastically reduced cell proliferation, whereas low doses of BMP-4 (0.01-0.1ng/mL) significantly increased culture cell content, cycling cells and reduced the number of apoptotic cells. Treatment of hASCs with low doses of BMP-4 did not modify the expression of Nanog or Oct4 or void their osteogenic or osteoblastic differentiation capacities. Natalina Q et al. demonstrated that FGF-2 treatment sustains the proliferative and osteogenic potential state of mASCs, while inhibiting their terminal osteogenic differentiation by antagonizing the retinoic-acid mediated up-regulation of BMPR-IB [96]. In their follow-up study, they further found that FGF ligand genes, such as FGF-2, FGF-4, FGF-8, and FGF-18, displayed a differential and dynamic profile during mouse ASC (mASC) osteogenesis[56]. Fgf-2 transcript was down-regulated, while Fgf-18 transcript level was strongly up-regulated. Also recent research has proven that the transfer of Runx2 or Osterix genes can enhance the in vitro and in vivo osteogenenic differentiation of ASCs [69, 71].

The culture conditions appeared to affect the osteogenic differentiation capacity in vitro, with more robust osteogenic differentiation seen in ASCs cultured in medium supplemented with human serum derivatives in or in SF conditions compared with FBS supplemented media [93, 94]. 17 beta-estradiol E(2) may stimulate the osteogenic differentiation of ASCs and therefore, can be used as an inducing agent to improve the efficiency of these cells in in vitro and in vivo studies [95]. Jing et al. demonstrated that VD3 induced the osteogenic differentiation of ASCs [96]. Song et al. suggested that vitamin D3 treatment, throughout the culture period with BMP-2, added in the later period is an effective and economical way of inducing the osteogenic differentiation of ASCs [87]. Gender differences were found to affect the osteogenic capacity of ASCs, with male ASCs differentiating more rapidly and more effectively than female ASCs in vitro [97]; the adipogenic potential was unchanged irrespective of age, while the osteogenic potential appears to decrease with increasing age [98]. These differences are likely due to the different steroid functions in males and females with hormone levels varying at different phases of life, which must be taken into account when designing clinical treatments for patients.

Osteoblastic differentiation of ASCs is still mainly used in the laboratory experiments or animal trials, and there are few studies about its clinical application. To date, two clinical case studies have been reported where the capacity of ASCs in bone tissue repair has been investigated [99, 56]. In the first case, the patient was a 7-year-old girl, who had sustained severe head injury after a fall that resulted in a closed multifragment calvarial fracture. The calvarial defect was treated with autologous ASCs that were isolated and applied in a single operative procedure in combination with milled autologous bone from the iliac crest. ASCs were supported in place with an autologous fibrin glue, and mechanical fixation was achieved with two large, resorbable macroporous sheets that acted as a soft tissue barrier. The new bone formation and near complete calvarial continuity was observed 3 months after the reconstruction. The harvesting of bone tissue or a composite microvascular flap is frequently followed by morbidity and a donor site defect despite. Furthermore, a large amount of autologous blood is needed for plasmapheresis, which may, in some cases, be difficult to obtain. It is known that ASCs can secrete angiogenic factors that promote neovascularization and vessel-like structure formation [100]. In the second case, K. Mesimäki et al. reported the reconstruction of maxillary defect of a 65-year-old male patient, who underwent a hemimaxillectomy due to a large keratocyst, with a microvascular flap using auto-ASCs, beta-tricalcium phosphate and bone morphogenetic protein-2 [56]. It was the first clinical case in which ectopic bone was produced using autologous ASCs in microvascular reconstruction surgery. The successful outcome of this clinical case paves the way for extensive clinical trials using ASCs in custom-made implants for the reconstruction craniofacial bone defects.

Because ASCs have bright prospects in clinical stem cell therapy, improved methods to assess safety, efficiency, reproducibility and quality of the vitro expanded or osteoblast differentiated stem cells are urgently called for. These methods must be not only safe in vitro, but also in vivo and in the clinical. The cell source, culturing components such as FBS and osteoinductive supplements, and the cell expansion time may have considerable effects on the cells at the gene level and may affect the quality and safety of the cell products. Furthermore, producing cells that are genetically stable and nontoxic is a step towards ensuring that the cells do not transform and lead to a genetically aberrated progeny or virus infection when transplanted into the recipient, especially tissues engineered ASCs with gene transfected by virus vectors. Few studies have been carried out on the mechanism of immunocharacteristic by ASCs. Therefore, assessing the immunogenic properties of the cells in vitro and in vivo is important to assure that anaphylactic reactions in the recipient are avoided. Reports have shown that the immunosuppressive capacity of the ASCs may, in some cases, favor the growth of tumor cells, but contradictory results exist [101, 102, 103]. These controversial results indicate that further studies are necessary to fully elucidate the true effect of ASCs on tumor formation. Hence, further pre-clinical safety and efficacy studies are required to assess and verify the safe outcome of the clinical procedure using in vitro expanded or osteoblastic differentiated stem cells.

6. References

[1] Vats A., Tolley N.S., Polak J.M., et al. Stem cells: sources and applications. Clin. Otolaryngol. Allied Sci.2002; 27, 227–232.

[2] Le B.K., Pittenger M. Mesenchymal stem cells: progress toward promise. Cytotherapy.2005; 7, 36–45.

[3] Zuk P.A., Zhu M., Ashjian P., et al. Human adipose tissue is a source of multipotent stem cells. Mol Cell Biol 2002;13,4279–4295.

[4] Ahn H.H., Kim K.S., Lee J.H., et al. In vivo osteogenic differentiation of human adipose - derived stem cells in an injectable in situ-forming gel scaffold, Tissue Eng. A. 2009;15, 1821 -1832.

[5] Rehman J.,Traktuev D.,Li J., et al. Secretion of angiogenic and antiapoptotic factors by human adipose stromal cells, Circulation. 2004;109,1292-1298.

[6] Dominici M., Le B.K, Mueller I.,et al. Minimal criteria for defining multipotent mesenchymal stromal cells. The International Society for Cellular Therapy position statement. Cytotherapy. 2006;8(4),315-317.

[7] Mitchell J.B., McIntosh K., Zvonic S., et al. Immunophenotype of human adipose-derived cells: temporal changes in stromal-associated and stem cell-associated markers. Stem Cells.2006; 24 (2),376-385.

[8] Lin C.S., Xin Z.C., Deng C.H., et al. Defining adipose tissue-derived stem cells in tissue and in culture. Histopathol.2010;25, 807–815.

[9] Dragoo J.L., Choi J.Y., Lieberman J.R., et al. Bone induction by BMP-2 transduced stem cells derived from human fat. J Orthop Res. 2003;21,622–629

[10] Li H, Dai K, Tang T, et al. Bone regeneration by implantation of adipose-derived stromal cells expressing BMP-2. Biochem Biophys Res Commun. 2007;356, 836 – 842

[11] Zhang X., Yang M., Lin L., et al. Runx2 overexpression enhances osteoblastic differentiation andmineralization in adipose-derived stem cells in vitro and in vivo. Calcif Tissue Int. 2006;79,169–178

[12] Wu L., Wu Y., Lin Y., et al. Osteogenic differentiation of adipose derived stem cells promoted by overexpression of osterix. Mol Cell Biochem. 2007;301,83–92

[13] Urist M. R. Bone: Formation by autoinduction. Science. 1965; 150,893.

[14] Ducy P., Zhang R., Geoffroy V., et al. Osf2/Cbfa1: a transcriptional activator of osteoblast differentiation.Cell. 1997; 89, 747–754.

[15] Shi Y.Y., Nacamuli R.P., Salim A., et al. The osteogenic potential of adipose-derived mesenchymal cells is maintained with aging. Plast. Reconstr. Surg.2005; 116, 1686–1696.

[16] Kang Q., Sun M.H., Cheng H., et al. Characterization of the distinct orthotopic bone-forming activity of 14 BMPs using recombinant adenovirus-mediated gene delivery. Gene Ther. 2004;11(17): 1312-1320.

[17] Urist M. R. .Bone morphogenetic protein: the molecularization of skeletal system development. J. Bone Miner. Res. 1997;12, 343–346

[18] Aono A., Hazama M., Notoya K., et al. Potent ectopic bone-inducing activity of bone morphogenetic protein-4/7 heterodimer. Biochem Biophys. Res. Commun. 1995; 210, 670 -677.

[19] Israel D.I., Nove J., Kerns K.M., et al. Heterodimeric bone morphogenetic proteins show enhanced activity in vitro and in vivo. Growth Factors. 1996;13, 291–300.

[20] Jadlowiec J.A., Celil A.B., Hollinger J.O.. Bone-tissuengineering: recent advances and promising therapeutic agents. Expe Opin. Biol. Ther. 2003;3, 409–423.
[21] Deregowski V., Gazzerro E., Priest L., et al. Notch 1 overexpression inhibits osteoblastogenesis by suppressing Wnt/beta-catenin but not bone morphogenetic protein signaling. J Biol Chem, 2006,281(10): 6203-6210.
[22] Nobta M., Tsukazaki T., Shibata Y., et al. Critical regulation of bone morphogenetic protein-induced osteoblastic differentiation by Delta1/Jagged1-activated Notch1 signaling. J Biol Chem, 2005;280(16), 15842 -15848.
[23] Mie M., Ohgushi H., Yanagida Y., et al. Osteogenesis coordinated in C3H10T1/2 cells by adipogenesis-dependent BMP-2 expression system. Tissue Eng . 2000;6,9–18.
[24] Saito A., Suzuki Y., Ogata S., et al. Accelerated bone repair with the use of a synthetic BMP-2-derived peptide and bone-marrow stromal cells. J Biomed Mater Res A.2005; 72,77–82.
[25] Knippenberg M., Helder M.N., Zandieh D.B., et al. Osteogenesis versus chondrogenesis by BMP-2 and BMP-7 in adipose stem cells. Biochem Biophys Res Commun. 2006; 342, 902 -908.
[26] Chiba S., Notch signaling in stem cell systems, Stem Cells. 2006;24, 2437–2447.
[27] Hilton M.J., Tu X.,Wu X., et al. Notch signaling maintains bone marrow mesenchymal progenitors by suppressing osteoblast differentiation, Nat. Med. 2008;14, 306–314.
[28] Shindo K.., Kawashima N., Sakamoto K., et al. Osteogenic differentiation of the mesenchymal progenitor cells is suppressed by Notch signaling, Exp. Cell Res. 2003;290, 370 -380.
[29] Sciaudone M., Gazzerro N., Priest L., et al, Notch 1 impairs osteoblastic cell differentiation, Endocrinology. 2003;144: 5631–5639.
[30] Nofziger D., Miyamoto A., Lyons K.M., et al, Notch signaling imposes two distinct blocks in the differentiation of C2C12 myoblasts. Development. 1999;126: 1689–1702.
[31] Shen Q., Christakos S. The vitamin D receptor, Runx2, and the Notch signaling pathway cooperate in the transcriptional regulation of osteopontin, J. Biol.Chem. 2005;280: 40589 -40598.
[32] Tezuka K, Yasuda M., Watanabe N., et al, Stimulation of osteoblastic cell differentiation by Notch, J. Bone Miner. Res. 2002;17, 231–239.
[33] Baron M. An overview of the Notch signaling. pathway. Semin. Cell Dev. Biol. 2003;14, 113–119.
[34] Miele L. Notch signaling. Clin. Cancer Res. 2006;12, 1074–1079.
[35] Miele L., Golde T., Osborne B. Notch signaling in cancer. Curr. Mol. Med. 2006;6, 905–918.
[36] Wu L., Griffin J.D.Modulation of Notch signaling by mastermind-like (MAML) transcriptional co-activators and their involvement in tumorigenesis. Semin. Cancer Biol.2004; 14, 348–356.
[37] Grottkau B.E., Chen X., Friedrich C.C., et al. DAPT Enhances the Apoptosis of Human Tongue Carcinoma Cells. Int J Oral Sci.2009; 1,81–89.
[38] Iso T., Chung G., Hamamori Y., et al. HERP1 is a cell type-specific primary target of Notch. J. Biol. Chem.2002;277, 6598–6607.

[39] Iso T., Kedes L., Hamamori Y. HES and HERP families: multiple effectors of the Notch signaling pathway. J. Cell. Physiol. 2003;194,237–255.
[40] Ohazama A., Hu Y., Schmidt.U.R, et al. A dual role for Ikk alpha in tooth development. Dev.Cell. 2004;6, 219–227.
[41] Nickoloff B.J., Qin J.Z., Chaturvedi V., et al. Jagged-1 mediated activation of notch signaling induces complete maturation of human keratinocytes through NF-kappaB and PPARgamma. Cell Death Differ.2002; 9, 842–855.
[42] Kadesch T. Notch signaling: the demise of elegant simplicity. Curr. Opin. Genet. Dev. 2004;14, 506–512.
[43] Engin. F, Yao Z., Yang T., et al, Dimorphic effects of Notch signaling in bone homeostasis, Nat. Med. 2008;14: 299–305.
[44] Canalis E., Notch signaling in osteoblasts, Sci. Signal 1 2008, pe17.
[45] Naganawa T., Xiao L., Abogunde E.et al. In vivo and in vitro comparison of the effects of FGF-2 null and haploin sufficiency on bone formation in mice. Biochem. Biophys. Res. Commun. 2006;339, 490–498.
[46] Zhao G., Monier-Faugere M. C., Langub, M. C., et al. Targeted overexpression of insulin-like growth factor I to osteoblasts of transgenic mice: increased trabecular bone volume without increased osteoblast proliferation. Endocrinology 2000;141, 2674–2682.
[47] Bikle D. D., Sakata T., Leary C., et al. Insulin-like growth factor I is required for the anabolic actions of parathyroid hormone on mouse bone. J. Bone Miner. Res. 2002;17, 1570–1578.
[48] Nevins M., Giannobile W. V., McGuire M. K., et al. Platelet-derived growth factor stimulates bone fill and rate of attachment level gain: results of a large multicenter randomized controlled trial. J. Periodontol. 2005;76, 2205–2215.
[49] Ferrari S.L., Pierroz D.D., Glatt V., et al .Bone response to intermittent parathyroid hormone is altered in mice null for {beta}-Arrestin2.Endocdnology. 2005;146(4):1854-1862.
[50] Gamradt S.C., Lieberman J.R. Genetic modification of stem cells to enhance bone repair. Ann Biomed Eng 2004;32,136-147.
[51] Virk M.S., Conduah A., Park S.H., et al. Influence of short-term adenoviral vector and prolonged lentiviral vector mediated bone morphogenetic protein-2 expression on the quality of bone repair in a rat femoral defect model. Bone 2008;42,921-931.
[52] Kumar S., Wan C., Ramaswamy G.,et al. Mesenchymal stem cells expressing osteogenic and angiogenic factors synergistically enhance bone formation in a mouse model of segmental bone defect. Mol Ther 2010;18,1026-1034.
[53] Prockop D.J. Repair of tissues by adult stem/progenitor cells (MSCs): controversies, myths, and changing paradigms. Mol Ther 2009;17,939-946.
[54] Rada T., Reis R.L., Gomes ME. Adipose tissue-derived stem cells and their application in bone and cartilage tissue engineering. Tissue Eng Part B Rev 2009;15,113-125.
[55] Levi B., James A.W., Nelson E.R., et al. Human adipose -derived stromal cells heal critical size mouse calvarial defects. PLos ONE. 2010; 5:11177.

[56] Mesimaki K., Lindroos B., Tornwall J., et al. Novel maxillary reconstruction with ectopic bone formation by GMP adipose stem cells. Int. J. Oral. Maxillofac. Surg. 2009; 38, 201–209.
[57] Follmar K.E., Decroos F.C., Prichard H.L., et al. Effects of glutamine, glucose, and oxygen concentration on the metabolism and proliferation of rabbit adipose-derived stem cells. Tissue Eng . 2006; 3525–3533.
[58] Miyazaki M., Zuk P.A., Zou J., et al. Comparison of human mesenchymal stem cells derived from adipose tissue and bone marrow for ex vivo gene therapy in rat spinal fusion model. Spine 2008;33,863–869.
[59] Hicok K.C., Du Laney T.V., Zhou Y.S., et al. Human adipose-derived adult stem cells produce osteoid in vivo. Tissue Eng. 2004;10, 371–380.
[60] Lee J.H., Rhie J.W., Oh D.Y. Osteogenic differentiation of human adipose tissue-derived stromal cells (hASCs) in a porous three-dimensional scaffold. Biochemical and Biophysical Research Communications.2008; 370: 456–460.
[61] Juthamas R. , Sorada K., Yasuhiko T. Growth and osteogenic differentiation of adipose-derived and bone marrow-derived stem cells on chitosan and chitooligosaccharide films. Carbohydrate Polymers. 2009;78: 873–878.
[62] Kang S.W., Kim J.S., Park K.S. Surface modification with fibrin/hyaluronic acid hydrogel on solid-free form-based scaffolds followed by BMP-2 loading to enhance bone regeneration. Bone 2001;48: 298–306.
[63] Lin Y.f., Wang T., Wu L. Ectopic and in situ bone formation of adipose tissue-derived stromal cells in biphasic calcium phosphate nanocomposite. Journal of Biomedical Materials Research Part A .2006;900-910.
[64] Heather L.P, Reichert W.M., Bruce K. Adult adipose-derived stem cell attachment to biomaterials. Biomaterials .2007;28 : 936–946.
[65] Yuan H., Yang Z., De Bruij J.D. Material dependent bone induction by calcium phosphate ceramics: A 2.5-year study in dog. Biomaterials 2001;22:2617–2623.
[66] Knop C., Sitte I., Canto F., et al. Successful posterior interlaminar fusion at the thoracic spine by sole use of beta-tricalcium phosphate. Arch Orthop Trauma Surg 2006: 126: 204–210.
[67] Chou Y.F., Zuk P.A., Chang T.L., et al. Adipose-derived stem cells and BMP2: part 1. BMP2-treated adipose-derived stem cells do not improve repair of segmental femoral defects. Connect Tissue Res 2011;52:109-118.
[68] Dupont K.M., Sharma K., Stevens H.Y., et al. Human stem cell delivery for treatment of large segmental bone defects. Proc Natl Acad Sci USA 2010; 107:3305-10.
[69] Lee S.J., Kang S.W., Do H.J. Enhancement of bone regeneration by gene delivery of BMP2/ Runx2 bicistronic vector into adipose-derived stromal cells. Biomaterials 2010;31 :5652-5659.
[70] Lin C.Y., Lin K.J., Kao C.Y. The role of adipose-derived stem cells engineered with the persistently expressing hybrid baculovirus in the healing of massive bone defects. Biomaterials 2011;32: 6505-6514.
[71] Lee J.S., Lee J.M., Im G. Electroporation-mediated transfer of Runx2 and Osterix genes to enhance osteogenesis of adipose stem cells. Biomaterials 2011;32: 760-768.

[72] Yoon E., Dhar S., Chun D.E., et al. In vivo osteogenic potential of human adipose-derived stem cells/ polylactide-coglycolic acid constructs for bone regeneration in a rat critical-sized calvarial defect model . Tissue Eng 2007 ;13 (3) 619-627.

[73] Di B.C, Farlie P., Penington A.J. Bone regeneration in a rabbit critical-sized skull defect using autologous adipose-derived cells. Tissue Eng Part A2008;14:483–490.

[74] Braccini A., Wendt D., Farhadi J., et al. The osteogenicity of implanted engineered bone constructs is related to the density of clonogenic bone marrow stromal cells. J Tissue Eng Regen Med 2007;1:60–65.

[75] Cui L., Liu B., Liu G., et al. Repair of cranial bone defects with adipose derived stem cells and coral scaffold in a canine model. Bio material 2007;28(36): 5477- 5486 .

[76] Cowan C.M., Shi Y.Y., Aalami O.O., et al. Adipose- derived adult stromal cells heal critical- size mouse calvarial defects . Nat Biotechno, 2004, 22 (5) : 560 - 567 .

[77] Dudas J.R., Marra K.G., Cooper G.M., et a. The osteogenic potential of adipose- derived stem cell s for the repair of rabbit calvarial defects. Ann Plast Surg, 2006 (5) : 543 - 548 .

[78] Natalina Q., Michael T.L. Differential expression of specific FGF ligands and receptor isoforms during osteogenic differentiation of mouse Adipose-derived Stem Cells (mASCs) recapitulates the in vivo osteogenic pattern. Gene 2008;424: 130–140.

[79] Gimble J.M., Katz A.J., Bunnell B.A. Adipose-Derived Stem Cells for Regenerative Medicine.Circ Res, 2007,100(9):1249-1260..

[80] Tobita M., Uysal A.C., Ogawa R., et al. Periodontal Tissue Regeneration with Adipose - Derived Stem Cells.Tissue Engineering. 2008;14: 945-953.

[81] Finka T., Jeppe G. R., Emmersen J., et al. Adipose-derived stem cells from the brown bear(Ursus arctos) spontaneously undergo chondrogenic and osteogenic differentiation in vitro. Stem Cell Research .2011; 7,89–95.

[82] Tommaso R., Gomes M.E., Reis R.L.. A novel method for the isolation of subpopulations of rat adipose stem cells with different proliferation and osteogenic differentiation potentials. Journal of tissue engineering and regenerative medicine .2011;5 (8): 655-664.

[83] Raabe O., Shell K., Würtz A., et al. Further insights into the characterization of equine adipose tissue-derived mesenchymal stem cells. Veterinary Research Communications. 2011; 35 (6): 355-365.

[84] Naghmeh A., Bahrami A.R., Ebrahimi M.,et al. Comparative Analysis of Chemokine Receptor's Expression in Mesenchymal Stem Cells Derived from Human Bone Marrow and Adipose Tissue. Journal of Molecular Neuroscience.2011;44, (3): 178-188.

[85] Esmat E., Goertzen A.L., Xiang Bo.Viability and proliferation potential of adipose-derived stem cells following labeling with a positron-emitting radiotracer. Eur Jour of Nuc Med and Mol Imag. 2011;38(7): 1323-1334.

[86] Carlori G.M., Donati D., DiBella C., et al. Bone morphogenetic proteins and tissue engineering: future directions. Injury 2009;40(Suppl. 3),67–76.

[87] Song I., Kim B.S., Kim C.S., et al. Effects of BMP-2 and vitamin D 3 on the osteogenic differentiation of adipose stem cells. Biochemical and Biophysical Research Communications. 2011;408: 126-131.

[88] Claudia K, Alexander F, Gerald Z, et al. Human adipose derived stem cells reduce callus volume upon BMP-2 administration in bone regeneration. Injury, Int. J. Care Injured.2011;42, 814–820.

[89] Friedman M.S., Long M.W., Hankenson K.D.. Osteogenic differentiation of human mesenchymal stem cells is regulated by bone morphogenetic protein-6, J. Cell. Biochem. 2006;98,538.

[90] Carly M.K, Ali V., Holly E.W, et al. Bone morphogenetic protein 6 drives both osteogenesis and chondrogenesis in murine adipose-derived mesenchymal cells depending on culture conditions. Biochemical and Biophysical Research Communications. 2010;401,20-25.

[91] Vicente Lopez Maria A; Vazquez Garcia Miriam N. Low doses of bone morphogenetic protein 4 increase the survival of human adipose-derived stem cells maintaining their stemness an multipotency. Stem cells and Dev. 2011; 20 (6): 1011 -1019.

[92] Quarto N., Longaker M.T.. Molecular mechanisms of FGF-2 inhibitory activity in the osteogenic context of mouse adipose-derived stem cells (mASCs). Bone.2008; 42: 1040–1052.

[93] Lindroos. B., Aho K. L., Kuokkanen H., et al. Differential gene expression in adipose stem cells cultured in allogeneic human serum versus fetal bovine serum. Tissue Engineering Part A, 2010;16, 2281–2294.

[94] Lindroos B., Boucher S., Chase L., et al. Serum-free, xeno-free culture media maintain the proliferation rate and multipotentiality of adipose stem cells in vitro. Cytotherapy, 2009;11, 958–972.

[95] Taskiran Dilek, Evren Vedat. Stimulatory effect of 17 beta-estradiol on osteogenic differentiation potential of rat adipose tissue-derived stem cells. General Physiology and Biophysics.2011,30 (2): 167-174.

[96] Jing W, Xiong Z.H., Cai X.X., et al. Effects of γ-secretase inhibition on the proliferation and vitamin D3 induced osteogenesis in adipose derived stem cells. Biochemical and Biophysical Research Communications.2010;392: 442–447.

[97] Aksu, A.E., Rubin, J.P., Dudas, J.R., et al. Role of gender and anatomical region on induction of osteogenic differentiation of human adipose-derived stem cells. Annals of Plastic Surgery, 2008;60: 306–322.

[98] Zhu M., Kohan E., Bradley J., et al. The effect of age on osteogenic, adipogenic and proliferative potential of female adipose-derived stem cells. Journal of Tissue Engineering and Regenerative Medicine, 2009;3, 290–301.

[99] Lendeckel S., Jodicke A., Christophis P., et al. Autologous stem cells (adipose) and fibrin glue used to treat widespread traumatic calvarial defects: case report. Journal of Cranio maxillofacial Surgery, 2004,32, 370–373.

[100] De Francesco F., Tirino V., Desiderio V., et al. Human CD34+/CD90+ ASCs are capable of growing as sphere clusters, producing high levels of VEGF and forming capillaries. PLoS ONE, 2009; 4, e6537.

[101] Kucerova L., Altanerova V., Matuskova M., et al. Adipose tissue-derived human mesenchymal stem cells mediated prodrug cancer gene therapy. Cancer Research,2007; 67: 6304–6313.

[102] Yu J. M., Jun E. S., Bae Y. C., et al. Mesenchymal stem cells derived from human adipose tissues favor tumor cell growth in vivo. Stem Cells and Development,2008; 17: 463-473.

[103] Cousin B., Ravet E., Poglio S., et al. Adult stromal cells derived from human adipose tissue provoke pancreatic cancer cell death both in vitro and in vivo. PLoS ONE, 2009;4, e6278.

7

Mechanotransduction and Osteogenesis

Carlos Vinícius Buarque de Gusmão,
José Ricardo Lenzi Mariolani and William Dias Belangero
State University of Campinas / Department of Orthopaedics and Traumatology, Brazil

1. Introduction

It is well known that mechanical stimulation induces osteogenesis. Consciously or not, everyday we use mechanical loading to incite osteogenesis: normal daily activities like walking, or physical activities like gymnastics. It is easy to comprehend how biochemical factors (for example, hormones) activate biological reactions (for example, bone formation). In opposite, it is not simple to understand how mechanical forces cause biological reactions. The aim of this chapter is to describe the current knowledge about how bone cells react to mechanical stimuli, and what bone cells have to sense mechanical forces.

According to Wolff's Law, mechanical loads determine changes in bone structure (Duncan & Turner). In 1964, Frost proposed the **mechanostat model**, which is an upgrade of Wolff's Law. Within this model, relative deformations of bone are sensed by bone cells, which, in turn, produce or resorb bone tissue. The relative deformation, or strain, represents the ratio between the lengthening or shortening of a body and its original length. Strain is dimensionless and can be expressed as decimal fraction, percentage or μstrain. For example, the strain of an 1 mm long body that - under action of an external load - lengthens or shortens 0.001 mm, is equal to 0.001 or 0.1% or 1000 μstrain. Deformations below 50-100 μstrain are in the **disuse** range, and result in bone resorption. Deformations between the ranges of 50-100 to 1000-1500 μstrain are in the **physiological** range. Physiological deformation can produce microfractures that are repaired; however, bone mass does not alter although the activation of osteogenesis. Deformations between the ranges of 1000-1500 to 3000 μstrain are in the **overuse** range, and produce microfractures, which are also repaired. Interestingly, in this case bone mass increases. There is no knowledge on how bone cells distinguish physiological and overuse deformations. Deformations above 3000 μstrain are in the **pathological overuse** range, and produce a number of microfractures that exceed bone repair capacity. As a result, microfractures accumulate, coalesce and weaken bone, ending in stress fractures (or fatigue fractures). Macroscopic fractures occur when relative deformation is over 25000 μstrain (Fig. 1) (Burr et al., 1998; Carter & Hayes, 1977; Frost, 2000, 2003; O'brien et al., 2005). In conclusion, the role of mechanostat is to avoid mechanical deformations above 3000 μstrain, which may cause bone fracture.

Further, in addition to Frost's mechanostat model, it was realized that mechanostat can sense other physical parameters not only relative deformation: frequency, number of cycles resting periods, relative deformation distribution and local gradients of relative deformation (Torcasio et al., 2008). Relative deformation, frequency, number of cycles and resting periods are the unique variables that can be controlled in mechanical assays. Moreover, there is no unit that encloses all these controllable variables. All of this impairs the analysis of bone cells response to mechanical stimulation, and may explain the difference in some values presented in this chapter.

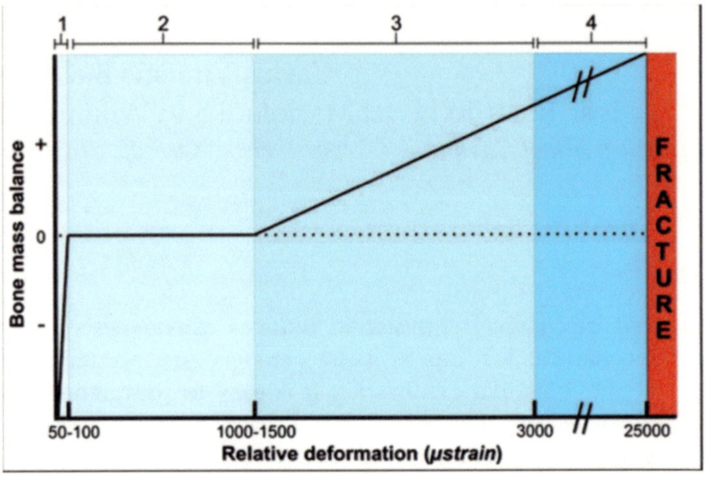

Fig. 1. *Bone mass balance as a function of relative deformation.* Within area 1, bone resorption rate is greater than bone formation rate, resulting in a negative balance (disuse range). Within area 2, bone resorption rate is equal bone formation rate, resulting in a neutral balance (physiological rate). Within area 3, bone resorption rate is lower than bone formation rate, resulting in a positive balance (overuse range). Within area 4, microfractures accumulate, resulting in decrease of bone resistance (pathological overuse range) that can lead to macroscopic bone fracture (area in red).

1.1 Frequency

The same strain applied on bone at 1-30 Hz frequencies increases osteogenesis. The opposite is not always true: different strains applied on bone at a fixed frequency may increase osteogenesis or not. Whether the strain will increase bone formation or not depends on the frequency of the stimulation. When the frequency is within the range of 5-10 Hz, bone exhibits the greatest osteogenesis rate. Above the range of 5-10 Hz, the osteogenesis rate decreases; probably, because mechanical loads at frequencies above 5-10 Hz exceed the capacity of bone cells to return to their previous shape like if bone tissue had become more rigid. If bone cells do not return to their not deformed shape, they will not undergo deformation; thus, they will not respond to mechanical deformation.

Curiously, vibratory mechanical loads induce bone formation at higher frequencies (17-90 Hz) and lower strain (5 *μstrain*). We hypothesize vibratory mechanical loads may stimulate a wider bone area, creating more local gradients of deformation; and hence, increasing mechanical stimulation on bone. Since various local gradients of deformation are created, more bone cells are incited to produce bone. In other words, there are more sites of osteogenesis; therefore, mechanical loads with lower strain at higher frequencies applied to bone will incite significant bone formation (Castillo et al., 2006; Fritton et al., 2000; Hsieh & Turner, 2001; Jacobs et al., 1998; Rubin et al., 2001; Torcasio et al., 2008; Warden & Turner, 2004; You et al., 2001).

1.2 Number of cycles

The product of the frequency and the duration of the stimulus is the number of cycles. As the number of cycles increases so does osteogenesis until a certain plateu (Burr et al., 2002; Umemura et al., 1997) (Fig. 2).

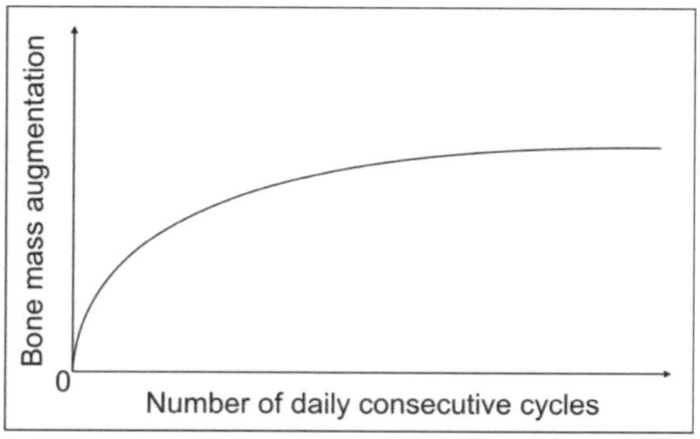

Fig. 2. *Bone mass augmentation as a function of the number of consecutive cycles per day.* After a certain number of consecutive cycles, which depends on the study design, bone mass augmentation ceases.

1.3 Resting periods

Continuous mechanical stimulation does not increase bone formation. Mechanical stimulation must have a pause otherwise bone cells osteogenic response will cease, because bone cells need a resting period to reorganize their cytoskeleton, recover ion concentration balance and dephosphorylate proteins to recover their mechanosensitivity. The resting period varies between studies from 8 to 48 hours. Since bone cells need a resting period to respond to mechanical deformation "at full strength", the first stimulus may be the most important to determine how much bone formation a certain treatment can induce. One study supports this idea: the authors compared bone formation rate in the ulnae of rats subjected to 3 different protocols of mechanical stimulation. The first group was stimulated with progressively decreasing strains; the second group was stimulated with progressively increasing strains; and the third group was stimulated with constant strains. Bone formation rate was greater in the first group, followed by the third group (Burr et al., 2002; Pavalko et al., 1998; Robling et al., 2001, 2006; Schriefer et al., 2005; Tang et al., 2006).

2. Amplification of mechanical stimulation

Our bones in the skeleton can be subjected to 400 to 3000 *μstrain* during usual locomotion; however, it rarely exceeds 1000 *μstrain*. Nevertheless, *in vitro* bone cells response to mechanical stimulation is observed only with ~10000-100000 *μstrain* range, which is 10 to 100 fold greater than the usual strain bone is subjected. Interestingly, if bone was subjected to the same strain range bone cells need to be activated (~10000-100000 *μstrain*), bone would undergo fracture. You et al (2001) proposed a mathematical model to explain the different intensities needed to induce osteogenesis in the skeleton and in bone cells, pointing the actin cytoskeleton and the bone canalicular system as strain amplifiers at the cellular level (Duncan & Turner, 1995; Fritton et al., 2000; Robling et al., 2006; Rubin & Lanyon, 1984; You et al., 2001).

2.1 Histological anatomy of bone

Schematically, long bones can be compared to a cylinder that contains several smaller cylinders (the Haversian canals), which intercommunicate via Volkmann's canals. Lamellae are the Haversian canals walls; disposed radially from each Haversian canal; composed of bone ECM (Table 1), which is basically hydroxyapatite (main inorganic component) and type I collagen (main organic component). Osteocytes are located within the lacunae, where they become imprisoned by the ECM synthesized during osteoblasts cellular differentiation. Osteocytes possess cytoplasmic processes (or dendrites) which are a prolongation of the cytoplasm. The cytoplasmic processes lacunae are called canaliculi (Fig 3).

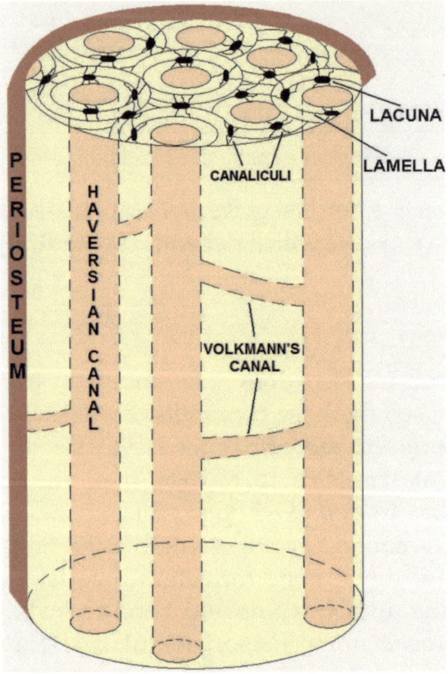

Fig. 3. Scheme of the histological anatomy of bone.

Between the canalicular wall and the cytoplasmic process is the pericellular space, whose diameter varies from 14 to 100 nm depending on the person age, osteocyte age, histological type of bone, and other features. Pericellular space diameter variation from 20 to 100 nm alters less than 40% the amplification of the mechanical stimulus within the cytoplasmic process. Within the pericellular space, there is a fluid with albumin and a PEM composed of proteoglycans and transverse fibrils. The osteocyte cytoplasmic process is anchored and centered in its canaliculus by these transverse fibrils. Within this system, You L et al., calculated that strains in the physiological range produce shear stresses from 0.5 to 3.0 Pa on cytoplasmic processes, but relative deformation from 8300 to 19700 *μstrain* at 1-20 Hz frequencies, which induce a cellular response. The larger the diameter of the space between glycosaminoglycans side chains, the lower is strain amplification. The calculation was based on the relationship between the albumin diameter (~7nm) and the space between the glycosaminoglycans side chains along a proteoglycan monomer. Within osteocytic cytoplasmic processes there are actin filaments arranged on the same axis of the process

Abbreviation	Meaning	Abbreviation	Meaning	Abbreviation	Meaning
AC	Adenylate Cyclase	GLAST	Glutamate/ Aspartate Transporter	NOS	Nitric Oxide Synthase
cAMP	Cyclic Adenosine Monophos-phate	cGMP	Cyclic Guanosine Monophosphate	OPG	Osteoprotegerin
AP	Activator Protein	GSK3b	Glycogen Synthase Kinase-3b	PDGF	Platelet-Derived Growth Factor
ATP	Adenosine Triphosphate	IGF	Insulin Growth-Like Factor	PEM	Pericellular Matrix
C/EBPβ	CCAAT-enhancer-binding protein	IGF-1R	IGF-1 Receptor	PI3K	Phosphatidylinos itol 3-Kinase
cox	Cyclooxy-genase	IP_3	Inositol Triphosphate	PIP2	Phosphatidyl-inositol 4,5-Bisphosphate
CREB	cAMP Response Element Binding	IRS	Insulin Receptor Substrate	PKA and C	Protein Kinase A and C
Cx	Connexin	LIPUS	Low-Intensity Pulsed Ultrasound	PLA and PLC	Phospholipase A and C
DAG	Diacylglycerol	Lrp	Low-Density Lipoprotein Receptor-Related Protein	PTH	Parathyroid Hormone
EAAT	Excitatory Amino-acid Transporter	MAPK	Mitogen-Activated Protein Kinase	PYK2	Proline-Rich Tyrosine Kinase-2
ECM	Extracellular Matrix	mGluR	Metabotropic Glutamate Receptor	RANK(L)	Receptor Activator of NF-κB (Ligand)
ERα	Estrogen Receptor α	NF-κB	Nuclear Factor-κB	SH2	Src-homology-2
ERK	Extracellular Signal-Regulated Kinase	NMDA	N-Methyl-D-Aspartate	VEGF	Vascular Endothelial Growth Factor
FAK	Focal Adhesion Kinase	NO	Nitric Oxide		

Table 1. Abbreviations

membrane. Fimbrin is a rigid cross-linking protein that keeps actin filaments separated from each other ~25 nm of distance. The larger that distance, the higher the strain amplification at cytoplasmic processes level (Buckwalter et al., 1996a, 1996b; Owan & Triffitt, 1976; Sauren et al., 1992; Tanaka-Kamioka et al., 1998; You et al., 2001) (Fig 4).

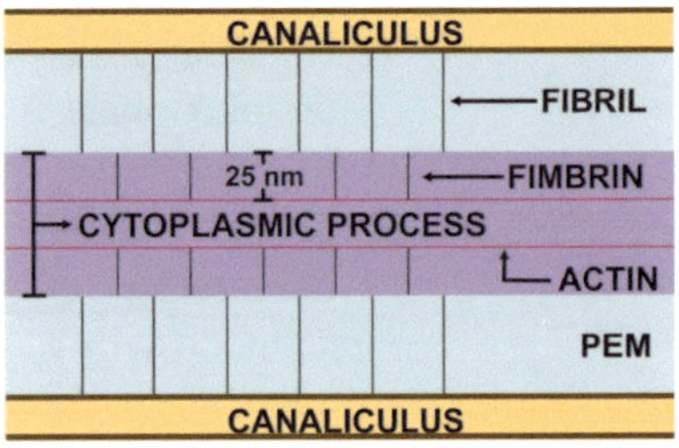

Fig. 4. *Actin cytoskeleton and fimbrins interaction.* Fimbrins keep actin filaments separated from each other ~25 nm of distance, which is optimum for mechanical stimulation amplification at the cytoplasmic process.

2.2 Drag force and shear stress

Bone deformation produces areas subjected to compression and tension stresses, creating pressure gradients within Haversian canals; and hence, forcing the fluid in canaliculi to flow from sites of compression stress (higher pressure) to sites of tension stress (lower pressure). This produces a fluid flow within the cytoplasmic processes pericellular space. The fluid flow imposes a drag force onto the PEM. Drag force is the resultant of the forces that oppose the relative motion of an object through a fluid. Considering 7 nm of diameter between the glycosaminoglycans side chains, You L et al (2001) calculated that,

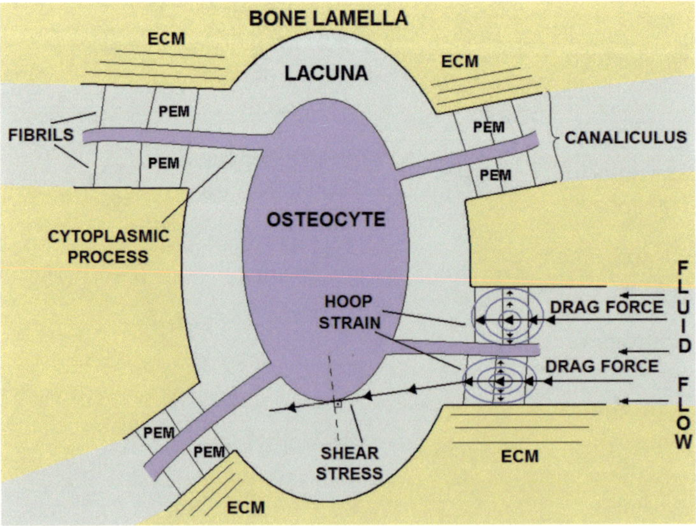

Fig. 5. *Mechanical stimulation amplification.* Mechanical deformation of bone tissue produces fluid flow, which, in turn, produces drag force on the cytoplasmic processes and the canaliculi walls. Besides, fluid flow produces a tangential force on the osteocyte cytoplasmic membrane, resulting in shear stress.

independently of the magnitude and frequency of the mechanical load, the drag force is 19.6 times larger than the shear force per unit length of cell process. Because of the histological anatomy of bone, mechanical deformations within the physiological range produce drag force that produces hoop strains on the membrane-cytoskeleton system of cytoplasmic processes, which are 20 to 100 times higher (or more) than the deformation experienced on the whole bone producing strains from 3000 to 50000 μstrain on the cytoplasmic process membrane. The larger the magnitude, or the frequency, of a mechanical loading, the higher is the strain amplification. Hoop strains are the normal tension forces on a body with circular symmetry. They produce compression and tension forces at the microscopic level (Fig. 5). According to the model proposed by You L et al, shear stress is not important for strain amplification *in* vivo. However, it does not mean that shear stress is disposable for the cellular response to mechanical load (Boutahar et al., 2004; Duncan & Turner, 1995; Hughes-Fulford, 2004; Kapur et al., 2003; Liedbert et al., 2006; Norvell et al., 2004; Scott et al., 2008; You et al., 2001).

3. The main mechanosensor cell

Osteoblasts, osteocytes and osteoclasts are the main bone cells. For decades, osteoblasts and osteoclasts were considered the protagonists of bone remodeling. For this reason, there are more reports with osteoclasts and osteoblasts than osteocytes, which comprise 90-95% of all bone cells. After realizing that osteocytes also respond to mechanical stimulation, authors inquire which is the main mechanosensor bone cell: osteoblasts or osteocytes (Bonewald, 2006; Buckwalter et al., 1996a).

Although there is no definitive proof, osteocytes are considered the cells that orchestrate bone remodeling through biochemical mediators that regulate the activity of osteoblasts and osteoclasts. Supporting this idea, it was demonstrated that osteocytes subjected to fluid flow stimulate osteoblasts to produce bone tissue; and that osteocytes produce prostaglandins faster than osteoblasts after mechanical stimulation. Prostaglandins mediate osteoclasts and osteoblasts activity. Moreover, it is more reasonable that osteocytes are the main mechanosensor bone cells since they comprise 90-95% of all bone cells and participate in the canalicular system for strain amplification proposed by You L et al whereas osteoblasts are located at the periosteum, where strain does not undergo amplification (Bonewald, 2006; Chen et al., 1999; Cherian et al., 2005; Duncan & Turner, 1995; Goldspink, 1999; Gupta & Grande-Allen, 2006; Hsu et al., 2007; Klein-Nulend et al., 1995; Li et al., 2004; Plotkin et al., 2005; Taylor et al., 2007).

4. Piezoelectricity or streaming potential?

Fukada E and Yasuda I (1957) observed that bone is a viscoelastic material which possesses piezoelectric activity, producing negative electric charge in compression sites, and positive electric charge in tension sites. Furthermore, bone undergoes deformation when subjected to electric potentials. Interested in the study of piezoelectricity, Anderson JC and Eriksson C (1970, 1986) investigated the cause of those authors' observation.

They knew piezoelectricity does not occur in symmetric crystalline materials, and is as greater as asymmetric is its crystalline structure. Since hydroxyapatite is a symmetric crystalline material, bone piezoelectric property cannot be attributed to hydroxyapatite. Unlike the dried collagen, wet collagen, which is the *in vivo* collagen form, is not piezoelectric because water molecules interact with the collagen structure which becomes symmetric. On the other hand, one third of the ECM collagen length interacts with hydroxyapatite, which blocks collagen interaction with some water molecules and impairs wet collagen structural changes, keeping the wet collagen asymmetric. With these data, one could hypothesize collagen is responsible for the electric potential detected after mechanical stimulation. Nevertheless, *in vivo* bone ECM collagen is embedded with a fluid containing high conductivity ions. As a result, the mechanically-induced fluid flow produces an electric potential, named streaming potential. Therefore, the electric potential observed after mechanical loading is the sum of the piezoelectric and the streaming potentials. Streaming potential depends on the type of the ion absorbed on a molecule surface (for example, collagen), inducing the formation of a diffuse layer composed of ions of the opposite charge. The fluid flow gives rise to a transport network of an ion type, determining a potential gradient (streaming potential), whose magnitude depends on the type of the molecule and the solution pH. Piezoelectric potential, in turn, depends only on the cellular mechanical deformation.

Anderson JC and Eriksson C observed that the molecule of collagen embedded within a fluid with pH 4.7 induces absorption of the same quantity of negative and positive charged ions, resulting in an isoelectric streaming potential; therefore, an electrode will detect only the piezoelectric potential of the molecule of collagen. In that experiment, the authors could not separate the bone ECM collagen from the hydroxyapatite; hence, they could not determine the streaming potential with pH 4.7 to 5.0. However, it was observed the lowest streaming potential within that pH range, suggesting the mechanically-induced electric potential in bone depends mainly on the streaming potential (Butcher et al., 2008; Qin et al., 2002) (Fig. 6).

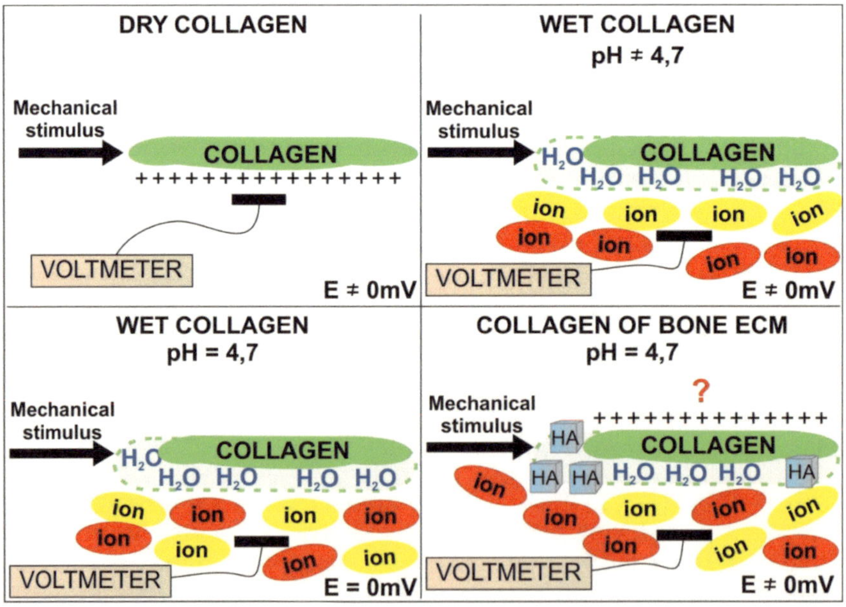

Fig. 6. *Piezoelectricity x Streaming potential.* Dried collagen is assymmetric and has piezoelectric activity. Hydrated collagen is symmetric and does not have piezoelectric activity. Streaming potential occurs when the fluid pH is different of 4.7; and does not occur when the fluid pH is 4.7. Bone ECM collagen is asymmetric although hydrated because it interacts with hydroxyapatite (HA). Therefore, collagen may exhibit piezoelectric activity and, principally, streaming potential.

Protein	Start of the event	Peak of event	Event duration
Akt	Increased activation: 5 minutes	15 minutes	At least 2 hours
ATP	Increased efflux: 1 minute	No data	No data
β-catenin	Increased activation: 1 hour	No data	3 hours
Actin cytoskeleton	Reorganization: 1 hour	No data	No data
Collagen I	Increased synthesis: 3 days	3 days	No data
cox-2	Increased synthesis: 30-60 minutes	3-6 hours	At least 9 hours
Cx43	Increased synthesis: 2 hours	2 hours	24 hours
ERK	Increased activation: 0-15 minutes	15-240 minutes	2-4 hours
Sclerostin	Decreased synthesis: 24 hours	No data	No data
FAK	Increased activation: 0-5 minutes	0-30 minutes	1-4 hours
Alkaline phosphatase	Increased synthesis: 24-48 hours	No data	No data
GLAST (mRNA)	Decreased transcription: 6 hours	No data	No data
Cx43 hemichannels	Increased activation: immediately	Immediately	8-24 hours
α2, α5, β1 and β3 integrins subunits	Increased synthesis: 20 minutes	3-6 hours	No data
NF-κB	Increased activation: 30 minutes	30-60 minutes	No data
NO	Increased synthesis: 5-15 minutes (2 works); 12 hours (1 work)	5-15 minutes	24 hours
Osteopontin	Increased transcription: 1-3 days	No data	No data
Osteocalcin	Increased synthesis: 3 days	3 days	No data
p38	Increased activation: 15 minutes	30 minutes	90 minutes
PGE_2	Increased synthesis: 1-6 hours (4 works); or 0-10 minutes (2 works)	18-24 hours	At least 24 hours
$PGF_{2\alpha}$	Increased synthesis: 5 minutes	5 minutes	10 minutes
PGI_2	Increased synthesis: 30 minutes	No data	At least 1 hour
PI3K	Increased activation: 5 minutes	15 minutes	1 hour
PYK2	Increased activation: 30 minutes	4 hours	No data
PYK2-FAK	Coupling: 30 minutes	30 minutes	No data
Src	Increased activation: immediately	Immediately	4 hours
Src-FAK	Coupling: immediately	Immediately	4 hours
VEGF	Increased synthesis: 6 hours	12 hours	No data

Table 2. Chronology of the mechanotransduction events

PROTEIN	EFFECTS RELATED TO MECHANOTRANSDUCTION
AP-1	Activates CREB; increases type I collagen, alkaline phosphatase, iNOS, ostepontin and osteocalcin synthesis; and determines 48% of cox-2 transcription.
ATP	Activates $P2Y_2$ and $P2X_7$; increases $P2Y_2$ synthesis; and determines 80% of PGE_2 synthesis.
C/EBP	Determines 59% of cox-2 transcription.
Calcium	Increases PYK2, ERK and p38 activation; determines 83% of PGE_2 synthesis via G protein/AC pathway; determines 50% of ATP synthesis; *activates PLA_2; *increases IGF-I and TGF-β synthesis; *complexes with calmodulin; and *releases ATP from vesicles.
calcium-calmodulin	Activates CREB, C/EBPβ, AC* and iNOS*.
β-catenin	Activates Lef/TCF; and increases cox-2, Cx43 and c-jun synthesis.
cox-2	Increases Runx-2 synthesis; determines 100% of alkaline phosphatase synthesis, cellular proliferation and bone formation; and synthesizes PGE_2 and PGI_2.
CREB	Determines 66% of cox-2 synthesis; and *increases c-fos synthesis.
Cx43	Determines 60% of PGE_2 efflux.
EP2/4	Activates AC.
ERK	Activates Lef/TCF, NF-kB and AP-1; Increases c-fos, c-jun and NO synthesis; determines 80% of osteocalcin synthesis, 80-100% of osteopontin synthesis, 100% of alkaline phosphatase and cox-2 synthesis, and 100% of cellular proliferation; and inhibits apoptosis.
Sclerostin	*Inhibits Wnt/β-catenin pathway.
FAK	Activates FAK-Src/Grb2/Sos/Ras/Raf/MEK/ERK-1/2 and FAK/PI3Kp85/Akt/NF-κB pathways; increases cox-2 synthesis; and *induces cellular migration.
c-fos	Complexes with c-jun, forming AP-1 heterodimer.
Alkaline phosphatase	Induces hydroxyapatite synthesis and ECM mineralization; and inhibits nucleation removers.
Frizzled proteins	*Activate G protein/PLC pathway; and compete with RANK*.
cGMP	*Closes sodium channels; and *induces vasodilatation.
GSK3b	*Degrades β-catenin.
IGF-1	*Activates Ras/MEK/ERK/Tcf-Lef and PI3K/Akt pathways; *activates IRS-1/2; *induces ECM synthesis, osteoblasts and osteoblasts precursors differentiation, and chondrocytes proliferation; and, in adipocytes, increases FAK autophosphorylation by 30%* and *PYK2 phosphorylation.
IRS-1/2	*Activates the pathways of Grb2 and PI3K.
Lrp5	Increases the cellular response to mechanical stimulation, and *frizzled proteins synthesis.
mGluR	*Activates G protein/PLC pathway.
NF-kB	Increases cox-2, *iNOS and *RANKL synthesis.

PROTEIN	EFFECTS RELATED TO MECHANOTRANSDUCTION
NO	Determines 100% of: cellular proliferation, alkaline phosphatase synthesis, and β1 integrin subunit and ERK activation; *decreases bone resorption induced by PTH and vitamin D3; *induces: osteoblast precursors differentiation, 94% of OPG synthesis, osteocalcin synthesis, and NF-κB activation; *inhibits: osteoclastic activity, NF-κB activation, and 70-82% of RANKL synthesis; and *synthesizes cGMP.
iNOS	Increases PGE_2 synthesis; determines 90% of VEGF synthesis; and *synthesizes NO.
OPG	*Decreases osteoclasts recruitment; competes with RANK.
Osteopontin	*Constitutes bone ECM; *sets osteoclasts at resorption sites through αvβ3 integrin binding; and *inhibits hydroxyapatite formation.
Osteocalcin	Captures calcium from the ECM; *inhibits ECM mineralization and hydroxyapatite formation.
$P2X_7$	Increases: osteoblasts activity, 31% of the sensitivity to mechanical stimulation, and 50% of ERK activation; determines 61-73% of the osteogenesis rate; inhibits osteoclast activity; allows PGE_2 efflux and calcium influx.
$P2Y_2$	Increases intracellular calcium concentration via G protein/PLC pathway; and allows calcium efflux.
p38	Determines 80% of osteopontin synthesis; and *phosphorylates C/EBP and CREB.
PDGF-β	*Induces: chondrocytes proliferation, osteoblast precursors differentiation and bone resorption.
PGE_2	*Activates EP2/4 and protein G/AC pathway; induces osteogenesis; induces osteoclast precursors and osteoblast precursors proliferation and differentiation; induces calcium influx; inhibits collagen and RANKL synthesis*, GSK3b activity*, osteoclast activity and osteoblast proliferation; recruits osteoblasts to bone surface; and enhances gap junctions intercellular communication.
PGI_2	*Activates protein G/AC pathway.
PI3K/Akt	Determines 100% of cox-2 synthesis; inhibits apoptosis; *activates β-catenin; and *inactivates GSK3b.
PKA	*Activates CREB and C/EBPβ; *induces osteoblast differentiation and IGF-1 synthesis; and *phosphorylates calcium and potassium channels, prolonging their action.
PKC	*Activates MEK/ERK pathway; and *activates CREB and C/EBPβ.
PLA_2	*Activates cox-1/2.
G protein	*Activates PLC/DAG and IP3/PKC pathway and AC/AMPc/PKA pathway; *activates voltage-dependent L-type calcium channels, Ras and PI3K; and *determines 83% of PGE_2 synthesis.
PTH	*Activates PI3K/Akt/Bad, G protein/AC and PKC/ERK pathways; *increases c-fos synthesis 2.5 fold, and IL-6 synthesis 11 fold; *decreases 90% of osteocalcin synthesis; and *induces RANK, RANKL, Runx2 and PGE_2 synthesis; and *induces bone resorption.

PROTEIN	EFFECTS RELATED TO MECHANOTRANSDUCTION
PYK2	Increases ERK-1/2 activation; and transphosphorylates FAK at Tyr-397, 576 and 925.
RANK	*Induces osteoclastogenesis and *inhibits osteoclast apoptosis; *RANKL activates RANK.
Runx2	*Decreases RANKL synthesis; and *induces alkaline phosphatase, ECM and OPG synthesis; *induces bone mineralization, and osteoblast precursors and osteoblasts differentiation.
Tcf/Lef	*Activates Runx2.
Vitamin D3	*Decreases OPG synthesis and bone resorption; and *induces RANK and RANKL synthesis.
VEGF	Increases alkaline phosphatase synthesis; and induces cellular and vascular proliferation*.
Wnt	*Activates β-catenin, nuclear ERK and nuclear Akt; *increases osteopontin synthesis; and *inhibits glutamine synthetase (enzyme that degrades glutamate) and GSK3b.
*Data obtained from study not related to mechanotransduction.	

Table 3. Role of proteins

PROTEIN	PROPAGATION SPEED	EFFICIENCY
Cx43 gap junctions	0,5 μm/s	5-15 cells/field in 15-20 seconds (maintained for 3 hours, when the analysis ended)
$P2Y_2$	10 μm/s	30-50 cells/field in 15-20 seconds

Table 4. Intercellular calcium transportation efficiency

1. Existence of NMDA channels in osteoblasts and osteoclasts.
2. Existence of mGluR4/8 in osteoblasts.
3. Mechanical stimulation decreases GLAST-1 expression.
4. NMDA channels absence decreases osteogenesis (without affecting osteoblasts life expectancy).
5. Calcium influx, which is critical to glutamate release from vesicles, increases markedly in response to mechanical loads.

Table 5. Features that support the memory system of bone existence

5. Mechanotransduction

In theory, mechanical deformation that reaches bone cells cytoplasmic membrane is transmitted to the nucleus through a complex network connecting the cytoplasmic membrane to the nucleus: the ECM/PEM-integrin-cytoskeleton-nucleus system. This system is supposed to activate various biochemical reactions that result in apoptosis inhibition, cellular proliferation, cell differentiation etc. This cascade of events, starting with mechanical deformation of bone cells, and ending with a cellular response (osteogenesis or bone resorption) is named mechanotransduction, which, we believe, is the upgrade of the mechanostat model (Tables 2 and 3).

5.1 The ECM/PEM-integrins-cytoskeleton-nucleus system

This system is thought to function as a lever system with various pivot points. The interactions between the molecules that participate in the ECM/PEM-integrins-cytoskeleton-nucleus system work as a pivot point of the lever system. The physicochemical characteristics of each pivot point can be altered accordingly to the molecules interacting within the system; therefore, leading to different responses to mechanical loads (Fig. 7) (Buckwalter et al., 1996a, 1996b; Duncan & Turner, 1995).

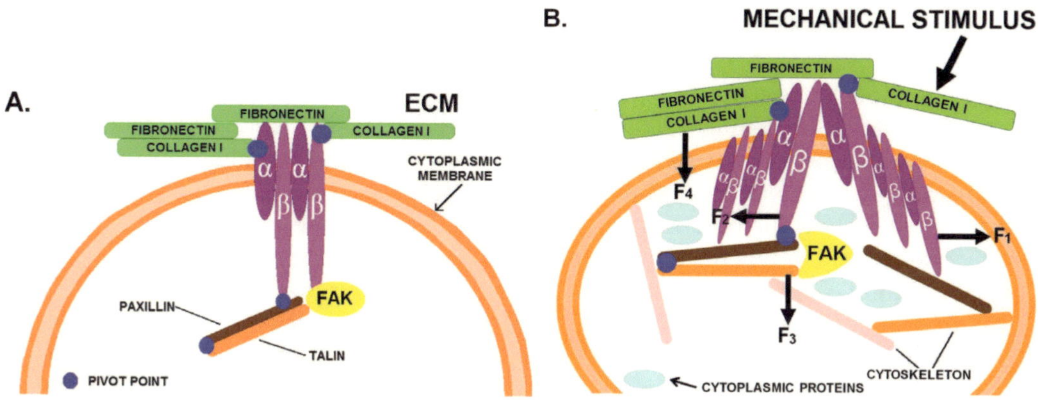

Fig. 7. *Model for the lever system of bone cells.* (A) Not stimulated bone cell. (B) The load is spread within the lever system via pivot points formed by interactions of the ECM/PEM-integrins-citoskeleton-nucleus system, resulting in forces (schematically, F1, F2, F3 and F4) that modify integrins and FAK conformational structure. At the same time, integrins cluster, the cytoskeleton reorganizes, and cytoplasmic proteins are attracted to the focal adhesions, where the first mechanically-induced biochemical reactions occur.

5.1.1 Integrins

Proteins interact with each component of the ECM/PEM-integrins-cytoskeleton-nucleus system. Within the constituents of the system, knowledge about integrins is greater. Integrins are considered the most important system component for mechanotransduction. Integrin refers to its role in integrating the intracellular environment (via cytoskeletal interactions) to the extracellular environment (ECM and PEM). Integrins are heterodimeric transmembrane glycoproteins of cellular adhesion. In humans, there are 24 types of integrins that result of the combination of the 18 types of α subunits and 8 types of β subunits. Different combinations of α and β subunits determine different interactions with ECM, cytoskeleton and cytoplasm components, as well as the affinity to a ligand. *In vitro*, osteoblasts express α2, α3, α4, α5, α6, β1, β3 and β5 subunits; *in vivo*, they express α3, α5, αv, β1 and β3 subunits. Of these subunits, α2, α5, β1 and β3 are responsive to mechanical load. Moreover, α5β1 and αvβ3 integrins are also responsive to mechanical loads (Bennett et al., 2001; Gronthos et al., 1997; Sinha & Tuan, 1996).

5.1.2 Focal adhesions

It is accepted that mechanical loading mobilizes the ECM/PEM-integrins-cytoskeleton-nucleus system, resulting in integrins structural changes that create high affinity sites for protein binding (for example, other integrins and cytoskeleton components). Mechanical deformation induces integrin clustering, which enhances integrin affinity to other molecules, and increases integrins expression. Integrins clusters anchor the components of the cytoskeleton; induce cytoskeleton reorganization; and give rise to the focal adhesion (or focal contact), which is a dynamic and specialized structure originated from the response to mechanical stimulation, and vanishes in the absence of mechanical stimulation. Focal adhesion is located near the cytoplasmic membrane and the ECM, and recruits various molecules involved in the mechanotransduction: tyrosine kinases, ion channels, PLC, MAPK etc (Fig. 7) (Boutahar et al., 2004; van der Flier & Sonnenberg, 2001; Lee et al., 2000; Pommerenke et al., 2002; Scott et al., 2008; Tang et al., 2006; Yang et al., 2005).

5.2 Ion channels

Mechanosensitive ion channels activation by fluid flow alters membrane potential, which can be positive or negative. Positive membrane potential results from membrane depolarization - usually when sodium channels activation predominates -, leading to bone resorption. Negative membrane potential results from membrane hyperpolarization - usually when calcium-dependent potassium channels activation predominates -, leading to osteogenesis. Fluid flow speed, streaming potentials, and the magnitude and frequency of mechanical stimulation are variables that regulate ion channels activity. This feature allows distinct responses to mechanical loads because (1) multiple channels can be activated in different combinations, (2) ion channels can be activated for different intervals, (3) and ion channels can be fully or partially activated. At the moment, however, there is no tool to help predicting ion channels activity based on that variables (Butcher et al., 2008; Genetos et al., 2005; Qin et al., 2002; Riddle & Donahue, 2009; Salter et al, 1997, 2000; Scott et al., 2008; Yokota & Tanaka, 2005). Besides, there is limited information about ion channels on the subject due to lack of studies.

5.2.1 Mechanism of activation

Reports indicate that ion channels are not activated directly by strain. Instead, it seems they are activated through the ECM/PEM-integrins-cytoskeleton-nucleus system. As examples, it was found that β1 and αv subunits of integrins, αvβ5 integrin and lack of the actin cytoskeleton impairs calcium-dependent potassium channels activation; and lack of β1 subunits of integrins and lack of the actin cytoskeleton impairs sodium channels activation (Desbois-Mouthon et al., 2001; Salter et al., 1997).

5.2.2 Calcium channels

Increased intracellular calcium concentration due to strain is crucial to enhance osteogenesis rate. Calcium intake depends on the activation of stretch-activated calcium channels, voltage-sensitive L-type calcium channels and endoplasmic reticulum IP_3 receptors. Endoplasmic reticulum IP_3 receptors are discussed to be the major responsible in determining intracellular calcium concentration. Therefore, it is speculated that an activator for the G protein/PLC/PIP2/DAG and IP_3 pathway (for example, mGLUR, Wnt5, frizzled proteins), integrins, or G protein is activated by strain, resulting in IP_3 synthesis, what leads to calcium release from endoplasmic reticulum and increases intracellular calcium concentration. Calcium forms complexes that activate AC, which, in turn, can phosphorylate voltage-sensitive L-type calcium channels and potassium channels through the G protein/AC/cAMP/PKA pathway. This event keeps these channels active for a longer time and perpetuates bone cells response to mechanical loading through a positive feedback mechanism (Champe & Harvey, 2000; Chen et al., 2004; Duncan & Turner, 1995; Genetos et al., 2005; Godin et al., 2007; Lent, 2001; Li et al., 2003; Liedbert et al., 2006; Ma et al., 1999; Reich et al., 1997; Yamamoto et al., 2007) (Fig. 8).

5.2.3 Potassium channels

As seen in endothelial cells, in bone cells potassium channels can be activated directly by mechanical stimulation; or may also be activated by calcium influx through calcium-dependent potassium channels. Potassium channels activation leads to potassium efflux, resulting in membrane hyperpolarization (Duncan & Turner, 1995; Liedbert et al., 2006) (Fig. 8).

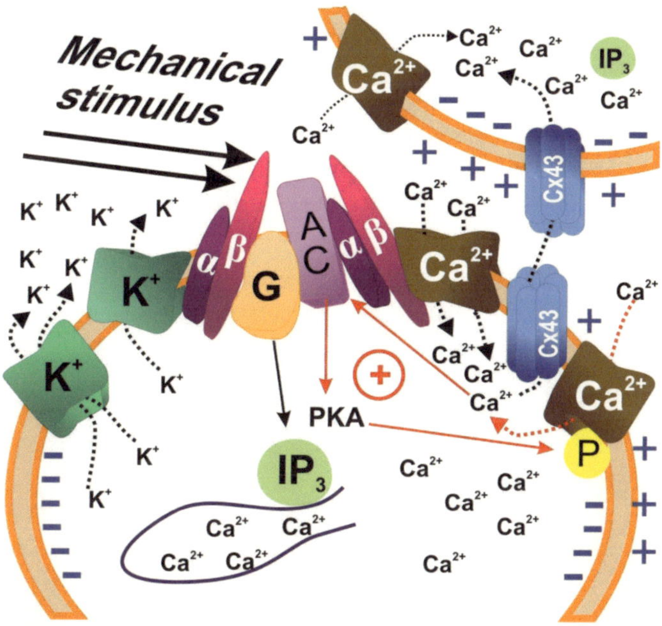

Fig. 8. *Ion channels activation*. Strain deforms the integrins, which may transmit the deformation to calcium (Ca^{2+}) and potassium (K^{+}) channels, producing calcium influx and potassium efflux, resulting in a negative action potential. At the same time, G protein (G) is activated by strain, and induces IP_3 synthesis. IP_3 is the main responsible for calcium influx. Calcium signaling pathways activate AC, resulting in PKA synthesis. PKA phosphorylates calcium and potassium channels (not showed) so that they remain active for longer, resulting in a positive feedback (arrows in red, and plus sign) that prolongs the cellular response to mechanical stimulation. Mechanical stimulation also activates Cx43 gap junctions, through which calcium, IP_3 and other molecules transit and transmit mechanical stimulation to neighboring cells, which can also deflagrate a negative action potential.

5.2.4 Sodium channels

We believe sodium channels are inhibited by strain at the beginning of the mechanical stimulation, probably by cGMP or another inhibitor; and activated posteriorly so that the intracellular homeostasis is restored (Duncan & Turner, 1995; Liedbert et al., 2006).

5.3 FAK pathways

Within all molecules that interact with integrins in focal adhesions, FAK is considered to be critical to mechanotransduction. FAK is an adaptor protein capable of interacting with various proteins to form different protein complexes. This feature may enable FAK to enhance the cellular response to mechanical loading, and may result in different responses to strain. It is not known whether this tyrosine kinase is always bound to integrins, or is recruited to the integrins clusters during focal adhesions formation, or both situations.

Following integrins deformation, FAK may be deformed and its molecular structure mechanically-modified, resulting in autophosphorylation of FAK's tyrosine-397 (Tyr-397) residue. This event activates FAK by creating high affinity binding sites for SH2-domain-containing proteins like Src and p85 subunit of PI3K. In sequence, FAK conjugates with Src or PI3K, activating their pathways. ERK-1/2 and Akt are effector proteins of these pathways. FAK, ERK-1/2 and Akt promote cellular migration, proliferation and differentiation, and apoptosis inhibition. It is speculated that these actions are enhanced when FAK, ERK-1/2 or Akt migrates to the nucleus. Investigations suggest that FAK, ERK-1/2 and Akt migration to the nucleus is regulated by the cytoplasmic concentration of these proteins and the concentration of their phosphorylated forms (Chen et al., 1999; Cornillon et al., 2003; Desbois-Mouthon et al., 2001; Duncan & Turner, 1995; Giancotti & Rouslahti, 1999;

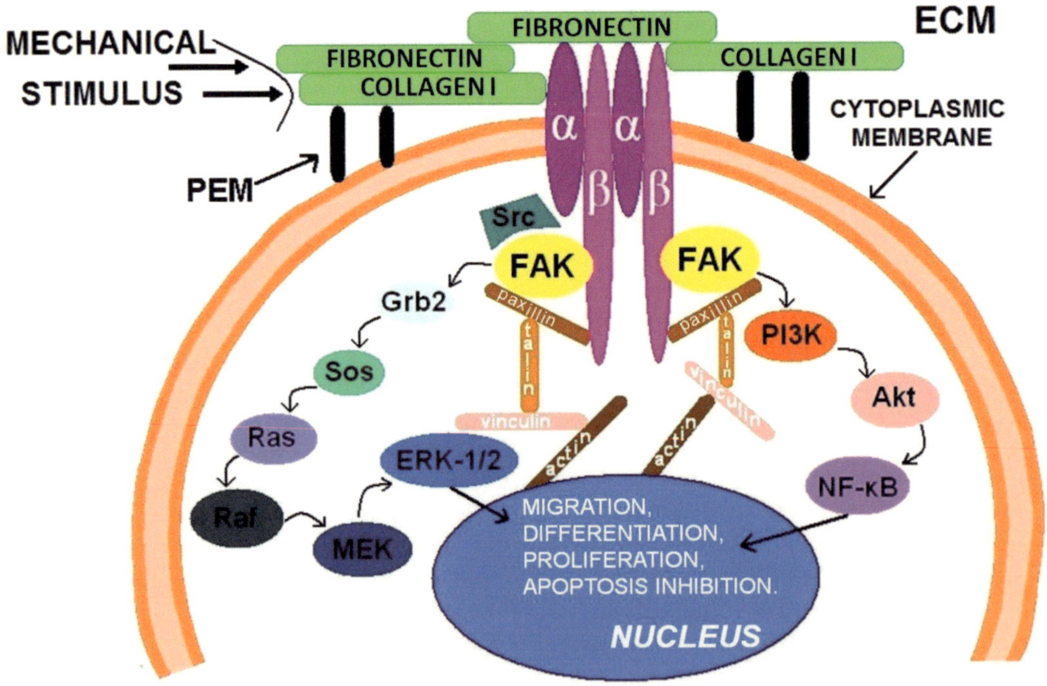

Fig. 9. *FAK signaling pathways.* FAK interacts with integrins and cytoskeleton components (actin, paxillin, talin and vinculin) - which also interact with the nucleus - and signal cellular mechanical deformation.

Hughes-Fulford, 2004; Kawamura et al., 2007; Liedbert et al., 2006; Mitra et al., 2005; Ogasawara et al., 2001; Raucci et al., 2008; Schlaepfer et al., 1998; Tang et al., 2006) (Fig.7 and Fig. 9).

5.3.1 Ion channels

Curiously, mechanical loads induce FAK ligation to calcium-dependent potassium channels without FAK autophosphorylation at Tyr-397. However, the effect of this event to the cellular response to strain is not known yet. For example, it is not known whether the potassium channel activity is altered by that ligation (Rezzonico et al., 2003).

5.3.2 PYK2

This protein is highly homologous to FAK. Through an unknown mechanism, strain induces a calcium-dependent phophorylation of PYK2 at Tyr-402, activating this protein. *In vitro*, PYK2 couples with FAK via SH2 and can transphosphorylate FAK at Tyr-397, Tyr-576 or Tyr-925. In opposite, FAK does not transphosphorylate PYK2. This indicates that PYK2 can enhance FAK tyrosine kinase activity because FAK phosphorylation at Tyr-397 gives rise to high affinity binding sites for SH2-containing-domain proteins. Supporting this hypothesis, it was found that PYK2 augments ERK-2 phosphorylation at Tyr-187 depending on PLC and calcium channels activity. Besides, PYK2 couples with Src like FAK, but this ligation does not depend on mechanical stimulation (Boutahar et al., 2004; Li et al., 1999; Liu et al., 2008).

5.3.3 p38

The activity of this MAPK increases with mechanical loads through an unknown mechanism. Within the pathways that result in p38 activation, FAK-Src/Grb2/Sos/Ras/PAK/MKK3/6 pathway may be deflagrated by strain because FAK is a mechanosensitive protein involved in this pathway. We found no study aiming to solve this issue (J. You et al., 2001).

5.4 Wnt pathways

Wnt is a family of 19 glycoproteins responsible for 88-99% of the mechanically-induced osteogenesis. Wnt1 class activates the canonical Wnt signaling pathway, in which complexes between Wnt1/3a, LRP5/6 and frizzled proteins are formed. Such complexes phosphorylate GSK3b, causing its inactivation; and hence, inhibit β-catenin degradation. Beta-catenin translocates to the nucleus where it accumulates, leading to Tcf/Lef transcription factor activation. Wnt also inhibits apoptosis via nuclear ERK and Akt activation. Wnt5a class participates in the non-canonical Wnt signaling pathway, and binds to frizzled proteins, leading to PLC activation via G proteins (Fig. 10).

There is exiguous information about Wnt pathways' relation to mechanotransduction. At the moment, it is known that (1) strain increases β-catenin activation and translocation to the nucleus, probably via PI3K activation, or decreasing sclerostin expression, which is an inhibitor of the canonical Wnt signaling pathway; (2) strain increases Wnt1, Wnt3a, Wnt5a and Lrp5 receptor expression; (3) and Lrp5 receptor hyperexpression increases the cellular response to mechanical loading, and decreases the strain needed to stimulate bone cells response to mechanical stimulation (Bonewals & Johnson, 2008; Johnson, 2004; Lau et al., 2006; Olkku & Mahonen, 2008; Robling et al., 2008; Turner, 2006; Yavropoulou & Yovos, 2007).

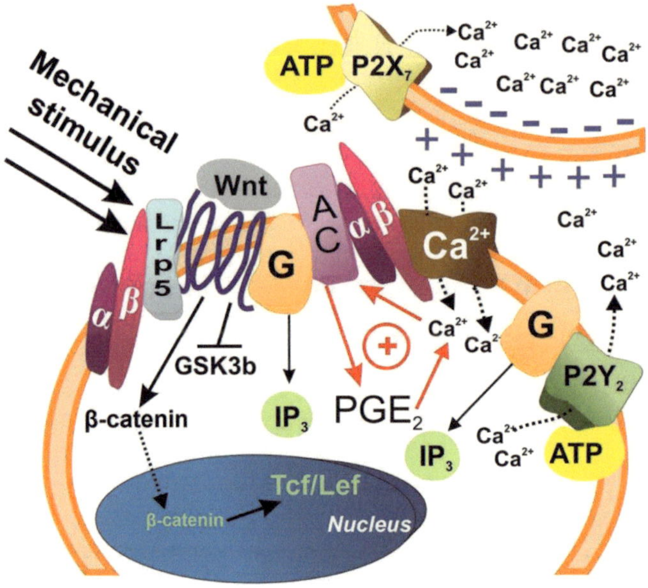

Fig. 10. *Not well known models of mechanical stimulation signaling*. Wnt complexes with the Lrp5 receptor and frizzled proteins (in blue), inhibiting GSK3b and activating Tcf/Lef (via β-catenin). The ATP produced after mechanical stimulation binds to its receptors ($P2X_7$ and $P2Y_2$), inside the cell where ATP was produced; or in the neighboring cells, when secreted by the stimulated cell (not showed). $P2X_7$ activation in a neighboring cell, alike Cx43 gap junctions, provokes calcium influx, which may result in a negative action potential that transmits strain biochemically. $P2Y_2$ and frizzled proteins stimulate IP_3 synthesis via G protein, increasing calcium concentration (not showed). PGE_2 produced in response to mechanical stimulation induces calcium influx, which activates AC that stimulates PGE_2 synthesis via a positive feedback mechanism (red arrows and plus sign). PGE_2 migrates to other cells through gap junctions or $P2X_7$.

5.5 Effector pathways

The signaling pathways activated by strain are part of bone mechanostat. Some products of these pathways are important to osteogenesis and are described below.

5.5.1 c-fos

Mechanical loads increase c-fos expression, which is a transcription factor that binds to c-jun, another transcription factor, forming the AP-1 heterodimer that induces osteogenesis (Judex et al., 2005; Mullender et al., 2004; Nomura & Takano-Yamamoto, 2000; Sikavitsas et al., 2001).

5.5.2 cox-1/2

Within cox isoforms, cox-2 (inducible cox) responds to mechanical stimulation with an increase in the amount of cox-2 mRNA. This protein participates in some mechanotransduction signaling pathways, and acts in the cytoplasm and nucleus of bone cells (Choudhary et al., 2008; Kapur et al., 2003; Ogasawara et al., 2001; Rouzer & Marnett, 2005; Tang et al., 2006).

5.5.3 Prostaglandins

The prostaglandins PGI_2, $PGF_{2\alpha}$ and PGE_2 are implicated in mechanically-induced osteogenesis. PGE_2 is responsible for 50-90% of the mechanically-induced osteogenesis; therefore, is pointed to be the most important prostaglandin in mechanotransduction. Besides, PGE_2 may be one of the regulators of the mechanostat because (1) its synthesis can increase via positive feedback (Fig. 10); (2) PGE_2 is transmitted to other cells through gap junctions, indicating that PGE_2 is involved in the intercellular transmission of mechanical stimulation; (3) and PGE_2 stimulates both osteogenesis and bone resorption. The underlying mechanism through which PGE_2 stimulates osteogenesis and bone resorption may be its intracellular concentration; however, this is a hypothesis. It is also possible that calcium concentration determines, indirectly, the cellular response to mechanical stimulation (osteogenesis or bone resorption) because this ion is responsible for 83% of PGE_2 synthesis. Additionally, the anabolic effects of PGE_2 are mediated by EP2 prostaglandin receptor and, mainly, by EP4 prostaglandin receptor, both located at the nuclear membrane (Cherian et al., 2005; Fortier et al., 2001; Genetos et al., 2005; Ke et al., 2003; Keila et al., 2001; Klein-Nulend et al., 1997; Li et al., 2005; Machwate et al., 2001; Mullender et al., 2004; Nomura & Takano-Yamamoto, 2000; Reich et al., 1997; Watanuki et al., 2002; Xu et al., 2007).

5.5.4 NO

Through an unknown mechanism, NO stimulates both osteogenesis and bone resorption. It participates in some osteogenesis pathways, and can decrease 50% of PTH-induced bone resorption and 68% of vitamin D-induced bone resorption (Fan et al., 2004; Kapur et al., 2003; Wang et al., 2004).

5.5.5 PDGF-β

It is described that PDGF-β stimulates chondrocytes proliferation, osteogenic cells differentiation into osteoblasts and bone resorption. The gene for PDGF-β has a shear stress response element (SSRE) region, which is present in the genes of other mechanosensitive proteins: cox-2, osteopontin, iNOS. For this reason, some authors believe PDGF-β has a role in the effector response to mechanical stimulation, although there is no report of PDGF-β involvement with mechanically-induced osteogenesis (Luo & Wang, 2004; Nomura & Takano-Yamamoto, 2000; Sikavitsas et al., 2001).

5.6 Biochemical transmission of mechanical stimulation

Each bone cell is subjected to different mechanical deformation intensities during one mechanical stimulation. But to produce significant bone mass, a great amount of bone cells may work together in response to mechanical stimulation. Besides, osteoblast precursor cells must be activated and migrate to the osteogenesis site; and osteoclasts must be inactive at the osteogenesis site. In order to these events occur bone cells are supposed to have means of intercellular communication.

5.6.1 Ion channels

Mechanical deformation activates ion channels (most importantly, calcium and potassium channels), generating a negative membrane potential. As the example of neuronal synapses, the negative membrane potential may be transmitted through the neighboring cells, which, in turn, activate biochemically their mechanotransduction pathways.

5.6.2 Cadherins

These single-chain transmembrane glycoproteins are expressed in the junction adherens of bone cells and link the cytoskeleton of adjacent cells through interactions between the extracellular segments of each cadherin. Like integrins, cadherins expression increases in response to strain. Both integrins and cadherins seem to have similar function: the first transmit the mechanical stimulation inside the deformed cell, and the latter transmit the mechanical stimulation to the adjacent cell (Pavalko et al., 2003).

5.6.3 Gap junctions

These specialized intercellular connections are pointed as the major contributor to intercellular transmission. Following mechanical stimulation, gap junctions allow the exchange of PGE_2 and other molecules smaller than 1 kDa (for example, calcium, IP_3 and cAMP) between adjacent cells (for example, osteocytes and periosteal cells). Each gap junction is composed of 2 hemichannels (each hemichannel belongs to each of the two adjacent cells). Each hemichannel allows communication between the cell and its ECM, and is composed of 6 connexins. Within the various types of connexins, Cx43 is the main constituent of the hemichannel, and is involved in the transmission of mechanical stimuli. In addition, mechanical loads increase Cx43 expression and phosphorylation, enhancing gap junctions intercellular communication; 60-100% of PGE_2 transmission to adjacent cells depends on Cx43; and calcium transmission between adjacent cells can occur via gap junctions (Cherian et al., 2005; Genetos et al., 2005; Miyauchi et al., 2006; Siller-Jackson et al., 2008; Stains & Civitelli, 2005; Yang et al., 2005) (Fig. 8).

5.6.4 ATP receptors

ATP binds to its transmembrane receptors $P2X_7$ and $P2Y_2$. The first receptor is a non-selective ion channel that complexes with various proteins like β2 subunits of integrins and α-actinin, suggesting the involvement of this receptor in mechanotransduction. $P2X_7$ receptor activation is responsible for about 61-73% of the mechanically-induced bone formation rate; increases bone tissue mechanosensitivity by 31%; and is responsible for 50% of the mechanically-induced ERK-1/2 activation. $P2Y_2$ receptor seems to activate G protein/PLC/PIP2/IP_3 pathway, which increases calcium intake; and promotes calcium efflux after mechanical loads, more efficiently than gap junctions (Table 4). On the other hand, $P2Y_2$ is not important for ERK-1/2 activation, and there are no reports showing $P2Y_2$ activation directly by strain (Cherian et al., 2005; Genetos et al., 2005; Jorgensen et al., 1997; Ke et al., 2003; Li et al., 2005; Liu et al., 2008; Reich et al., 1995) (Fig. 10).

5.7 Memory system of bone

Some reports suggest that bone cells possess a memory system that prolongs the cellular response to mechanical stimulation. For example, it was documented *in vitro* that mechanically-induced calcium influx was greater when bone cells were subjected to a second load, 30 minutes after the first load. The underlying mechanism of this memory system is unknown. The positive feedbacks of PGE_2 production and calcium influx (described above) may be part of the underlying mechanism because they are positive feedbacks. In memory cells of the central nervous system, the action potential can be prolonged by glutamate activation of voltage-dependent calcium channels (NMDA-type channels). This is called long-term potentiation. In those cells, it is described that following voltage-dependent calcium channels opening, calcium enters the neuron and binds to glutamate-containing vesicles releasing glutamate to the extracellular environment where glutamate binds to NMDA-type channels and mGluR. The activation of potassium channels and some classes of mGluR inhibit voltage-dependent calcium channels activation, blocking glutamate release. Glutamate actions end when GLAST (also called EAAT) takes glutamate from the extracellular environment and returns it back to the intracellular vesicles.

Based on the long-term potentiation mechanism, we believe there are five conditions in bone that makes possible the existence of a memory system in this tissue (Table 5). In addition, GLAST stops working when the extracellular concentration of sodium is low and the extracellular concentration of potassium is high. This situation is consistent with the available data: when extracellular potassium concentration is high, the cytoplasmic membrane hyperpolarizes (the calcium-dependent potassium channels open and the sodium channels close), leading to osteogenesis. Unfortunately, there are no reports about the NMDA channels and metabotropic receptors activation in bone cells subjected to mechanical loads (Godin et al., 2007; Hinoi et al., 2003; Lent, 2001; Mason, 2004; Nomura & Takano-Yamamoto, 2000; Spencer et al., 2007; Taylor, 2002).

5.8 Hormones and mechanotransduction

Some hormones and growth factors like PTH and IGF-1 have synergistic effect with mechanical loads to induce osteogenesis. The underlying mechanism that produces the synergistic effect is unknown. On the other hand, it is known that such hormones and growth factors, and mechanical loads activate ERK, which is hyperactivated when double phosphorylated, resulting in ERK migration to the nucleus where ERK's action is potentialized. Therefore, we hypothesize that the stimuli from mechanical loads and biological factors hyperphosphorylate ERK, leading to a greater osteogenesis rate (Ebisuya et al., 2005; Yee et al., 2008).

5.8.1 PTH

Increases 1.53-6 fold bone formation rate when associated with mechanical loads. The synergistic effect of PTH and mechanical loading depends 68-74% on voltage-dependent L-type calcium channels activation, probably because the synergistic effect of PTH may occur via PYK2-FAK/ERK, which is a calcium-dependent signaling pathway involved in mechanotransduction. Curiously in the presence of PTH, NO production augmentation is abolished even in the presence of mechanical stimulation (the study evaluated NO concentration until 30 minutes after mechanical loading) (Bakker et al., 2003; Chen et al., 2004; Choudhary et al., 2008; Fan et al., 2004; Ma et al., 1999; Ogasawara et al., 2001; Yamamoto et al., 2007).

5.8.2 IGF-1

When associated with mechanical loading, cellular proliferation increases 1.8-3.8 fold, IGF-1R phosphorylation increases 7.5 fold, and ERK activation increases 2-9.5 fold. IGF-1 activity depends totally on the presence of integrins, and Akt activation rate is not altered by mechanical stimulation in the presence of IGF-1 (Desbois-Mouthon et al., 2001; Kapur et al., 2005; Nomura & Takano-Yamamoto, 2000; Sakata et al., 2004; Sekimoto et al., 2005; Sikavitsas et al., 2001).

5.8.3 Estrogen

It was not found any report about the synergistic effect of estrogen and mechanical loading. On the other hand, it is documented that ER-α absence decreases 70% of the mechanically-induced bone formation rate, and inhibits 100% of the mechanically-induced cellular proliferation (Lee et al., 2003).

5.9 Mechanotransduction *in vivo*

The majority of the reports about mechanically-induced osteogenesis are based on *in vitro* experimental models, probably because it is difficult to obtain bone cells and their proteins after *in vivo* experimental procedures. The beneficial effect of LIPUS stimulation (mechanical stimulation) has already been documented in lesioned bones, which exhibited early consolidation[70]. We developed an *in vivo* experimental model to assess the effect of the mechanical stimulation on bone proteins of intact tibia and fibula of rats. LIPUS was used to subject the animals to a daily 20-minute treatment for 7, 14 or 21 days. At the end of the treatment, we evaluated the expression and activation of FAK, ERK-1/2 and IRS-1 by immunoblotting assays. It was found that FAK, ERK-1/2 and IRS-1 expression increased in a non-cumulative manner indicating that the mechanostat blocks LIPUS osteogenic effects after a period of continuous stimulation. Increased FAK and ERK-1/2 activation was detected 15 hours after the last LIPUS stimulation at seven days of treatment, supporting the theory of the memory system of bone.

Additionally, LIPUS increased IRS-1 expression and activation (data not published) after one week of treatment. Since IRS-1 is involved in growth factors signaling pathways, those results suggest mechanical stimulation also acts in signaling pathways activated by growth factors. This hypothesis may serve as an explanation for the synergistic effect of some hormones with mechanical loading. There are few investigations on this issue *in vivo* and *in vitro*.

The sham LIPUS stimulation (device turned off) increased FAK activation after one week of treatment, indicating the muscle contraction of the stressed animals also possesses osteogenic effects, possibly because of the vibratory load on bone, which is a mechanical load of high frequency and low magnitude; or because of a paracrine stimulus from muscle to bone cells (Gusmão et al., 2007, 2010; Naruse et al., 2003; Warden et al., 2001).

6. Future directions

We consider that bone is not merely a structure for locomotion. It is a complex organ that also responds to mechanical stimulation. The underlying mechanism of mechanically-induced osteogenesis is not fully understood, and many questions need to be answered. Therefore, further studies shall investigate how bone cells distinguish physiological from overuse deformations; the regulatory activity of osteocytes on other bone cells; the mechanically-induced activity of ion channels, intercellular communication of bone cells and the memory system of bone; the physicochemical properties of the ECM/PEM-integrins-cytoskeleton-nucleus system components; the events that trigger FAK, ERK and Akt mechanically-induced migration to the nucleus; the synergistic effect of growth factors and hormones with mechanical loads; and so on.

In addition, the current data about mechanically-induced osteogenesis are not linked. For example, a little is known about the activation of FAK pathways, integrins, and ion channels by mechanical loading; however, we do not know how they work together, how their combined activity influences bone response to mechanical stimulation, and how that bone response to mechanical stimulation macroscopically affects the skeleton. Therefore, we believe that studies shall be carried out to understand the events triggered by mechanical loading as a whole, because bone functions as a whole as well as the human body.

7. References

Anderson JC & Eriksson C. Electrical properties of wet collagen. Nature. 1968;218:166-8.

Anderson JC & Eriksson C. Piezoelectric properties of dry and wet bone. Nature. 1970;227:491-2.

Bakker AD, Joldersma M, Klein-Nulend J & Burger EH. Interactive effects of PTH and mechanical stress on nitric oxide and PGE2 production by primary mouse osteoblastic cells. Am J Physiol Endocrinol Metab. 2003;285:608-13.

Bennett JH, Carter DH, Alavi AL, Beresford JN & Walsh S. Patterns of integrin expression in a human mandibular explant model of osteoblast differentiation. Arch Oral Biol. 2001;46:229-38.

Bonewald LF. Mechanosensation and transduction in osteocytes. Bonekey Osteovision. 2006;3:7-15.

Bonewald LF & Johnson ML. Osteocytes, mechanosensing and Wnt signaling. Bone. 2008;42:606-15.

Boutahar N, Guignandon A, Vico L & Lafage-Proust MH. Mechanical strain on osteoblasts activates autophosphorylation of focal adhesion kinase and proline-rich tyrosine kinase 2 tyrosine sites involved in ERK activation. J Biol Chem. 2004;279:30588-99.

Buckwalter JA, Glimcher MJ, Cooper RR & Recker R. Bone biology. I: Structure, blood supply, cells, matrix, and mineralization. Instr Course Lect. 1996;45:371-86.

Buckwalter JA, Glimcher MJ, Cooper RR & Recker R. Bone biology. II: Formation, form, modeling, remodeling, and regulation of cell function. Instr Course Lect. 1996;45:387-99.

Burr DB, Turner CH, Naick P, Forwood MR, Ambrosius W, Hasan MS & Pidaparti R. Does microdamage accumulation affect the mechanical properties of bone? J Biomech. 1998;31:337-45.

Burr DB, Robling AG & Turner CH. Effects of biomechanical stress on bones in animals. Bone. 2002;30:781-6.

Butcher MT, Espinoza NR, Cirilo SR & Blob RW. In vivo strains in the femur of river cooter turtles (Pseudemys concinna) during terrestrial locomotion: tests of force-platform models of loading mechanics. J Exp Biol. 2008;211:2397-407.

Carter DR & Hayes WC. Compact bone fatigue damage: a microscopic examination. Clin Orthop Relat Res. 1977;127:265-74.

Castillo AB, Alam I, Tanaka SM, Levenda J, Li Jiliang, Warden SJ & Turner CH. Low-amplitude, broad-frequency vibration effects on cortical bone formation in mice. Bone. 2006;39:1087-96.

Champe PC & Harvey RA. Bioquímica ilustrada. São Paulo: ARTMED, 2000:85-91.

Chen C, Koh AJ, Datta NS, Zhang J, Keller ET, Xiao G, Franceschi RT, D'Silva NJ & McCauley LK. Impact of the Mitogen-activated protein kinase pathway on parathyroid hormone-related protein actions in osteoblasts. J Biol Chem. 2004;279:29121-9.

Chen K-D, Li Y-S, Kim M, Li S, Yuan S, Chien S & Shyy JY-J. Mechanotransduction in response to shear stress. Roles of receptor tyrosine kinases, integrins, and Shc. J Biol Chem. 1999;274:18393-400.

Cherian PP, Siller-Jakson AJ, Gu S, Wang X, Bonewald LF, Sprague E & Jiang JX. Mechanical strain opens connexin 43 hemichannels in osteocytes: a novel mechanism for the release of prostaglandin. Mol Biol Cell. 2005;7:3100-6.

Choudhary S, Huang H, Raisz L & Pilbeam C. Anabolic effects of PTH in cyclooxygenase-2 knockout osteoblasts in vitro. Biochem and Biophys Res Comm. 2008;372:536-41.

Cornillon J, Campos L & Guyotat D. Focal adhesion kinase (FAK), a multifunctional protein. Med Sci (Paris). 2003;19:743-752.

Desbois-Mouthon C, Cadoret A, Eggelpoël M-J B-V, Bertrand F, Cherqui G, Perret C & Capeau J. Insulin and IGF-1 stimulate the β-catenin pathway through two signalling cascades involving GSK-3β inhibition and Ras activation. Oncogene. 2001;20:252-9.

Duncan RL & Turner CH. Mechanotransduction and the functional response of bone to mechanical strain. Calcif Tiss Int. 1995;57:344-58.

Ebisuya M, Kondoh K & Nishida E. The duration, magnitude and compartmentalization of ERK MAP kinase activity: mechanisms for providing signaling specificity. J Cell Sci. 2005;118:2997-3002.

Fan X, Roy E, Zhu L, Murphy TC, Ackert-Bicknell C, Hart CM, Rosen C, Nanes MS & Rubin J. Nitric oxide regulates receptor activator of nuclear factor-kB ligand and osteoprotegerin expression in bone marrow stromal cells. Endocrinology. 2004;145:751-9.

van der Flier A & Sonnenberg A. Functions and interactions of integrins. Cell Tiss Res. 2001;305:285-98.

Fortier I, Patry C, Lora M, Samadfan R & de Brum-Fernandes AJ. Immunohistochemical localization of the prostacyclin receptor (IP) human bone. Prostaglandins Leukot Essent Fatty Acids. 2001;65:79-83.

Fritton SP, Kenneth JM & Rubin CT. Quantifying the strain history of bone: spatial uniformity and self-similarity of low-magnitude strains. J Biomech. 2000;33:317-25.

Frost HM. The Utah paradigm of skeletal physiology: an overview of its insights for bone, cartilage and collagenous tissue organs. J Bone Miner Metab. 2000;18:305-16.

Frost HM. Bone's mechanostat: A 2003 update. Anat Rec A Discov Mol Cell Evol Biol. 2003;275:1081-101.

Fukada E & Yasuda I. On the piezoeletric effect of bone. J Phys Soc Japan. 1957;12:1158-62.

Giancotti FG & Rouslahti E. Integrin signaling. Science. 1999;285:1028-32.

Genetos DC, Geist DJ, Liu D, Donahue HJ & Duncan RL. Fluid shear-induced ATP secretion mediates prostaglandin release in MC3T3-E1 osteoblasts. J Bone Miner Res. 2005;20:41-9.

Godin LM, Suzuki S, Jacobs CR, Donahue HJ & Donahue SW. Mechanically induced intracellular calcium waves in osteoblasts demonstrate calcium fingerprints in bone cell mechanotransduction. Biomech Model Mechanobiol. 2007;6:391-8.

Goldspink G. Changes in muscle mass and phenotype and the expression of autocrine and systemic growth factors by muscle in response to stretch and overload. J Anat. 1999;194:323-334.

Gronthos S, Stewart K, Graves SE, Hay S & Simmons PJ. Integrin expression and function on human osteoblast-like cells. J Bone Miner Res. 1997;12:1189-97.

Gupta V & Grande-Allen KJ. Effects of static and cyclic loading in regulating extracellular matrix synthesis by cardiovascular cells. Cardiovasc Res. 2006;72:375-83.

Gusmão CVB, Pauli JR & Belangero WD. Efeito do ultra-som de baixa potência na expressão da FAK (*focal adhesion kinase*), ERK-2 (*extracellular signal-regulated kinase-2*) e IRS-1 (*insulin receptor substrate-1*) no osso *in vivo*. In: Anais do XVI Congresso Médico Acadêmico da Unicamp; 2007;

de Gusmão CV, Pauli JR, Saad MJ, Alves JM & Belangero WD. Low-intensity ultrasound increases FAK, ERK-1/2, and IRS-1 expression of intact rat bones in a noncumulative manner. Clin Orthop Relat Res. 2010;468(4):1149-56.

Hinoi E, Fujimori S & Yoneda Y. Modulation of cellular differentiation by N-methyl-D-aspartate receptors in osteoblasts. FASEB J. 2003;17:1532-4.

Hsieh Y-F & Turner CH. Effects of loading frequency on mechanically induced bone formation. J Bone Miner Res. 2001;16:918-24.

Hsu H-C, Fong Y-C, Chang C-S, Hsu C-J, Hsu S-F & Lin J-G, et al. Ultrasound induces cyclooxygenase-2 expression through integrin, integrin-linked kinase, Akt, NF-κB and p300 pathway in human chondrocytes. Cell Signal. 2007;19:2317-28.

Hughes-Fulford M. Signal transduction and mechanical stress. Sci STKE. 2004;2004:RE12.

Jacobs CR, Yellowley CE, Davis BR, Zhou Z, Cimbala JM & Donahue HJ. Differential effect of steady versus oscillating flow on bone cells. J Biomech. 1998;31:969-976.

Johnson ML. The high bone mass family - the role of Wnt/Lrp5 signaling in the regulation of bone mass. J Musculoskelet Neuronal Interact. 2004;4:135-8.

Jorgensen NR, Geist ST, Civitelli R & Steinberg TH. ATP- and gap junction-dependent intercellular calcium signaling in osteoblastic cells. J Cell Biol. 1997;139:497-506.

Judex S, Zhong N, Squire ME, Ye K, Donahue LR, Hadjiargyrou M & Rubin CT. Mechanical modulation of molecular signals which regulate anabolic and catabolic activity in bone tissue. J Cell Biochem. 2005;94:982-94.

Kapur S, Baylink D & Lau K-HW. Fluid flow shear stress stimulates human osteoblast proliferation and differentiation through multiple interacting and competing signal transduction pathways. Bone. 2003;32:241-51.

Kapur S, Mohan S, Baylink DJ & Lau K-H W. Fluid shear stress synergizes with insulin-like growth factor-I (IGF-I) on osteoblast proliferation through integrin-dependent activation of IGF-I mitogenic signaling pathway. J Biol Chem. 2005;280;20163-70.

Kawamura N, Kugimiya F, Oshima Y, Ohba S, Ikeda T, Saito T et al. Akt1 in osteoblasts and osteoclasts controls bone remodeling. PLoS ONE. 2007;2:e1058.

Ke HZ, Qi H, Weidema AF, Zhang Q, Panupinthu N, Crawford DT, Grasser WA, Paralkar VM, Li M, Audoly LP, Gabel CA, Jee WSS, Dixon J, Sims SM & Thompson DD. Deletion of the $P2x_7$ nucleotide receptor reveals its regulatory roles in bone formation and resorption. Mol Endocrinol. 2003;17:1356-67.

Keila S, Kelner A & Weinreb M. Systemic prostaglandin E2 increases cancellous bone formation and mass in aging rats and stimulates their bone marrow osteogenic capacity in vivo and in vitro. J Endocrin. 2001;168:131-9.

Klein-Nulend J, Burger EH, Semeins CM, Raisz LG & Pilbeam CC. Pulsating fluid flow stimulates prostaglandin release and inducible prostaglandin G/H synthase mRNA expression in primary mouse bone cells. J Bone Miner Res. 1997;12:45-51.

Klein-Nulend J, van der Plas A, Semeins CM, Ajubi NE, Frangos JA, Nijweide PJ & Burger EH. Sensitivity of osteocytes to biomechanical stress in vitro. FASEB J. 1995;9:441-5.

Lau K-HW, Kapur S, Kesavan C & Baylink DJ. Up-regulation of the Wnt, estrogen receptor, insulin-like growth factor-I, and bone morphogenetic protein pathways in C57BL/6J osteoblasts as opposed to C3H/HeJ osteoblasts in part contributes to the differential anabolic response to fluid shear. J Biol Chem. 2006;281:9576-88.

Lee HS, Millward-Sadler SJ, Wright MO, Nuki G & Salter DM. Integrin and mechanosensitive ion channel-dependent tyrosine phosphorylation of focal adhesion proteins and beta-catenin in human articular chondrocytes after mechanical stimulation. J Bone Miner Res. 2000;15:1501-9.

Lee K, Jessop H, Suswillo R, Zaman G & Lanyon L. Endocrinology: Bone adaptation requires oestrogen receptor-α Nature. 2003;424:389.

Lent R. Cem bilhões de neurônios: conceitos fundamentais. São Paulo: Atheneu, 2001:121-6 e 151-9.

Li J, Duncan RL, Burr DB, Gattone VG & Turner CH. Parathyroid hormone enhances mechanically induced bone formation, possibly involving L-type voltage-sensitive calcium channels. Endocrinology. 2003;144:1226-33.

Li J, Liu D, Ke HZ, Duncan RL & Turner CH. The $P2X_7$ nucleotide receptor mediates skeletal mechanotransduction. J Biol Chem. 2005;280:42952-9.

Li X, Dy RC, Cance WG, Graves LM & Earp HS. Interactions between two cytoskeleton-associated tyrosine kinases: Calcium-dependent tyrosine kinase and focal adhesion tyrosine kinase. J Biol Chem. 1999;274:8917-24.

Li Z, Yang G, Khan M, Stone D, Woo SL-Y & Wang JH-C. Inflammatory response of human tendon fibroblasts to cyclic mechanical stretching. Am J Sports Med. 2004;32:435-40.

Liedbert A, Kaspar D, Blakytny R, Claes L & Ignatius A. Signal transduction pathways involved in mechanotransduction in bone cells. Biochem Biophys Res Comm. 2006;349:1-5.

Liu D, Genetos DC, Shao Y, Geist DJ, Li J, Ke HZ, Turner CH & Duncan RL. Activation of extracellular-signal regulated kinase (ERK1/2) by fluid shear is Ca2+- and ATP-dependent in MC3T3-E1 osteoblasts. Bone 2008;42:644-52.

Luo QF & Wang X. The effects of PL-derived growth factor on osteogenesis and skeletal reconstruction. Shanghai Kou Qiang Yi Xue. 2004;13:207-10.

Ma Y, Jee WS, Yuan Z,WeiW, Chen H, Pun S, Liang H & Lin C. Parathyroid hormone and mechanical usage have a synergistic effect in rat tibial diaphyseal cortical bone. J Bone Miner Res. 1999;14:439-48.

Machwate M, Harada S, Leu CT, Seedor G, Labelle M, Gallant M, Hutchins S, Lachance N, Sawyer N, Slipetz D, Metters KM, Rodan SB, Young R & Rodan GA. Prostaglandin receptor EP(4) mediates the bone anabolic effects of PGE_2. Mol Pharmacol. 2001;60:36-41.

Mason DJ. Glutamate signalling and its potential application to tissue engineering of bone. Eur Cell Mater. 2004;7:12-25.

Mitra SK, Hanson DA & Schlaepfer DD. Focal adhesion kinase: in command and control of cell motility. Nature. 2005;6:56-68.

Miyauchi A, Gotoh M, Notoya HKK, Sekiya H, Yoshimoto YTY, Ishikawa H, Takano-Yamamoto KCT & Mikuni-Takagaki TFY. $\alpha_V\beta 3$ integrin ligands enhance volume-sensitive calcium influx in mechanically stretched osteocytes. J Bone Miner Metab. 2006;24:498-504.

Mullender M, El Haj AJ, Yang Y, van Duin MA, Burger EH & Klein-Nulend J. Mechanotransduction of bone cells in vitro: mechanobiology of bone tissue. J Med Biol Eng Comput. 2004;42:14-21.

Naruse K, Miyauchi A, Itoman M & Mikuni-Takagaki Y. Distinct anabolic response of osteoblast to low-intensity pulsed ultrasound. J Bone Miner Res. 2003;18:360-9.

Nomura S, Takano-Yamamoto T. Molecular events caused by mechanical stress in bone. Matrix Biology. 2000;19:91-6.

Norvell SM, Alvarez M, Bidwell JP & Pavalko FM. Fluid shear stress induces β-catenin signaling in osteoblasts. Calcif Tiss Int. 2004;75:396-404.

O'brien FJ, Hardiman DA, Hazenberg JG, Mercy MV, Mohsin S, Taylor D & Lee TC. The behaviour of microcraks in compact bone. Eur J Morphol. 2005;42:71-9.

Ogasawara A, Arakawa T, Kaneda T, Takuma T, Sato T, Kaneko H, Kumegawa M & Hakeda Y. Fluid shear stress-induced cyclooxygenase-2 expression is mediated by C/EBP beta, cAMP-response element-binding protein, and AP-1 in osteoblastic MC3T3-E1 cells. J Biol Chem. 2001;276:7048-54.

Olkku A & Mahonen A. Wnt and steroid pathways control glutamate signalling by regulating glutamine synthetase activity in osteoblastic cells. Bone. 2008;43:483-93

Owan M & Triffitt JT. Extravascular albumin in bone tissue. J Phisyol. 1976;257:293-307.

Pavalko FM, Chen NX, Turner CH, Burr DB, Atkinson S, Hsieh Y-F, Qiu J & Duncan RL. Fluid shear-induced mechanical signaling in MC3T3-E1 osteoblasts requires cytoskeleton-integrin interactions. Am J Physiol Cell Physiol.1998;275:1591-601.

Pavalko FM, Norvell SM, Burr DB, Turner CH, Duncan RL & Bidwell JP. A model for mechanotransduction in bone cells: the load-bearing mechanosomes. J Cell Biochem. 2003;88:104-12.

Plotkin LI, Mathov I, Aguirre JI, Parfitt AM, Manolagas SC & Bellido T. Mechanical stimulation prevents osteocyte apoptosis: requirement of integrins, Src kinases, and ERKs. Am J Physiol Cell Physiol. 2005;289:633-43.

Pommerenke H, Schmidt C, Dürr F, Nebe B, Lüthen F, Muller P & Rychly J. The mode of mechanical integrin stressing controls intracellular signaling in osteoblasts. J Bone Miner Res. 2002;17:603-11.

Qin YX, Lin W & Rubin C. The pathway of bone fluid flow as defined by in vivo intramedullary pressure and streaming potential measurements. Ann Biomed Eng. 2002;30:693-702.

Raucci A, Bellosta P, Grassi R, Basilico C & Mansukhani A. Osteoblast proliferation or differentiation is regulated by relative strengths of opposing signaling pathways. J Cell Physiol. 2008;215:442-51.

Reich KM, McAllister TN, Gudi S & Frangos JA. Activation of G proteins mediates flow-induced prostaglandin E2 production in osteoblasts. Endocrinology. 1997;138:1014-8.

Rezzonico R, Cayatte C, Bourget-Ponzio I, Romey G, Belhacene N, Loubat A, Rocchi S, van Obberghen E, Girault J-A, Rossi B & Schmid-Antomarchi H. Focal adhesion kinase pp125FAK interacts with the large conductance calcium-activated hSlo potassium channel in human osteoblasts: potential role in mechanotransduction. J Bone Miner Res. 2003;18:1863-71.

Riddle RC & Donahue HJ. From streaming-potentials to shear stress: 25 years of bone cell mechanotransduction. J Orthop Res. 2009;27:143-9.

Robling AG, Burr DB & Turner CH. Recovery periods restore mechanosensitivity to dynamically loaded bone. J Exp Biol.2001; 204:3389-99.

Robling AG, Castillo AB & Turner CH. Biomechanical and molecular regulation of bone remodeling. Annu Rev Biomed Eng. 2006;8:455-98.

Robling AG, Niziolek PJ, Baldridge LA, Condon KW, Allen MR, Alam I, Mantila SM, Gluhak-Heinrich J, Bellido TM, Harris SE & Turner CH. Mechanical stimulation of bone in vivo reduces osteocyte expression of Sost/sclerostin. J Biol Chem. 2008;283:5866-75.

Rouzer CA & Marnett LJ. Structural and functional differences between cyclooxygenases: fatty acid oxygenases with a critical role in cell signaling. Biochem Biophys Res Commun. 2005;338:34-44.

Rubin CT & Lanyon LE. Regulation of bone formation by applied dynamic loads. J Bone Joint Surg Am. 1984;66:271-80.

Rubin C, Turner AS, Bain S, Mallinckrodt C & McLeod K. Low mechanical signals strengthen long bones. Nature 2001;412:603-4.

Sakata T, Wang Y, Halloran BP, Elalieh HZ, Cao J & Bikle DD. Skeletal unloading induces resistance to insulin-like growth factor-I (IGF-I) by inhibiting activation of the IGF-I signaling pathways. J Bone Miner Res. 2004;19:436-46.

Salter DM, Robb JE & Wright MO. Electrophysiological responses of human bone cells to mechanical stimulation: evidence for specific integrin function in mechanotransduction. J Bone Miner Res. 1997;12:1133-41.

Salter DM, Wallace WH, Robb JE, Caldwell H & Wright MO. Human bone cell hyperpolarization response to cyclical mechanical strain is mediated by an interleukin-1 beta autocrine/paracrine loop. J Bone Miner Res. 2000;15:1746-55.

Sauren YMHF, Mieremet RHP, Groot CG & Scherft JP. An electron microscopic study on the presence of proteoglycans on the mineralized matrix of rat and human compact lamellar bone. Anat Rec. 1992;232:36-44.

Schlaepfer DD, Jones KC & Hunter T. Multiple Grb2-mediated integrin-stimulated signaling pathways to ERK2/mitogen-activated protein kinase: summation of both c-Src- and focal adhesion kinase-initiated tyrosine phosphorylation events. Mol Cell Biol. 1998;18:2571-85.

Schriefer JL, Warden SJ, Saxon LK, Robling AG & Turner CH. Cellular accommodation and the response of bone to mechanical loading. J Biomech. 2005;38:1838-45.

Scott A, Khan KM, Duronio V & Hart DA. Mechanotransduction in human bone in vitro cellular physiology that underpins bone changes with exercise. Sports Med. 2008;38:139-60.

Sekimoto H, Eipper-Mains J, Pond-Tor S & Boney CM. αvβ3 integrins and Pyk2 mediate iInsulin-like growth factor I activation of Src and mitogen-activated protein kinase in 3T3-L1 cells. Mol Endocrinol. 2005;19:1859-67.

Siller-Jackson AJ, Burra S, Gu S, Xia X, Bonewald LF, Sprague E & Jiang JX. Adaptation of connexin 43-hemichannel prostaglandin release to mechanical loading. J Biol Chem. 2008;283:26374-82.

Sinha RK & Tuan RS. Regulation of human osteoblast integrin expression by orthopaedic implant materials. Bone. 1996;18:451-7.

Sikavitsas VI, Temenoff JS & Mikos AG. Biomaterials and bone mechanotransduction. Biomaterials. 2001;22:2581-93.

Spencer GJ, McGrath CJ & Genever PG. Current perspectives on NMDA-type glutamate signalling in bone. Int J Biochem Cell Biol. 2007;39:1089-104.

Stains JP & Civitelli R. Gap junctions in skeletal development and function. Biochim Biophys Acta. 2005;1719:69-81.

Tanaka-Kamioka K, Kamioka H, Ris H & Lim SS. Osteocyte shape is dependent on actin filaments and osteocyte processes are unique actin-rich proections. J Bone Miner Res. 1998;13:1555-68.

Tang CH, Yang RS, Huang TH, Lu DY, Chuang WJ, Huang TF & Fu WM. Ultrasound stimulates cyclooxygenase-2 expression and increases bone formation through integrin, FAK, phosphatidylinositol 3-kinase and Akt pathway in osteoblasts. Mol Pharmacol. 2006;69:2047-57.

Taylor AF. Functional osteoblastic ionotropic glutamate receptors are a prerequisite for bone formation. J Musculoskel Neuron Interact. 2002;2:415-22.

Taylor AF, Saunders MM, Shingle DL, et al. Mechanically stimulated osteocytes regulate osteoblastic activity via gap junctions. Am J Physiol Cell Physiol. 2007; 292:C545-52.

Torcasio A, van Lenthe GH & Van Oosterwyck H. The importance of loading frequency, rate and vibration for enhancing bone adaptation and implant osteointegration. Eur Cell Mater. 2008;16:56-68.

Turner CH. Bone strength: current concepts. Ann NY Acad Sci. 2006;1068:429-46.

Umemura Y, Ishiko T, Yamauchi T, Kurono M & Mashiko S. Five jumps per day increase bone mass and breaking force in rats. J. Bone Miner. Res. 1997;12:1480-5.

Wang F-S, Kuo Y-R, Wang C-J, Yang KD, Chang P-R, Huang Y-T, Huang H-C, Sun Y-C, Yang Y-J & Chen Y-J. Nitric oxide mediates ultrasound-induced hypoxia-inducible factor-1a activation and vascular endothelial growth factor-A expression in human osteoblasts. Bone. 2004;35:114-23.

Warden SJ, Favaloro JM, Bennell KL, McMeeken JM, Ng KW, Zajac JD & Wark JD. Low-intensity pulsed ultrasound stimulates a bone-forming response in UMR-106 cells. Biochem Biophys Res Commun. 2001;286:443-50.

Warden SJ & Turner CH. Mechanotransduction in the cortical bone is most efficient at loading frequencies of 5-10 Hz. Bone. 2004;34: 261-270.

Watanuki M, Sakai A, Sakata T, Tsurukami H, Miwa M, Uchida Y, Watanabe K, Ikeda K & Nakamura T. Role of inducible nitric oxide synthase in skeletal adaptation to acute increases in mechanical loading. J Bone Miner Res. 2002;17:1015-25.

Xu Z, Choudhary S, Okada Y, Voznesenskyl O, Alander C, Raisz L & Pilbeam C. Cyclooxygenase-2 gene disruption promotes proliferation of murine calvarial osteoblasts in vitro. Bone. 2007;41:68-76.

Yamamoto T, Kambe F, Cao X, Lu X, Ishiguro N & Seo H. Parathyroid hormone activates phosphoinositide 3-kinase-Akt-Bad cascade in osteoblast-like cells. Bone. 2007;40:354-9.

Yang R-S, Lin W-L, Chen Y-Z, Tang C-H, Huang T-H, Lu B-Y & Fu W-M. Regulation by ultrasound treatment on the integrin expression and differentiation of osteoblasts. Bone. 2005;36:276-83.

Yavropoulou MP & Yovos JG. The role of the Wnt signaling pathway in osteoblast commitment and differentiation. Hormones. 2007;6:279-94.

Yee KL, Weaver VM & Hammer DA. Integrin-mediated signalling through the MAP-kinase pathway. IET Syst Biol. 2008;2:8-15.

Yokota H & Tanaka SM. Osteogenic potentials with joint-loading modality. J Bone Miner Metab. 2005;23:302-8.

You J, Reilly GC, Zhen X, Yellowley CE, Chen Q, Donahue HJ & Jacobs CR. Osteopontin gene regulation by oscillary fluid flow via intracellular calcium mobilization and activation of mitogen-activated protein kinase in MC3T3-E1 osteoblasts. J Biol Chem. 2001;276:13365-71.

You L, Cowin SC, Schaffler MB & Weinbaum S. A model for strain amplification in the actin cytoskeleton of osteocytes due to fluid drag on pericellular matrix. J Biomech. 2001;34:1375-1386.

8

Biological Response of Osteoblasts and Osteoprogenitors to Orthopaedic Wear Debris

Richard Chiu and Stuart B. Goodman
Stanford University Medical School, Department of Orthopaedic Surgery, USA

1. Introduction

Total joint replacements are one of the most commonly performed orthopaedic procedures worldwide, with over 700,000 surgeries performed annually in the US to treat arthritic conditions of the hip and knee. One of the major complications of total joint replacement is implant wear and osteolysis, a process that involves continuous shedding of micron- and submicron-sized particles from implant components. Implant particles elicit cascades of inflammatory, osteolytic, and granulomatous reactions from macrophages, osteoclasts, and fibroblasts, causing the prosthesis to become unstable. Since the mid 1990s, in vitro studies have shown that wear debris particles inhibit the osteogenic function of osteoblasts and osteoprogenitor cells of human and rodent species. Osteolysis and implant loosening involve not only increased bone resorption by osteoclasts and inflammatory cells, but also reduced bone formation by osteoblasts and their progenitors. This disruption of proliferation, differentiation, function, and survival of osteoblasts prevents the implant from properly integrating with surrounding bone.

The inhibitory effects of implant wear debris on osteoblasts and osteoprogenitors have been demonstrated using particles of metallic (titanium, cobalt chrome), polymeric (polyethylene, PMMA), and ceramic (alumina, zirconia) implants. Human and rodent primary osteoblasts and osteoblast cell lines, such as MG-63 cells, treated with titanium and polyethylene particles in culture, uniformly show reduced type I collagen synthesis with evidence of particle phagocytosis and morphological changes consistent with cell injury and cytoskeletal disorganization on microscopy. Selected studies also show that particles impair osteoblast viability, proliferation, adhesion, extracellular matrix production, and osteogenic protein expression (e.g., alkaline phosphatase). Implant particles uniformly stimulate expression of NF-κB and IL-6, IL-8, PGE_2, RANKL, M-CSF, and MCP-1, pro-inflammatory factors known to recruit monocyte-macrophages or induce osteoclast differentiation and activity. These studies also indicate that the effect of particles on osteoblasts depends on particle size and composition and the maturational state of the cell. Metal implants such as cobalt chromium and titanium alloys pose an additional risk of metal ion toxicity.

Wear debris particles also inhibit the osteogenic activity of osteoprogenitors and marrow stromal cells (MSCs). Human bone marrow-derived MSCs exposed to titanium particles exhibit reduced proliferation, type I collagen expression, viability, and matrix mineralization with evidence of particle phagocytosis and structural and biochemical changes indicative of apoptosis. The exposure of human MSCs to BMP-6, FGF-2, IGF-1, and TGF-β1, factors with trophic, osteogenic, and prosurvival effects, partly mitigates the inhibitory effects of titanium particles. Studies have shown that PMMA particles inhibit the osteogenic differentiation of mouse and human bone marrow-derived MSCs and murine MC3T3-E1 pre-osteoblasts. When exposed to PMMA particles, these cells show a dose-dependent decrease in proliferation, alkaline phosphatase expression, and matrix mineralization. MC3T3-E1 cells also show reduced viability and expression of osteogenic transcription factors Runx2, osterix, and Dlx5, and changes in expression patterns of MAP kinase signaling molecules. Treating MC3T3-E1 cells with OP-1 (BMP-7) partly mitigates the inhibitory effect of PMMA particles. Polyethylene particles (ultrahigh molecular weight) also inhibit the osteogenic differentiation of mouse MSCs and MC3T3-E1 cells in a similar fashion. Phagocytosis of implant particles by MSCs and osteoprogenitors mediates the inhibitory effects and causes morphological changes indicative of cell damage.

Biological responses of osteoblasts and osteoprogenitors to orthopaedic wear debris have been studied in vitro and in vivo. In vitro studies have used osteoblast cell lines or primary osteoblasts isolated from human trabecular bone or rat calvarium, and MSCs and osteoprogenitors derived from bone marrow of human or mouse femur and tibia. Orthopaedic particles are obtained from commercial sources or extracted from membrane tissues or synovial fluids of failed hip or knee replacements or serum of in vitro wear simulator tests. In vivo tissue responses to wear debris particles have been studied with the femoral intramedullary injection model or the bone harvest and drug test chambers. Clinically, the inhibition of osteoblast function and differentiation by implant wear debris reduces bone formation in the prosthetic bed and predisposes the implant toward accelerated osteolysis. The inhibitory effects of wear particles appear to be partly mitigated by growth factors with trophic and osteogenic effects. Prevention strategies and therapies for osteolysis and implant loosening will involve development of wear-resistant biomaterials and pharmagolocial modalities for increasing bone formation in the implant.

2. Total joint arthroplasty

Total joint arthroplasty is the surgical replacement of a diseased, dysfunctional joint with a prosthetic joint. In the United States alone, over 400,000 total knee and 300,000 total hip replacements are performed annually to treat joint diseases such as osteoarthritis, rheumatoid arthritis, osteonecrosis, and arthritic conditions caused by autoimmunity, trauma, crystal deposits, or hip dysplasia. In arthritis, the layer of articular cartilage in the joint is worn away by the disease process, exposing the underlying bone to friction and causing the joint to become inflamed, painful, and stiff. When conservative measures such as anti-inflammatory drugs, corticosteroids, physical therapy, and joint preserving procedures fail to relieve pain and restore function, joint replacement is considered the next line of treatment. The procedure effectively alleviates pain and restores joint function, and is associated with an implant survival rate of at least 90% at 10 years. Elderly and middle-aged persons constitute the great majority of patients and are considered better candidates than younger persons given that lower physical activity prolongs the longevity of the implant. Since the introduction of the modern arthroplasty in the 1960s, the procedure has benefited millions of patients in the United States and worldwide.

The modern arthroplasty is a modular system composed of separable components. This modularity allows the surgeon to tailor the prosthesis to match the patient's requirements, or to replace components without removing the entire implant when the need for revision surgery arises. The current orthopaedic market offers a large range of prosthetic components based on different surgeon preferences for implant materials, designs, wear properties, and fixation techniques, and considerations for patient age, anatomy, bone stock, and activity level. The modern arthroplasty is based on a prototypical design in which two metal units articulate with an intervening cushion that is a plastic spacer that serves as a low-friction surface. Using total hip arthroplasty as an example, the prosthesis generally consists of four components: a round, highly polished femoral head made of cobalt chromium alloy that articulates with a concave acetabular liner made of ultrahigh molecular weight polyethylene in a "ball and socket" fashion; a femoral stem made of cobalt chromium or titanium alloy inserted into the medullary canal of the femur; and a dome-shaped acetabular shell made also of cobalt chromium or titanium alloy that provides a platform for fixing the acetabular liner to the acetabulum via screws, pegs, and roughened, coated, or porous surfaces. The sizes and diameters of the modular components are chosen such that the acetabular liner fits precisely in the acetabular shell and the femoral head in the concavity of the acetabular liner. Implant materials must withstand cyclic forces and not fail under load, meaning they must have appropriately high tensile, compressive, yield, shear, and fatigue strengths.

Metals commonly used in joint implants include pure titanium, titanium alloy with 6% aluminium and 4% vanadium (Ti-6Al-4V), and cobalt alloy with 27-30% chromium and 5-7% molybdenum (Co-Cr-Mo). These metals are chosen based on their light weight, biocompatibility (lack of reaction to body fluids and tissues), corrosion resistance, and ability to integrate with adjacent bone. Cobalt chromium alloy is additionally characterized by high tensile strength, toughness, and resistance to wear, fatigue, and fracture, which makes it a highly suitable material for articulating surfaces. The incorporation of molybdenum into the cobalt chromium alloy increases its strength and corrosion resistance. Titanium metals are relatively light (density 4.5 g/cm^3) and are also corrosion resistant due to a protective oxide layer (TiO_2) that forms on its surface. However, because of their lower shear strength, surface hardness, and wear resistance than cobalt chromium alloys, titanium metals are used mainly for the femoral stem and acetabular shell, while cobalt chromium is used for the femoral head. Stainless steel grades 316 and 316L are also used in joint replacements, but mainly as screws, plates, and rods for implant fixation due to their greater tendency to corrode and leach toxic substances than cobalt chromium or titanium alloys. Cobalt chromium alloy and titanium metals have served as successful femoral implants since their introduction in the 1960s. Newer alloys are currently available and hope to improve on the properties of conventional alloys. Issues exist however, regarding wear debris production, which is the focus of this chapter.

Ultrahigh molecular weight polyethylene (UHMWPE) is the main polymer used in joint implants (Kurtz, 2004). Polyethylene molecules of this molecular weight range are 3 to 6 million daltons, approximately 10 times that of conventional polyethylene molecules. UHMWPE solid is characterized by low friction, biocompatibility, and high toughness, impact and tensile strength, and wear resistance. Because of these qualities, UHMWPE is used as the articulating material in almost all joint prostheses, including those of the shoulder, elbow, and ankle. UHMWPE derives it strength from its large molecules which exert a vast degree of van der Waals forces between its linearly aligned molecules. In addition, the large size of UHMWPE molecules causes less efficient packing, which yields lower density and crystallinity. These properties are also beneficial to its clinical performance since lower density decreases weight, and lower crystallinity increases resistance to cracks and wear. The strength and wear properties of UHMWPE are also affected by cross-linking between molecules, with greater cross-linking improving strength, toughness, and wear resistance. This has led to the development of highly cross-linked UHMWPE, which consists of highly branched polyethylene molecules. Cross-linking between the branched molecules is induced by irradiation of the material at high gamma doses (50,000 to 150,000 Gy), often followed by annealing. Different cross-linking protocols exist, resulting in variance in mechanical properties. Wear experiments have shown that cross-linked material has significantly lower wear rates compared to conventional UHMWPE; however clinical studies are needed to evaluate its performance in patients in the long term. Ten year wear rates have been extremely encouraging. Conventional UHMWPE has served as an excellent load-bearing material in the past four decades. Despite its excellent wear properties, however, it continues to be the main source of wear debris particles that elicit chronic inflammation and osteolysis.

Polymethylmethacrylate (PMMA) bone cement is used as a grout for fixing prosthetic components such as the femoral stem or acetabular shell to adjacent bone. Prostheses can be anchored to bone by cementless or cemented techniques. Although the choice of cementless versus cemented fixation is dependent on the surgeon, cementless fixation is generally preferred for younger patients with good bone stock, while cemented fixation is preferred by some older patients with poor bone stock. Cementless prostheses employ roughened or porous surfaces for long-term bone ingrowth and implant stability. The porous coating in a femoral stem, for instance, may extend over the entire length of the implant or only over the metaphyseal and proximal diaphyseal areas. Bone ingrowth into porous coatings takes place over weeks or months to achieve fixation. In cemented arthroplasties, powder is mixed with a monomer solution to form a polymer. The cement fills spaces between implant and bone and then solidifies in an exothermic process. Bone cement is most commonly applied to the femoral stem to achieve fixation with surrounding bone. PMMA is usually mixed with radiopacifiers such as barium sulfate to make it visible on radiograph, and sometimes with antibiotics to prevent infection. Although highly successful as a grouting agent, PMMA has good compressive strength but relatively poor fatigue and shear strength under load. PMMA may also leach monomers and cause surrounding thermal necrosis that can induce formation of fibrous tissue layer at the bone implant interface.

Ceramic materials, alumina (aluminum oxide Al_2O_3) and zirconia (zirconium oxide ZrO_2), have been used as alternatives to metal alloys and polyethylene for weight-beaing surfaces because of their high wear resistance, low friction, hardness, and biocompatibility. Interest in ceramics has arisen from the issue of wear debris production from conventional metal-on-polyethylene surfaces and the search for better wear-resistant materials. Experiments have shown that ceramics outperform metals and polyethylene in this respect. Ceramic-on-ceramic articulations show significantly lower coefficients of friction and wear rates than conventional metal-on-polyethylene articulations. Ceramic wear debris particles are also reported to be less bioreactive and inflammatory than metal or polyethylene debris. Despite their low wear and friction, ceramics are brittle and prone to fracture or cracking. For this reason, ceramic implants are considered mainly for younger patients because they benefit more from the reduced rates of wear debris production. Alumina is now the main ceramic available in the orthopaedic market. Alternative bearing combinations reported to have lower wear rates are ceramic-on-polyethylene and metal-on-metal articulations, though the long-term clinical performance of these implants need to be assessed, particularly with respect to wear, osteolysis, metal ion toxicity, and adverse tissue reactions.

The modern total knee arthroplasty is modular and consists of distal femoral and proximal tibial components made of cobalt chromium or titanium alloy, and a UHMWPE tibial insert in between that articulates with the femoral component. The distal femoral component is round-ended resembling the shape of the femoral condyles; the proximal tibial component has a flat top which holds the UHMWPE tibial insert, and a stemmed bottom for insertion in the tibial medullary cavity. Like hip arthroplasties, knee implants can be cementless or cemented, the choice of which is surgeon-dependent, and older patients > 70 years of age have longer implant survival than young patients due to lower physical activity. Cementless knee implants contain porous coatings that allow bone ingrowth. However, unlike hip arthroplasties, cementless knee implants are less desirable than cemented ones due to the higher incidence of tibial loosening and polyethylene wear. Total shoulder arthroplasties are designed much like the hip prosthesis: they consist of modular units and are based on a humeral stem that articulates with a glenoid implant in a "hemisphere-socket" fashion. The shoulder prosthesis can also take form of a normal or reverse shoulder design. In the normal shoulder design, the humeral stem is connected to convex humeral head, which articulates with a concave glenoid implant. In the reverse shoulder design, the humeral stem is connected to a humeral neck with a concave surface that articulates with a convex "glenoid sphere," which in turn is linked to a glenoid fixation implant. In both designs, a low-friction UHMWPE insert is cushioned between the articulating "concave-convex" units, similar to the hip and knee prostheses. The humeral stem and neck and glenoid fixation devices are made of cobalt chromium or titanium metal, while the highly polished humeral head and glenoid sphere are made of cobalt chromium. The glenoid fixation device is attached to glenoid cavity with compression screws. Like hip and knee prostheses, shoulder implants can be cementless or cemented. Cementless shoulder implants have porous coatings for bone ingrowth or holes for screw fixation. Cement may be applied to humeral and glenoid implants when bone is fragile. Arthroplasties of other joints such as the elbow and ankle employ the same design of two metal components articulating on a UHMWPE insert.

Clinical complications that are common to all total joint arthroplasties include implant fracture, infection, dislocation, nerve palsy, vascular injury, thromboembolism, and most importantly, *osteolysis and aseptic loosening* caused by biological reactions to *particulate debris* produced from *implant wear*. The rest of this chapter will be devoted to issues concerning wear, osteolysis, and implant loosening, which are the most common and important reason arthroplasties are brought in for revision surgery. Currently, 10% of all total hip and knee replacements succumb to this complication at 10 years. Revision arthroplasties are much more difficult to perform and have a substantially lower implant survival rate than the primary arthroplasty.

3. Implant wear and osteolysis

One of the most significant clinical complications of total joint arthroplasty is implant loosening and osteolysis associated with wear debris (Wright & Goodman, 2001). This scenario accounts for the majority of revision surgeries performed for failed hip and knee implants. Approximately 80,000 revision surgeries are performed annually in the United States for loosening and osteolysis of the hip and knee. Symptoms associated with osteolysis such as pain and decreasing function usually do not appear until the lesion is fairly advanced radiographically. Revision surgery is aimed at replacing loose implant units, removing diseased tissues and debris particles, repairing bone defects caused by osteolysis, thus relieving pain and restoring function. Revision surgeries are more costly, harder to perform, and less successful than the primary surgery.

Osteolysis is caused by particulate debris generated from wear between implant components, particularly by those of load-bearing, articulating surfaces such as the UHMWPE acetabular liner and cobalt chromium femoral head of a hip prosthesis, or the tibial UHMWPE insert and cobalt chromium femoral components of a knee prosthesis. Wear at these articulating surfaces can produce up to hundreds of millions of submicron particles each year. Wear particles migrate through interfaces between implant, cement, and bone, screw holes, or crevices in these materials to enter surrounding tissue. Osteolysis of the hip, for instance, occurs in the acetabulum behind the acetabular shell where wear particles can access peri-implant tissues through screw holes or interfaces of the polyethylene liner, and along the endosteal margins of the femoral medullary canal directly exposed to particles. Wear debris is also produced from non-articulating surfaces, such as backside wear between UHMWPE insert and acetabular shell or tibial tray, micro-movements at sheared or fractured cement interfaces with implant or bone, or friction around loosened metallic stems or screws. Wear is also accelerated by corrosion, oxidation, or fracture.

The main source of wear debris particles is the UHMWPE insert or liner at the surface of articulation. Although UHMWPE has low friction, high wear resistance, and good impact strength, conventional polyethylene wears at an average linear rate of 0.1-0.2 mm/year, or volumetric wear rate of 50-100 mm^3/year, against cobalt chromium femoral heads. The great majority of UHMWPE wear debris is submicron-sized, more than 90% of which are less than 1.0 μm in diameter, the mean being 0.5 μm. Ceramic particles are on also on the order of 0.5-0.7 μm in diameter. Cobalt chromium and titanium metal wear debris are mostly on the nanometer scale, averaging 50 nm in size, roughly 1/10 the average size of polyethylene debris. Volumetric wear rate of metals is an order of magnitude lower than that UHMWPE, but because the particles are also much smaller in size, the number of particles produced is still significantly greater than that of polyethylene. New bearing surfaces such as highly crosslinked polyethylene, metal-on-metal (cobalt chromium), and ceramic-on-ceramic (alumina), have substantially reduced wear rates as shown by simulator tests and implant retrievals. However, particulate debris of the same size, whether it is polymeric or ceramic, and in most cases of metallic debris, elicits similar biological reactions. The concentration of particles appears to be the strongest factor dictating the degree of inflammation.

Wear debris particles infiltrate surrounding tissue and elicit a cascade of biologic events involving pro-inflammatory factor secretion, fibrous membrane formation, and bone resorption, processes that may culminate in loosening of the prosthesis. These events are mediated by macrophages, osteoclasts, fibroblasts, osteoblasts, and their progenitors (Tuan et al., 2008). The majority of wear particles are submicron to nanometer in size, and the size range of particles capable of activating and being phagocytosed by these cells is about 0.3 to 10 μm. Macrophages resident in peri-prosthetic tissue, also called histiocytes, are the primary cells to react to particles. These cells phagocytose particles and release a multitude of pro-inflammatory cytokines, chemokines, arachidonic acid metabolites, and degradative enzymes. The major cytokines that mediate inflammation and bone destruction are TNF-α, IL-1α, and IL-1β, but others that directly or indirectly increase bone resorption are IL-6, IL-8,

PGE_2, RANKL, M-CSF, GM-CSF, and MCP-1. These cytokines recruit distant inflammatory cells such as neutrophils and monocytes (via IL-8 and MCP-1 respectively), directly stimulate osteoclasts to resorb bone (via IL-6, RANKL, M-CSF), induce the activity of macrophages (via IL-1, GM-CSF, M-CSF), kill bone forming cells (via TNF-α), participate in matrix degradation (via MMP-2, MMP-9), or induce other cells such as osteoblasts to release RANKL, MMPs, collagenases (via IL-1, TNF-α). Macrophage release of proinflammatory factors after particle phagocytosis is mediated by transcription factor NF-κB, which is activated by the upstream MAPK (mitogen-activated protein kinase) pathway. Studies have

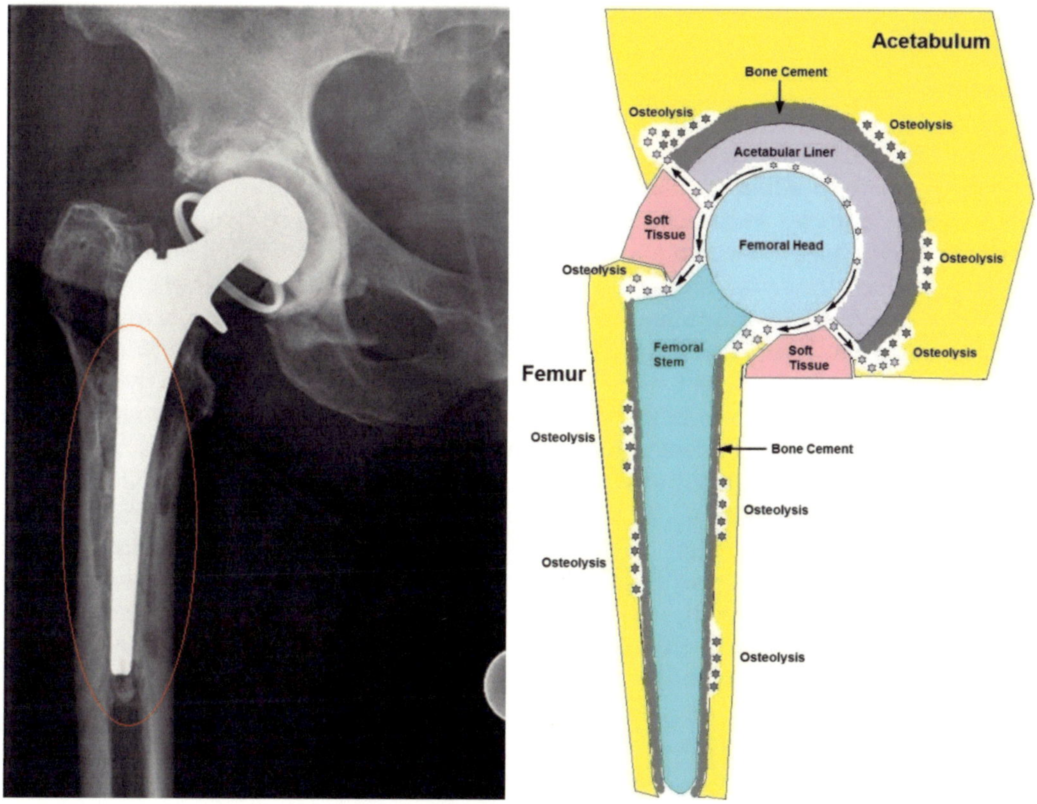

(a) (b)

Fig. 1. (a) Radiograph of a cemented hip prosthesis with osteolysis around the femoral stem due to cement fragmentation (radiolucent areas within the red circled area surrounding the femoral stem). (b) Diagram of a cemented hip prosthesis with osteolysis around the acetabular and femoral implants. Wear particles are represented by small hexagonal stars, and in the illustration, are produced primarily from the acetabular liner (light gray stars liberated from the inner, articulating surface) and bone cement around the acetabular liner and femoral stem (dark gray stars liberated from fragmented cement). Interfaces between implant, bone, and cement serve as conduits for particle migration, as represented by the arrows. Particles can also be produced by the femoral head and stem, which are respectively made of cobalt chromium and titanium alloys. The acetabular liner is most often made of UHMWPE, and in most cases is the main source of wear particles.

shown that surface contact of macrophage membrane with particles of non-phagocytosable size (> 20 μm) is sufficient to trigger an inflammatory response; however, the response elicited is much smaller than that triggered by particle phagocytosis. Other cells recruited to the site of osteolysis include migrated monocyte/macrophages, neutrophils, and lymphocytes; however, it is the macrophage that plays the dominant role in this inflammatory response. In vitro studies have used macrophages from primary sources such as murine peritoneal macrophages and human peripheral blood monocytes, or immortalized cell lines such as Raw267.4 and J774 macrophages. Macrophages are activated by all particle types including titanium, polyethylene, and PMMA, and have in nearly all cases been documented to release cytokines in a dose-dependent manner, with particles in the size range of 0.5 to 10 μm yielding the highest inflammatory response.

Besides invoking inflammation, wear debris particles also indirectly promote the formation and activity of osteoclasts, the primary cells that mediate bone resorption. After phagocytosing particles, macrophages secrete the osteoclastogenic factors RANKL and M-CSF. Furthermore, fibroblasts, osteoblasts, and marrow stromal cells are also capable of phagocytosing particles and releasing RANKL and M-CSF. These two factors stimulate monocyte-macrophage precursors of hematopoietic lineage to differentiate into pre-osteoclasts, which then fuse to become mature osteoclasts capable of resorbing bone and showing phenotypes such as multinucleation and expression of TRAP (tartrate resistant acid phosphatase). Monocytes respond to RANKL via the surface receptor RANK. Monocytes may be resident in peri-implant tissue or recruited from peripheral blood. The ability of monocytes to form bone-resorbing osteoclasts after being challenged with wear debris particles has been well documented with human peripheral blood monocytes and mouse peritoneal macrophages exposed directly to particles in vitro, treated with RANKL and M-CSF, cocultured with particle-treated macrophages, osteoblasts, or marrow stromal cells, or grown in conditioned medium taken from these particle-treated cell cultures. This osteoclastogenic effect is seen with all particle materials, including polyethylene, titanium, and PMMA. A series of studies has shown that osteoclast differentiation from mouse monocytes co-cultured with UMR-106 osteosarcoma cells is potentiated by PMMA particles, as indicated by increased numbers of TRAP-positive cells and resorbed pits in co-cultured bone slices, compared to control monocytes not exposed to PMMA particles (Sabokbar et al., 1996, 1997, 1998). This enhanced osteoclastogenic response was also documented in a similar study which showed that mouse monocytes grown in osteoclastogenic medium containing M-CSF and RANKL yielded higher numbers of TRAP-positive multi-nucleated cells and resorbed pits in co-cultured bone slices when treated with PMMA particles, compared to monocytes grown in the same system but not exposed to PMMA particles (Zhang et al., 2008). Another series of studies has shown that enhanced osteoclastogenesis of mouse monocytes in medium containing M-CSF and RANKL after exposure to PMMA particles involves increased expression and activity of NF-κB (Clohisy et al., 2006), MAP kinases p38, ERK, and JNK (Abbas et al., 2003; Yamanaka et al., 2006), and the transcription factor NFAT (Yamanaka et al., 2008); these enhanced osteoclastogenic responses were respectively abrogated by inhibitors against NF-κB, the MAP kinases, and NFAT. A similar study has also demonstrated that titanium particles enhance NFAT expression in monocyte-derived osteoclasts in medium containing M-CSF and RANKL, a process that was also disrupted using an inhibitor against NFAT (Liu et al., 2009). Osteoclasts are also regulated by osteoblasts, which are a major source of OPG (osteoprotegerin), a soluble receptor that binds to RANKL and prevents it from binding RANK on monocytes. OPG is normally secreted by osteoblasts to inhibit osteoblast formation and activity. TNF-α, IL-1, and PGE_2 increase expression of RANK on monocytes and reduce expression of OPG in osteoblasts. The intracellular effects of RANKL-RANK binding are mediated by the master transcription factor NF-κB. The prevention of RANKL-RANK interactions by knockout methods in mice or by administration of a RANKL antagonist abolishes the osteolytic response to orthopaedic wear particles. IL-1 is another factor important for formation and activity of osteoclasts. Knockout of IL-1 receptors, IL-1RI and IL-1RII, in mice or administration of IL-1 receptor antagonists, also abolishes osteolytic response to particles.

Wear debris also causes the formation of a fibrous, granulomatous tissue membrane around the loosened prosthesis (Goodman, 1994). The membrane stroma is formed from fibroblasts and serves as a support structure for macrophages, osteoblasts, osteoclasts, lymphocytes, and multinucleated/foreign body giant cells. This fibrous membrane is formed from micro-movements at the bone-implant interface, and not only harbours these cells, but serves as a conduit for particle migration and inflammatory mediators. Granulomas in the membrane are clusters of macrophages and fibroblasts mixed within collagen deposits, and represent an attempt to wall off foreign material that it cannot destroy. Tissues retrieved from failed implants and cultured in vitro release high quantities of TNF-α, IL-1, IL-6, IL-8, PGE_2, RANKL, M-CSF, MCP-1, MMPs, collagenases, the same factors released by macrophages, osteoblasts, osteoclasts, and fibroblasts when treated individually with particles in vitro. In vitro fibroblast studies have been conducted with primary human or mouse foreskin and synovial fibroblasts, mouse calvarial and neonatal fibroblasts, and fibroblast cell lines. Fibroblasts produce the same inflammatory and osteoclastogenic factors as macrophages and osteoblasts, such as IL-6, RANKL, PGE_2, which are capable of stimulating osteoclast formation in co-cultures with monocytes.

Metal particles can potentially exert a toxic ion effect on cells. Unlike polyethylene and ceramics, metals such as titanium, cobalt chromium, and stainless steel potentially dissolve into metal ions, albeit very slowly. The high surface area-volume ratio of the predominantly nanometer-sized metal particles facilitates their dissolution into ions. Metals can also undergo corrosion and oxidation, especially in the physiological environment of the body. Aluminium, vanadium, and nickel in alloys also have the potential to produce small particles and ions. High concentrations of metal ions have been detected in joint fluid and tissues retrieved from failed implants. These metal ions may trigger a cytotoxic or hypersensitivity reaction from tissues in vivo. Metal hypersensitivity has been reported to be as high as 50-60% in patients with failed implants, whereas it is only 10-15% in the general population. Metal ion toxicity has been demonstrated in vitro with metal salts such as $CoCl_2$, $CrCl_3$, and $CrCl_6$, on murine macrophages and osteoblasts, which show reduced cell viability. In these studies, cobalt ions have proven to be the most toxic, while ions of titanium, chromium, and aluminum are relatively well tolerated. Metal ions can remain in body fluid as soluble ions, precipitate as insoluble metal salts or oxides, chelate with organic anions to form organometallic complexes, or be stored and transported by carriers like hemosiderin. Elevated ion levels may be detected in local tissue, serum, and urine; they may also be transported to distant organs via the bloodstream. The organs of patients with failed implants show high levels of cobalt and chromium in serum, liver, spleen, kidney, and lymphatic tissues. Cobalt chromium alloy is most resistant to wear and corrosion (it dissolves at a linear rate of about 50 nm per year), while stainless steel corrodes more easily. Titanium alloy is softer and wears more easily, hence it is not used as articulating surface but as stem components. Inflammation and osteolysis of implants yields a locally acidic environment which accelerates the rate of wear and corrosion. Although in vivo studies in rats and dogs have shown that cobalt chromium and stainless steel implants yield a slightly higher incidence of sarcomas, this has not been demonstrated in humans. Chronic metal ion toxicity may be exacerbated in the presence of renal failure.

Immune reactions associated with wear debris particles can be augmented by the presence of bacterial lipopolysaccharides (LPS) or endotoxin, which are molecules that can independently induce inflammation (Greenfield et al., 2008). Endotoxin adheres to implant surfaces, and may be introduced into the joint by contaminated implants or via circulation from distant sites of infection. Endotoxin may accumulate on the implant and accelerate the process of inflammation and osteolysis. Monocyte macrophages, in particular, respond to endotoxin by releasing pro-inflammatory mediators and inducing osteoclast formation and activity. Osteoblasts respond to endotoxin with diminished proliferation, collagen synthesis, and differentiation. Endotoxin has been found in tissues of failed implants, more frequently in patients with inflammatory arthritis such as rheumatoid arthritis.

4. Biological response of osteoblasts

Osteoblasts in peri-implant tissue deposit bone and are responsible for ensuring osseointegration of the implant. Continual exposure of osteoblasts to wear particles impairs their function and shifts bone metabolism in favor of increased bone resorption and decreased bone formation. In vitro studies have shown that implant wear debris not only induces inflammatory, osteolytic, and granulomatous reactions, but also affects osteoblasts by disrupting their proliferation, survival, adhesion, extracellular matrix synthesis, and cytokine release profile. These results have been demonstrated with metal, polyethylene, cement, and ceramic particles on osteoblasts from primary sources and osteoblast cell lines. Osteoblasts can phagocytose particles less than 10 μm in size. Internalized particles cause damage to intracellular organelles and disrupt cytoskeletal networks, leading to cell death and loss of ability to proliferate and synthesize matrix proteins such as collagen and proteoglycans. Osteoblasts normally interact with osteoclasts in a delicate balance via secreted factors RANKL and OPG, but during inflammatory states induced by particles, they secrete higher levels of RANKL, inflammatory mediators such as IL-6 and PGE_2, and chemokines such as IL-8 and MCP-1. The response of osteoblasts to particles differs according to particle size, shape, material composition, and number, and the maturational state of the osteoblast. Table 1 summarizes the findings of selected in vitro osteoblast studies.

Orthopaedic wear particles less than 10 μm in size are universally phagocytosed by osteoblasts. Although cell surface contact with particles of non-phagocytosable size (e.g., > 20 μm) is reported to elicit some degree of inflammation from osteoblasts, the adverse reactions of osteoblasts to phagocytosable particles is much greater. Particle phagocytosis is generally regarded as the first step for triggering adverse reactions from these cells, as all studies involving osteoblasts and implant particles less than 10 μm have reported phagocytosis (Pioletti et al., 1999, 2002; Vermes et al., 2001; Yao et al., 1997). Particle

Author	Year	Particle (Size)	Cell Type	Outcomes
Allen	1997	CoCr (14.37 ± 5.89 μm) Co (4.75 ± 4.16 μm) Cr (1.89 ± 1.58 μm)	MG63, SaOS-2	alkaline phosphatase (↓), osteocalcin (↓), viability (↓ for Co only), collagen I (↓ for Co only)
Yao	1997	Ti (91% < 3 μm) Ti (21-85 μm)* PolS (1.14 ± 0.007 μm) PolS (21.1 ± 4.09 μm)*	MG63, HOS	procollagen I and III (↓), collagen I (↓), proliferation (-), viability (-), particle phagocytosis(+)
Martinez	1998a	UHMWPE (20-200 μm)*	PHO	procollagen I (↓), alkaline phosphatase (↑), osteocalcin (↑)
Martinez	1998b	UHMWPE (< 160 μm)*	PHO	proliferation (↓)
Zambonin	1998	PMMA (70% < 10 μm)	PHO	proliferation (↓), collagen I (↓), osteocalcin (↑), IL-6 (↑)
Dean	1999a	UHMWPE (90% < 1.5 μm)	MG63	proliferation (↑), collagen (↓), alkaline phosphatase (↓), osteocalcin (↓), proteoglycan (↓), PGE2 (↑
Dean	1999b	UHMWPE (1.0 ± 0.96 μm)	MG63	proliferation (↑), alkaline phosphatase (↓), proteoglycan (↓), PGE2 (↑), TGFβ1 (↓), osteocalcin (-)
Pioletti	1999	Ti (3.1 ± 3.6 μm)	RatNC	viability (↓), particle phagocytosis (+), apoptosis (+), soluble cytotoxic factors
Heinemann	2000	Ti6Al4V (1-3 μm)	PHO, MG63	particle phagocytosis (+)
Kwon	2000	Ti (80% < 5 μm, 1-10 μm)	RatNC	adhesion (↓)
Lohmann	2000	Ti (0.84 ± 0.12 μm) Ti6Al4V (1.35 ± 0.09 μm) CoCr (1.21 ± 0.16 μm) UHMWPE (1.0 ± 0.96 μm)	MG63, PHO	alkaline phosphatase (↓), PGE2 (↑), intracellular organelle damage (+), proliferation (↑ for MG63)
Shida	2000	Ti (1-3 μm)	MG63	IL-6 (↑), particle phagocytosis (+), NF-κB and NF-IL-6 binding (+)
Takei	2000	Ti (80% < 5 μm)	MG63, SaOS-2	proliferation (↓), alkaline phosphatase (↓), IL-6 (↑), conditioned medium effect (-)
Vermes	2000	Ti (1-3 μm) Ti6Al4V (90% < 3 μm) UHMWPE (90% < 3 μm) PolS (1.14 ± 0.01 μm) Ti (21-85 μm)* PolS (21.1 ± 4.1 μm)*	MG-63, PHO SaOS-2, HOS	procollagen I and III (↓), collagen I (↓), IL-6 (↑), particle phagocytosis (+), NF-κB binding (↑), TNF-α (-), IL-1α (-), IL-1β (-), osteonectin (-), osteocalcin (-), alkaline phosphatase (-)
Dean	2001	UHMWPE (0.46-1.26 μm)	MG63	proliferation (↑), PGE2 (↑), alkaline phosphatase (↓)
Kwon	2001	Ti (80% < 5 μm, 1-10 μm)	RatNC	adhesion (↓), proliferation (↓)
Roebuck	2001	Ti (94% < 3 μm)	MG63	NF-κB binding (↑), PTK activity (↑)
Rodrigo	2001	UHMWPE (20-200 μm)**	PHO	procollagen (↓), alkaline phosphatase (-)
Vermes	2001	Ti (1-3 μm) Ti6Al4V (90% < 3 μm) UHMWPE (90% < 3 μm) PolS (1.14 ± 0.01 μm)	MG63	procollagen I (↓), proliferation (↓), IL-6 (↑), viability (-), particle phagocytosis (+), TNF-α (-), IL-1 (-), osteonectin (-), osteocalcin (-), alkaline phosphatase (-)
Fritz	2002	Ti (94% < 3 μm)	MG63, PHO	IL-8 (↑), MCP-1 (↑), NF-κB binding (↑)
Lohmann	2002a	UHMWPE (1.0 ± 0.96 μm)	MG63, OCT-1, MLO-Y4	PGE2 (↑), osteocalcin (-), proliferation (↑ for MG63, - for OCT1, ↓ for MLO-Y4), NO production (- for MG63, ↑ for OCT1, ↑ for MLO-Y4)
Lohmann	2002b	PMMA (2.22 ± 007 μm) Al2O3 (1.09 ± 0.15 μm) ZrO2 (1.84 ± 0.04 μm)	MG63	PGE2 (↑), proliferation (↓ for Al2O3, ↑ for ZrO2 and PMMA), alkaline phosphatase (↓ for Al2O3, ↑ for ZrO2 and PMMA)
Pioletti	2002	Ti (10% < 10 μm)* PMMA (10% < 10 μm)*	MG63, SaOS2, RatNC	apoptosis (+), particle phagocytosis (+), cytoskeletal disruption (+)
Rodrigo	2002	HDPE (< 5 μm) Al2O3 (< 5 μm)	PHO	IL-6 (↑)
Granchi	2004	UHMWPE (0.1-1.0 μm) Al2O3 (1.0 μm mean)	PHO	IL-6 (↑), RANKL (↑), OPG (↓ for UHMWPE, ↑ for Al2O3), GM-CSF (-), TNF-α (-), viability (-)
O'Conner	2004	Ti (< 1.5, 1.5-4, 5-9 μm)	RatNC	proliferation (↓), viability (↓), particle phagocytosis (+), cytoskeletal disruption (+)
Pioletti	2004	Ti (4.5 μm mean)	PHO	RANKL and CSF-1 (↑), OPG (-)
Ciapetti	2005	FeAlCr (3.4-7.5 μm) Ti6Al4V (150 μm mean)	SaOS-2	particle phagocytosis (+), viability (↓), proliferation (↓), Al and Cr ion (+)
Fritz	2005	Ti (94% < 3 μm)	MG63	NF-κB binding (↑), ERK1/2 and JNK 1/2 activation (↑)
Granchi	2005	UHMWPE (0.1-1.0 μm) Al2O3 (1.0 μm mean)	PHO	RANKL (↑ for UHMWPE only), OPG (↓ for UHMWPE only)
Peter	2005	Ti (4.5 μm mean)	MG63, MC3T3E1	alkaline phosphatase (↓)
Friz	2006	Ti (94% < 3 μm)	MG63, PHO	IL-8 (↑), MCP-1 (↑), NF-κB binding (↑)
Ramachandran	2006	Ti (4-10 μm) PMMA (1-10 μm)	MG63	NO production (-), viability (-), alkaline phosphatase (-), osteocalcin (-)
Valles	2008	Ti (3.32 ± 2.39 μm) TiO2 (0.45 ± 0.26 μm)	PHO	IL-6 (↑), PGE2 (↑), RANKL (-), OPG (+/-), GM-CSF (+/-), viability (-)
Kanaji	2009	CoCrMo (0.5-10 μm)	MLO-Y4	TNF-α (↑), IL-6 (↓), caspase-3 and caspase-7 (↑)
Lenz	2009	Ti (3 μm mean) ZrO2 (1.75 ± 4.66 μm) Ti6Al7Nb (3.46-4.44 μm mean) CoCrMo (2.81-3.24 μm mean)	PHO	viability (↓), collagen I (↓)

Table 1. Summary of implant particle effects on osteoblasts. Studies are listed in in chronological order. Abbreviations: Ti = titanium particles, Ti6Al4V = titanium alloy particles, UHMWPE = ultrahigh molecular weight polyethylene particles, PMMA = polymethylmethacrylate particles, CoCr (CoCrMo) = cobalt chromium alloy particles, PolS= polystyrene particles, Al2O3 = aluminium oxide/alumina particles, ZrO2 = zirconium oxide/zirconia particles, FeAlCr= iron alloy particles, HDPE = high density polyethylene particles, TiO2 = titanium oxide (rutile) particles, RatNC = neonatal rat calvarial osteoblasts, PHO = primary human osteoblasts. Osteoblast cell lines are represented as MG-63, SaOS-2,

HOS, OCT-1, MLO-Y4. Signs: (↓) indicates decrease, (↑) indicates increase, (+) indicates presence of, (-) indicates no change, (+/-) indicates small increase, asterix * indicates particles are of non-phagocytosable size.

internalization can be visualized using fluoresceinated particles such as Fluoresbrite (polystyrene-based fluorescent particles). Fluoresbrite particles have been used to demonstrate that phagocytosis occurs mostly within 24 hours of in vitro exposure, and that cells become saturated with these particles (0.926 ± 0.027 μm in size) at 40-60 particles/cell, a quantity that can be determined by plotting the fluorescence of particles extracted from lysed cells against a fluorescence intensity standard curve of known Fluoresbrite numbers (Vermes et al. 2001). Fluorescence and transmission electron microscopy and energy-dispersive x-ray analysis have been used to reveal that osteoblasts with internalized particles have evidence of damage to cell membranes, mitochonrdria, endoplasmic reticulum, and Golgi bodies, and ultrastructural changes indicative of cytotoxicity (Lohmann et al., 2000, 2002b). These morphological changes have been observed with titanium, titanium alloy, cobalt chromium alloy, UHMWPE, PMMA, and alumina particles. Fluorescence microscopy has been used to visualize the organization of actin filaments stained with rhodamine phalloidin assembled around internalized implant particles, as compared to healthy cells in which actin filaments organize around the nucleus (Kwon et al., 2000). The requirement of phagocytosis is proven with the use of cytochalasin D, a fungal substance that prevents actin filament assembly, a process required for cell division, phagocytosis, and formation of cytoplasmic extensions. Osteoblasts pre-treated with cytochalasin D at 1-5 μM are prevented from phagocytosing particles and show lower degrees of IL-8 release (Fritz et al., 2006), cytotoxicity and apoptosis (Pioletti et al., 1999), and inhibition of procollagen type I expression (Vermes et al., 2000, 2001) compared to particle-treated osteoblasts not exposed to cytochalasin D. Phagocytosed particles can also be visualized by confocal microscopy (Valles et al., 2008; Yao et al., 1997); light and phase contrast microscopy can be used to crudely visualize particles floating within individual cells in cell culture or suspension. Particles of non-phagocytosable sizes induce lower degrees of adverse effects from osteoblasts. Titanium particles > 20 μm for instance do not effectively inhibit collagen and procollagen synthesis as particles < 10 μm (Vermes et al., 2000; Yao et al., 1997). Studies have indicated that particles 0.1-1.0 μm are most deleterious to osteoblasts. Scanning electron microscopy has revealed that particulate materials generated from implant wear vary more greatly in shape than commercially produced particles, and are more detrimental or inflammatory to osteoblasts. UHMWPE debris particles generated from wear simulator tests or retrieved from failed hip arthroplasties for instance, can be round, oblong, or thin and fibril-like, with irregular grainy surfaces (Dean et al., 1999b), while commercially produced polymeric particles such as PMMA or polystyrene, are mostly spherical.

Depressed type I collagen synthesis is universally observed in osteoblasts exposed to implant wear debris in MG-63, SaOS-2, human osteogenic sarcoma, and primary human osteoblasts treated with titanium, titanium alloy, cobalt chromium, PMMA, UHMWPE, or polystyrene particles (Dean et al., 1999a; Lenz et al., 2009; Vermes et al., 2000, 2001; Yao et al., 1997; Zambonin et al., 1998). These studies reveal a clear dose-dependent decrease in collagen mRNA and protein synthesis over at least a 72 hour period. The inhibitory effects on collagen are related to particle size and dose, but not to the material composition of the particles. Particles are reported to affect the production of other osteoblast proteins, though these reports differ in whether particles inhibit or stimulate this process. A series of studies has reported that submicron-sized UHMWPE particles dose-dependently inhibit the production of alkaline phosphatase, osteocalcin, and proteoglycans (Dean et al., 1999a, 1999b, 2001). Another study with metal particles including titanium, titanium alloy, or cobalt chromium has shown that these materials dose-dependently reduce alkaline phosphatase activity in MG-63 and primary human osteoblasts (Lohmann et al., 2000). However, another series of studies did not report that particles of titanium, titanium alloy, UHMWPE, or polystyrene affected the production of alkaline phosphatase, osteocalcin, or osteonectin in MG-63, SaOS-2, or primary human osteoblasts (Vermes et al., 2000, 2001). Yet other studies have shown that these responses vary with particle material composition; for instance, these studies have shown that PMMA particles increase production of alkaline phosphatase and osteocalcin respectively in MG-63 cells and primary human osteoblasts (Lohmann et al., 2002b; Zambonin et al., 1998), and that alumina particles decrease while ziconia particles increase alkaline phosphatass production in MG-63 cells (Lohmann et al., 2002b).

Orthopedic wear particles are reported to affect the proliferation of osteoblasts. However, reports differ as to whether particles inhibit or stimulate their proliferation. One study reported that proliferation of MG-63 osteoblasts was inhibited dose-dependently when treated with titanium, titanium alloy, UHMWPE, and polystyrene particles (Vermes et al., 2001); other studies showed that titanium particles dose-dependently inhibited the proliferation of neonatal rat calvarial osteoblasts (Kwon et al., 2001) and MG-63 and SaOS-2 osteoblasts over a 72 hr period (Takei et al., 2000). The inhibitory effects of titanium particles were stronger on SaOS-2 cells than MG-63 cells (Takei et al., 2000), suggesting that different maturational states affected the degree of sensitivity to particles. PMMA particles were also shown to decrease proliferation of primary human osteoblasts (Zambonin et al., 1998). Some studies however, reported that wear particles stimulated osteoblast proliferation. A series of studies demonstrated that submicron-sized UHMWPE wear particles from failed hip arthroplasties and GUR 4150 wear tests increased dose-dependently the proliferation of MG-63 cells (Dean et al., 1999a, 1999b, 2001). Another study demonstrated that titanium, titanium alloy, cobalt chromium, and UHMWPE particles increased proliferation of MG-63 osteoblasts in a dose-dependent manner (Lohmann 2000). Yet other studies showed that the effects of particles on proliferation varied with particle composition and size, and cell type and maturational state. One such study showed that when challenged with submicron-sized UHMWPE debris, proliferation increased for MG-63 (immature osteoblasts), remained unaffected for OCT-1 (mature secretory osteoblasts), and decreased for MLO-Y4 (osteocytes) cells (Lohmann et al., 2002a). Another study showed that proliferation of MG-63 cells was dose-dependently decreased by alumina particles and increased by PMMA and zirconia particles (Lohmann et al., 2002b). Yet another study showed that UHMWPE particles of higher molecular weight induced proliferation of MG-63 cells more readily than those of lower molecular weight (Dean et al., 2001). The different results for particle effects on proliferation may be due to differences in cell type, maturational state, passage number, health condition, and particle material, size, shape, and dose, as well as specific protocols for the experiments by different groups.

Wear particles are reported to impair osteoblast viability and adhesion. One study has shown that titanium particles dose-dependently decrease the viability of neonatal rat calvarial osteoblasts over 72 hrs (O'Conner et al., 2004; Pioletti et al., 1999, 2002), with evidence of elevated caspase-3 activity and DNA fragmentation indicative of apoptosis (Pioletti et al., 1999, 2002). When cytochalasin D is applied to these cells, the inhibition of particle phagocytosis reduces the amount of cytotoxic cell death (Pioletti et al., 1999). Other studies have shown that cobalt chromium particles cause elevated caspase-3 and -7 activity in MLO-Y4 osteocytes after 24 hrs (Kanaji et al., 2009), and titanium and iron alloy particles cause reduced viability and proliferation in SaOS-2 cells after 48 hrs. However, some studies did not detect significant reductions in viability in MG-63 or primary human osteoblasts exposed to titanium, UHMWPE, polystyrene, or alumina particles (Granchi et al., 2004; Valles et al., 2008; Vermes et al., 2001; Yao et al., 1997). Titanium particles are also reported to impair the adhesion of neonatal rat calvarial osteoblasts in a dose-dependent manner, conducted at the single cell level using a micropipette system to measure detachment force (Kwon et al., 2000), and the strength of osseointegration of titanium alloy rods in the rat tibia (Choi et al., 2005).

Implant wear debris induces osteoblasts to secrete inflammatory cytokines, chemokines, and osteoclastogenic factors, while downregulating growth factors that promote osteoblast growth or inhibit osteoclastogenesis. Osteoblasts exposed to implant particles release factors that promote the following processes: (1) inflammation mediated by IL-6, and PGE_2, upregulated by transcription factor NF-κB activated after particle phagocytosis; (2) chemoattraction of inflammatory cells by IL-8 and MCP-1, which recruit neutrophils and monocyte-macrophages respectively (the latter are precursors to osteoclasts); (3) osteoclast formation and activation induced by M-CSF and RANKL, (the latter binding to the receptor RANK on monocytes, promoting their differentiation into osteoclasts) and diminished expression of OPG (osteoprotegerin) and TGF-β1, factors which suppress osteoclast activity; and (4) matrix degradation by matrix metalloproteinases MMP-2 and MMP-9, and collagenases. IL-6 released by osteoblasts potentiates bone resorption by recruiting osteoclasts and promoting their differentiation and activation. Implant particles activate NF-κB through increased degradation of IκBα, an inhibitor that binds to and prevents NF-κB from translocating from cytosol into the nucleus. Particles decrease osteoblast expression of TGF-β1, a growth factor that stimulates osteoblast proliferation and procollagen I expression and inhibits osteoclastogenesis (Dean et al., 1999b).

Studies universally show that osteoblasts release cytokines that promote inflammation and osteoclastogenesis after exposure to wear particles. RANKL and CSF-1 production by primary human osteoblasts is induced by titanium particles after 24-48 hours of treatment (Pioletti et al., 2002). IL-6 and PGE_2 are released from primary human osteoblasts after exposure to titanium and titanium alloy (Valles et al., 2008; Vermes et al., 2000, 2001), PMMA (Zambonin et al., 1998), and alumina (Rodrigo et al., 2002) particles. Two series of studies have confirmed that UHMWPE particles induce the release of PGE_2 from MG-63 (Dean 1999a, 1999b, 2001), OCT-1, and MLO-Y4 cells (Lohmann et al., 2002a). One of these series has also shown that MG-63 cells release PGE_2 in a dose-dependent manner after exposure to titanium, titanium alloy, cobalt chromium, PMMA, alumina, and zirconia particles (Lohmann et al., 2000, 2002b). Chemokines IL-8 and MCP-1 are dose-dependently released from MG-63 and primary human osteoblasts treated with titanium particles (Fritz et al., 2002, 2006). Some studies, however, have reported that osteoblasts challenged with titanium particles do not release IL-1 or TNF-α (Vermes et al., 2000, 2001) or show no changes in secretion of GM-CSF, RANKL, or OPG unless at high particle doses (Valles et al., 2008). Studies have shown that adherent peripheral blood mononuclear cells (PBMCs) grown in conditioned media taken from osteoblasts treated with UHMWPE particles, are associated with greater numbers of TRAP-positive, multinucleated cells indicative of osteoclasts compared to PBMCs grown in media from control cells not treated with particles, or in media from cells treated with alumina particles (Granchi et al., 2004, 2005). Medium from control cells also induces osteoclast formation, albeit to a lesser extent. ELISA analysis indicates that the OPG-to-RANKL ratio is significantly lower in medium from UHMWPE-treated cells (lower OPG-to-RANKL ratio favors osteoclast formation) compared to that from alumina-treated cells, which is about the same as the OPG-RANKL ratio from control cell medium (Granchi et al., 2004). This induction of osteoclast formation by conditioned media is blocked by anti-RANKL antibodies. OPG levels were negligible (below detectable limits) in UHMWPE-challenged cultures, but remained high in control cell and alumina-treated cultures (Granchi et al., 2004).

Wear debris activates NF-κB and protein tyrosine kinase (PTK) in osteoblasts as the pathway to inflammation and inhibition of collagen synthesis. Titanium particles activate NF-κB nuclear translocation and binding to gene promoters, and induce phosphorylation of PTK at 2 hours post-exposure to titanium particles, as indicated by presence of NF-κB binding complexes and tyrosine-phosphorylated proteins on western blot (Vermes et al., 2000). These studies did not reveal the involvement of alternate pathways such as protein kinase A or C in particle-mediated effects, as inhibitors of these pathways did not affect gene expression. On the other hand, inhibitors of PTK such as genistein, and of NF-κB such as PDTC (pyrrolidine dithiocarbamate), abolish the inhibitory effect of titanium particles on collagen expression in MG-63 and primary human osteoblasts, indicating that PTK and NF-κB mediate particle suppressive effects (Vermes et al., 2000). Large, non-phagocytosable particles (> 20 μm) also cause some degree of NF-κB binding, confirming the original observation that cell surface contact mediates minor adverse effects. Another series of studies has shown that NF-κB activates IL-8 expression in MG-63 and primary human osteoblasts after titanium particle exposure (Fritz et al., 2002, 2005). Titanium particles induce expression of NF-κB subunit p65 (RelA) and to a minor extent subunit p50 (NF-κB1). Gel shift mobility assays reveal binding of p65 and p50 to the IL-8-specific promoter an hour after particle exposure. The addition of an inhibitor of NF-κB, N-acetyl-L-cysteine, prevents p65 and p50 binding to the IL-8 promoter and leads to decreased production of IL-8. Titanium particles also activate the mitogen-activated kinase (MAPK) pathways ERK1/2 (p44/p42) and JNK1/2 (p54/p46) within minutes of particle challenge (Fritz et al., 2005). The pre-treatment of osteoblasts with MAPK inhibitors U0126 and SB203580 abolished the activity of ERK and p38, and concomintantly reduced the production of IL-8 (Fritz et al., 2005). Another study confirmed the role of NF-κB and PTK in reduction of collagen synthesis in MG-63 cells challenged with titanium particles (Roebuck et al., 2001). Titanium particle exposure led to upregulation of p65 and p50 and activation of PTK pathway, concurrent with suppressed type I collagen synthesis. Addition of the NF-κB inhibitor PDTC, or the PTK inhibitor genistein or herbimycin A, reduced the inhibitory effects expression and established the role of these pathways in mediating particle effects. On the other hand, inhibitors of protein kinase A and C did not influence the effects of particles on collagen expression, indicating that these pathways were not involved. These studies revealed the role of NF-κB and PTK as the mediators of downstream events of inflammation and diminished collagen synthesis that follow particle phagocytosis.

Metal wear debris has the additional issue of ion toxicity due to its potential to dissolve and corrode with time. Metal wear debris is on the scale of nanometers in size (mean, 50 nm), which is about 10x smaller than the average size of polyethylene particles (mean, 0.5 μm). The smaller size of metal particles increases their surface area for dissolution. Studies have shown that titanium and iron alloy (Ti-Al-V, Fe-Al-Cr) particles liberate aluminum and chromium ions into culture media in a dose-dependent manner, in addition to impairing viability and proliferation of tested SaOS-2 cells after phagocytosis (Ciapetti et al., 2005). A study evaluating the comparative cytotoxicity of cobalt, chromium, and cobalt-chromium alloy particles on MG-63 and SaOS-2 cells has shown that all three particle types inhibit alkaline phosphatase and osteocalcin expression, but cobalt particles inhibit these parameters to a much greater extent and are the only particles toxic enough to impair cell viability and type I collagen synthesis (Allen et al., 1997). Another study has shown that cobalt (Co^{2+}, 0-10 ppm) and chromium (Cr^{3+}, 0-150 ppm) ions generated from $CoCl_2$ and $CrCl_3$ are cytotoxic to MG-63 cells in a dose- and time-dependent manner over 72 hours, as

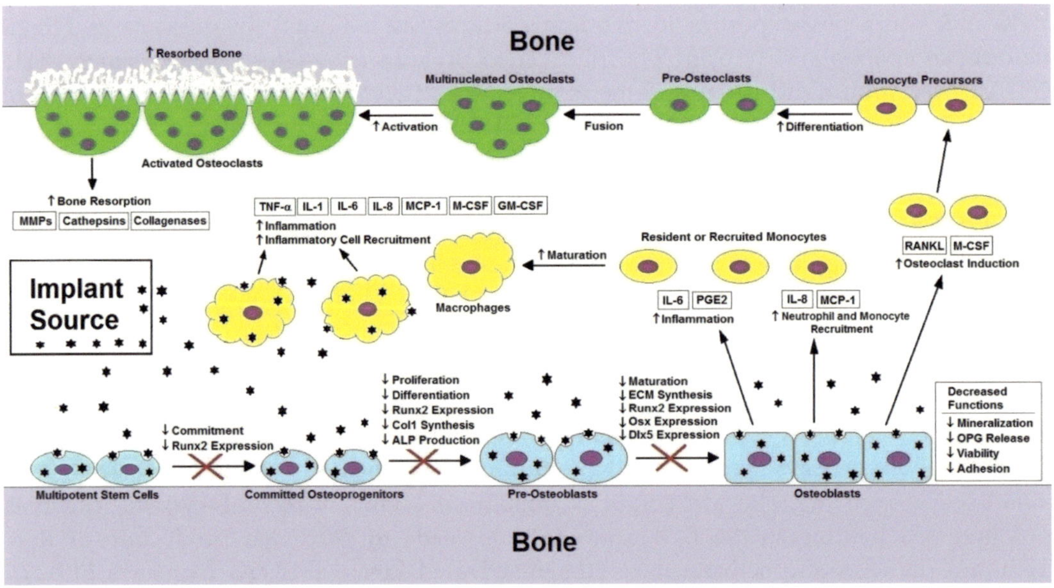

Fig. 2. Osteoblast-Osteoclast-Macrophage interactions during wear particle-induced inflammation and osteolysis. Small black hexagonal stars represent wear particles produced from the implant source. Bone-lineage cells (multipotent stem cells, osteoprogenitors, pre-osteoblasts, osteoblasts) are inhibited at each stage of development after phagocytosing wear particles. Osteoblasts release pro-inflammatory cytokines (IL-6, PGE_2), chemoattractants (IL-8, MCP-1), and osteoclastogenic factors (RANKL, M-CSF) after exposure to particles. Resident macrophages also phagocytose particles and release a wide range of factors that mediate inflammation, osteoclast activation, and cell recruitment. Monocytes resident in local tissue or recruited from bloodstream mature into macrophages or differentiate into osteoclasts. RANKL and M-CSF produced from osteoblasts induce osteoclast formation and bone resorption. Activated osteoclasts produce matrix metalloproteinases, cathepsins, and collagenases, which degrade bone. ALP = alkaline phosphatase, Col1 = collagen I, Osx = osterix, ECM = extracellular matrix.

measured by MTT viability assay and cell count, with Co^{2+} being more cytotoxic than Cr^{3+} (Fleurry et al., 2006). Ion concentrations in this experiment however, are in the ppm range, and most likely beyond the physiological relevant range of ppb in fluids surrounding metal-on-metal prostheses. Another study, however, has shown that SaOS-2 cells incubated with Co^{2+}, Cr^{3+}, and Cr^{6+} ions from chloride salts for 72 hrs, exhibited reduced viability only at doses far greater than physioloigical ranges in blood circulation (0.005 μM, or 0.25 μg/L). Specifically, SaOS-2 cells have shown decreased survival starting at 10 μM for Cr^{6+} (the most potent of the three ions), 100 μM for Co^{2+}, and 450 μM for Cr^{3+} (Andrews et al., 2011). All three ion types have reduced alkaline phosphatase production and mineralization, but only at doses > 100 μM. Whether these ion doses are close to elevated levels of cobalt and chromium in synovial fluid of metal-on-metal prostheses needs to be determined. Yet another study has shown that Co^{2+} ions from $CoCl_2$ induce primary human osteoblasts to release IL-8 and MCP-1, which causes the migration of neutrophils and macrophages in transwell experiments (Queally et al., 2011). Co^{2+} ions also significantly inhibit alkaline phosphatase production and calcium deposition in osteoblasts (Queally et al., 2011). These studies reveal that cobalt and chromium ions can be detrimental to osteoblasts, especially at elevated doses in peri-implant fluids of failed prostheses.

5. Biological response of osteoprogenitors

Bone formation involves bone and osteoid matrix deposition by osteoblasts and their differentiation from osteoprogenitors and multipotent stem cells, the latter being capable of differentiating along osteogenic, chondrogenic, and adipogenic pathways. These multipotent stem cells are often referred to as mesenchymal stem cells, which are defined as positive for mesenchymal markers CD27, CD44, CD90, CD105, CD166, and negative for hematopoietic markers CD34, CD45, and CD14. The term marrow stromal cells refers to the heterogeneous bone marrow cell population that remains adherent in tissue culture plates after removal of non-adherent blood cells. Within this marrow stromal cell population are multipotent stem cells, committed osteoprogenitors, fibroblasts, monocyte-macrophages, endothelial cells, and other undefined stromal support cells (Peister et al., 2004; Phinney et al., 1999). Upon exposure to osteoinductive factors, stem cells in this adherent culture commit to the osteogenic lineage. The osteoprogenitors undergo an initial period of proliferation, aggregation, and condensation, forming colonies that serve as the basis for subsequent osteoid matrix deposition (Lian & Stein, 2001). Osteoid production involves synthesis of type I collagen, proteoglycans, and glycosaminoglycans, and incorporation of osteonectin, osteocalcin, bone sialoprotein, and bone morphogenetic proteins (BMPs) into the matrix. Throughout this process, osteoprogenitors differentiate into pre-osteoblasts, which then mature into osteoblasts that can produce hydroxyapatite and bone. Once encased in bone matrix, osteoblasts turn into terminally differentiated, quiescent osteocytes. Osteoprogenitor differentiation is guided by the master transcription factor Runx2, which is required for expression of alkaline phosphatase, osteocalcin, collagen type 1, ostepontin, osteonectin, and bone sialoprotein. Another crucial transcription factor required for osteogenic differentiation is osterix (Osx), which is expressed by pre-osteoblasts and is downstream of Runx2 (Komori, 2006). Absence of Runx2 or osterix results in complete lack of osteogenesis (Komori, 2006). Two homeobox domain transcription factors, Dlx5 and Msx2, also regulate osteogenesis (Komori, 2006). Dlx5 promotes osteogenic differentiation, while Msx2 acts as a functional antagonist or repressor of Dlx5-mediated osteogenesis (Chiu et al., 2010; Komori, 2006). Signaling pathways that mediate osteogenic differentiation include the mitogen-activated protein kinase (MAPK) system, which involves p38, ERK1/2, and JNK as the main signalling molecules, and the BMP/Smad system, which involves Smad proteins 1, 5, and 8 as the tranducers of extracellular signals from BMPs (Lian & Stein, 2001). In summary, osteogenic differentiation involves an initial period of progenitor cell proliferation, an intermediate stage of extracellular matrix production, and a final stage of mineralization. Throughout this process, stem cells differentiate sequentially into osteoprogenitors, pre-osteoblasts, osteoblasts, and osteocytes. Multiple signalling pathways such as those of the MAP kinases and Smad signalling molecules, mediate downstream expression of the transcription factors Runx2 and osterix, which are required for osteogenesis. Orthopaedic wear debris has been shown to inhibit the osteogenic differentiation of osteoprogenitors and stem cells with respect to proliferation, viability, transcription factor expression, and osteogenic protein production. Given that osteogenesis requires the production of functional osteoblasts from osteoprogenitors, the inhibition of osteoprogenitor differentiation and proliferation by implant wear debris also reduces bone formation.

The effects of orthopaedic wear debris on osteogenic differentiation have been demonstrated using human or mouse marrow stormal cells and pre-osteoblast cell lines. A series of studies has assessed the effects of titanium particles on human marrow stromal cells (hMSCs, called mesenchymal stem cells in these studies) taken from patients undergoing primary hip or knee arthroplasty (Okafor et al., 2006; Wang et al., 2002, 2003). The hMSCs are heterogeneous populations containing multipotent stem cells with osteochondrogenic potential. When grown in osteogenic medium containing ascorbic acid, dexamethasone, β-glycerophosphate, and vitamin D_3, hMSCs undergo osteogenesis in 12 days and divide at a much greater rate than those grown in non-osteogenic medium. In these studies, hMSCs exposed to titanium particles showed a dose-dependent decrease in proliferation, type I collagen and bone sialoprotein synthesis, mineralization, and viability (Wang et al., 2002). Titanium particles induced apoptosis in hMSCs, as evidenced by DNA fragmentation, upregulation of tumor suppressor proteins p53 and p73, and nuclear condensation (Wang et al., 2003). Like osteoblasts, hMSCs phagocytosed particles and showed evidence of disrupted cytoskeletal network. Zirconia particles also reduced proliferation, mineralization, and viability of hMSCs in a dose-dependent manner, but to a lesser degree than titanium particles, and did not affect collagen and BSP production, indicating that zirconia was less detrimental than titanium (Wang et al., 2002, 2003). Titanium particles also inhibited alkaline phosphatase production and impaired adhesion after particle phagocytosis; pre-treating hMSCs with cytochalasin D, an inhibitor of actin polymerization, prevented phagocytosis and apoptosis, and reversed the detrimental effects on adhesion and alkaline phosphatase production (Okafor et al., 2006). Another study showed that cobalt chromium particles inhibited the proliferation of multipotent stem cells purified from human marrow stromal cells by flow cytometry (positive for CD44, CD90, CD105, and negative for CD34, CD45, CD14), and that these cells also phagocytosed particles (Schofer et al., 2008).

The inhibitory effects of wear particles on osteogenic differentiation have also been demonstrated with mouse marrow stromal cells (mMSCs) isolated from mouse long bones, and the MC3T3-E1 pre-osteoblast cell line. Like hMSCs, mMSCs are heterogeneous and harbour a subpopulation of multipotent stem cells with osteochodrogenic ability. PMMA particles dose-dependently inhibited the proliferation, alkaline phosphatase production, and mineralization of mMSCs, with complete suppression of these parameters observed throughout the entire culture period at particle doses ≥ 0.150% vol (Chiu et al., 2006, 2007). Exposure of mMSCs to PMMA particles for 5 days in either osteogenic or non-osteogenic medium was sufficient to make the inhibitory effects permanent; that is, removal of particles on or after 5 days of treatment did not halt or mitigate the inhibitory effects (Chiu et al., 2006, 2007). However, if particles were removed from culture before day 5 (e.g., on day 1 or 3), the inhibition of osteogenesis was partially mitigated (Chiu et al., 2007). In addition, PMMA particles were significantly less inhibitory when added to mMSC cultures at later days or stages of differentiation (e.g., days 5, 10, or 15 of culture) when the cells had mostly matured into osteoblasts (Chiu et al., 2006). PMMA particles also dose-dependently inhibited the proliferation, type I collagen and alkaline phosphatase expression, and mineralization of human multipotent stem cells purified from human bone marrow by flow cytometry (selected positively for CD27, CD44, CD106, CD166, and negatively for CD34, CD45, and CD14), with evidence of particle phagocytosis (Chiu et al., 2010b). MC3T3-E1 pre-osteoblasts challenged with PMMA particles exhibited a dose-dependent decrease in proliferation, alkaline phosphatase production, and mineralization (Chiu R et al., 2008; Ma et al., 2010). These effects were accompanied by particle phagocytosis, cytotoxic cell death, and importantly, the dose-dependent inhibition of osteogenic transcription factors Runx2, osterix, and Dlx5 (Chiu R et al., 2010a). Given that Runx2, osterix, and Dlx5 regulate osteogenesis, their inhibition likely caused downstream loss of osteoblast phenotype such as mineralization and alkaline phosphatase production. Interestingly, production of osteocalcin and expression of transcription factor Msx2 in MC3T3-E1 cells were not affected by PMMA particles. Msx2 is documented by certain studies as a reciprocal antagonist or repressor of Dlx5-mediated osteogenesis; hence, its lack of response to PMMA particles is consistent with the observed inhibition of Dlx5 and other osteoblast phenotypes. Another study investigated the pattern of mitogen-activated protein kinases (MAPKs), particularly p38, in MC3T3-E1 cells exposed to PMMA particles (Ma et al., 2010). MC3T3-E1 cells normally showed p38 activation on day 8 of osteogenic differentiation, but when exposed to PMMA particles, p38 was not activated on day 8, but instead on days 1 and 4 (Ma et al., 2010). The reasons for this changed pattern of p38 activation are unclear, but may involve a switch from an osteogenic program (p38 activation on day 8) to an inflammatory or apoptotic program (activation on days 1 and 4) given that p38 is involved in multiple signalling pathways. Lastly, MC3T3-E1 cells treated with titanium particles of nanometer size (mean size < 100 nm) showed upregulated M-CSF production at about 3x the control levels within 48 hrs of particle exposure (Seo et al., 2007). This was accompanied by activation of another MAP kinase, ERK1/2, within 5 min of exposure to particles. Pre-treating MC3T3-E1 cells with an inhibitor of ERK1/2, PD98059, prevented ERK1/2 activation and concomitantly restored M-CSF secretion to control levels, which indicated that M-CSF expression was mediated by ERK1/2 signalling (Seo et al., 2007).

The exposure of osteoprogenitors inhibited by implant particles to trophic or osteogenic growth factors moderately improved their osteogenic capacity. hMSCs inhibited by titanium particles, when exposed to IGF-1, FGF-2, BMP-6, and TGF-β1 at ng/mL concentrations, showed slightly enhanced proliferation, viability, and osteogenesis (Jeong et al., 2008). FGF-

Author	Year	Particle (Size)	Cell Type	Outcomes
Wang	2002	Ti (0.939 ± 0.380 μm) ZrO2 (0.876 ± 0.540 μm)	hMSC	collagen I (↓), BSP (↓), viability (↓), proliferation (↓), mineralization (↓), particle phagocytosis (+), cytoskeletal disruption (+)
Wang	2003	Ti (0.939 ± 0.380 μm) ZrO2 (0.876 ± 0.540 μm)	hMSC	viability (↓), apoptosis (+)
Chiu	2006	PMMA (1-10 μm)	mMSC	proliferation (↓), alkaline phosphatase (↓), mineralization (↓)
Okafor	2006	Ti (0.519 ± 0.125 μm)	hMSC	proliferation (↓), viability (↓), adhesion (↓), alkaline phosphatase (↓), particle phagocytosis (+)
Chiu	2007	PMMA (1-10 μm)	mMSC	proliferation (↓), alkaline phosphatase (↓), mineralization (↓)
Seo	2007	Ti (< 100 nm)	MC3T3E1	M-CSF (↑), ERK1/2 (↑)
Chiu	2008	PMMA (1-10 μm)	MC3T3E1	proliferation (↓), alkaline phosphatase (↓), mineralization (↓), osteocalcin (-)
Jeong	2008	Ti (1.46 ± 0.20 μm)	hMSC	slight to non-significant decreases in proliferation, viability, and collagen I, alkaline phosphatase, and osteocalcin; BSP (-)
Schofer	2008	CoCrMo (1.6-9.1 μm)	hMSC	proliferation (↓), particle phagocytosis (+)
Chiu	2009	UHMWPE (0.5 ± 0.2 μm)	mMSC MC3T3E1	proliferation (↓), alkaline phosphatase (↓), osteocalcin (↓), mineralization (↓)
Chiu	2010	PMMA (1-10 μm)	MC3T3E1	proliferation (↓), viability (↓), Runx2 (↓), osterix (↓), Dlx5 (↓), Msx2 (-), particle phagocytosis (+)
Chiu	2010	PMMA (1-10 μm)	hMSC	proliferation (↓), alkaline phosphatase (↓), collagen I (↓), mineralization (↓), particle phagocytosis (+)
Kann	2010	PMMA (1-10 μm)	MC3T3E1	alkaline phosphatase (↓), mineralization (↓)
Ma	2010	PMMA (1-10 μm)	MC3T3E1	mineralization (↓), alkaline phosphatase (↓), osteocalcin (-)

Table 2. Summary of orthopaedic particle effects on osteogenic differentiation of osteoprogenitor and marrow stromal cells. Studies are listed in in chronological order. Abbreviations: Ti = titanium particles, UHMWPE = ultrahigh molecular weight polyethylene particles, PMMA = polymethylmethacrylate particles, CoCrMo= cobalt-chromium-molybdenum alloy particles, ZrO2 = zirconium oxide particles, hMSC = human marrow stromal cells, mMSC = mouse marrow stromal cells, MC3T3E1 = MC3T3-E1 preosteoblasts. Signs: (↓) indicates decrease, (↑) indicates increase, (+) indicates presence of, (-) indicates absence of change.

2 and IGF-1 respectively enhanced proliferation and viability most effectively, increasing these two parameters in particle-treated cultures by 30-50% more than those not exposed to growth factors, and at levels beyond the control. FGF-2, IGF-1, and BMP-6 enhanced expression of type I collagen, alkaline phosphatase, osteocalcin, and BSP in the presence or absence of particles, with BMP-6 being most effective. However, titanium particles in this study had only slightly inhibited proliferation (by 10-15% relative to control), viability (by a non-significant 7%), and expression of collagen type I (38%), alkaline phosphatase (24%), and osteocalcin (15%), while not affecting expression of BSP (Jeong et al., 2008). The study also showed that TGF-β1 did not increase alkaline phosphatase, osteocalcin, or BSP expression and was the weakest of the four growth factors in terms of overall trophic effects on hMSCs. In another study, osteogenic protein-1 (OP-1), also known as BMP-7, improved the mineralization and alkaline phosphatase production of MC3T3-E1 pre-osteoblasts treated with PMMA particles. MC3T3-E1 cells exposed to PMMA particles showed a dose-dependent decrease in mineralization and alkaline phosphatase production, while the addition of OP-1 at 200 ng/mL to cultures significantly boosted these parameters by 30-170% at all time periods of treatment (days 1-20, 1-4, or 4-20 out of a 20-day culture period) and all particle doses tested (Kann et al., 2010). This increase in osteogenesis by OP-1 was significant whether particles were added to MC3T3-E1 cultures on the first or fourth day of growth. However, one study showed that the bisphosphonate zoledronate did not improve proliferation of MC3T3-E1 pre-osteoblasts or MG-63 osteoblasts in the presence of titanium particles (at 0.01% wt, the highest dose the cells could endure without showing signs of decreased proliferation relative to controls) throughout a 28 day period and over a wide dose range of zoledronate tested (0.1 to 100 μM by increasing orders of magnitude) (Peter et al., 2005).

6. *In Vitro* experimental methods

Most of our current knowledge of osteoblast and osteoprogenitor responses to orthopaedic wear debris comes from in vitro studies. These studies involve at a minimum, purifying and sterilizing particles and characterizing them with respect to size and shape, isolating and expanding cells and treating them with particles, and conducting various outcome measurements with respect to cell proliferation, differentiation, mineralization, viability, gene expression, protein or cytokine production, adhesion, or particle phagocytosis. With respect to gene expression and protein or cytokine production, commonly utilized methods include quantitative PCR after reverse transcription, Northern blot, in situ hybridization, and gene microarray analysis for mRNAs, and ELISA, western blot, immunohistochemistry, and enzyme reaction assays for proteins. Osteoblast proteins such as osteocalcin, bone sialoprotein, osteonectin, and osteopontin are commonly measured by ELISA or western blot. Alkaline phosphatase is commonly measured by enzyme kinetic reaction of cell lysates with para-nitrophenyl phosphate, its substrate, with spectrophotometric quantitation of chromogenic substrate release (p-nitrophenol) at 405 nm, or by immunohistochemistry given it is a cell surface protein. Secreted cytokines such as IL-6, IL-8, RANKL, M-CSF, and MCP-1 are often measured by ELISA of supernatant samples. All of these proteins can be measured by Q-PCR for mRNA expression. Transcription factors such as Runx2, osterix, Dlx5, and Msx2, are often measured by Q-PCR, while their binding to promoter elements in DNA is assessed by mobility shift electrophoresis, which separates protein-DNA complexes on gel. Mobility shift electrophoresis is also used to study the promoter binding activity of NF-κB subunits (RelA, NF-κB1), the transcription factor regulating particle-induced inflammation, cytokine production, and inhibition of collagen expression. Particle phagocytosis and ensuing morphological and cellular changes can be visualized by confocal, transmission electron, fluorescence, and light or phase contrast microscopy. Intracellular actin networks can be fluorescently visualized by staining with rhodamine or TRITC-conjugated phalloidin.

Calcium phosphate mineralization can be visualized by Alizarin Red S or von Kossa staining, measured by radioactive ^{45}Ca incorporation, or by spectrophotometric quantification of o-cresolphthalein complexed with Ca^{2+} ions extracted from mineral nodules by 0.6 N HCl. Mineralized nodules in culture stained by the von Kossa method (incubation of fixed cultures in 5% silver nitrate under UV light for 30-60 min) can be quantified by NIH Imaging software and expressed as a percentage (total stained area over total culture well area) (Chiu et al., 2009). Mineralized nodules stained by Alizarin Red S can be quantified by spectrophotometrically measuring Alizarin Red dye extracted from mineralized nodules with 10% acetic acid (Gregory et al., 2004). Matrix collagen and proteoglycan content can be measured respectively by radioactive ^{3}H-proline and ^{35}S-sulfate incorporation.

Viability and proliferation are commonly measured outcomes of osteoblasts and osteoprogenitors in particle experiments. A variety of methods are used to assess viability: trypan blue exclusion, MTT assay, fluorescein diacetate uptake, Annexin V stain, LDH (lactate dehydrogenase) assay, and TUNEL or caspase-3 and 7 assays for apoptosis. Proliferation is assessed by cell counting, ^{3}H-thymidine incorporation, BrdU uptake, and Ki67 antigen detection. Commercial sources also have proprietary kits/methods of assessing viability or proliferation (e.g., Alamar Blue, CCK-8 assay). Many of these assays are based on the ability of viable cells to metabolize substrates (e.g., MTT, fluorescein diacetate, Alamar Blue) into chromogenic or fluorescent products for spectrophotometric measurement, or the ability of dividing cells to incorporate artificial nucleotides (e.g., BrdU, ^{13}H-thymidine) which can then be detected. Other assays are based on the leakage of intracellular proteins during necrosis or cell injury (e.g., LDH), or specific events occurring in apoptosis (e.g., DNA fragmentation, phosphotidylserine inversion, caspase production). Many of these assays are available as commercial kits.

One of the initial steps of in vitro experimentation is obtaining a pure, sterile source of implant particles, either commercially or by isolating them from tissues of patients with failed hip or knee arthroplasties or wear simulator tests. Most studies with titanium, PMMA, or polystyrene particles have obtained these materials from commercial sources, most often Polysciences (Warrington, PA, USA) for PMMA and polystyrene particles, and Alfa Aesar (Ward Hill, MA, USA), now a part of Johnson Matthey, for titanium particles. Polysciences also produces fluorescent (Fluoresbrite) and color-dyed polystyrene particles, while Sigma-Aldrich (St. Louis, MO, USA) produces titanium oxide (rutile) particles. These particles are available in micron and submicron size ranges of phagocytosable size. Several studies have reported use of UHMWPE particles or powder from Hoechst-Celanese (Dallas, TX, USA) or its affiliated company Ticona (Florence, KY, USA), or Stryker-Howmedica-Osteonics (Kalamazoo, MI, USA) in various medical grades, such as GUR 4150. However, the UHMWPE powders obtained from these sources may be predominantly non-phagocytosable (i.e., 20-200 μm in size) and must be filtered or subject to sedimentation to isolate particles of smaller size, with subsequent characterization by scanning electron microscopy to validate their actual size range. These particles can be sterilized by washing in 70% ethanol, autoclaving (for metal particles only), overnight UV light exposure, gamma irradiation, or ethylene oxide treatment.

UHMWPE wear debris is more often obtained from granulomatous membrane tissues or synovial fluid collected respectively from failed hip and knee arthroplasties during revision surgery or from serum lubricant in wear simulator tests (Campbell et al., 1995). Membranes are freshly stored in buffered formalin after retrieval, then minced into mm^3 sized pieces, washed thoroughly with water, and digested in papain solution (3 mg papain in 10 mL of 50 mM phosphate buffer, pH 6.5, with 2 mM N-acetyl-L-cysteine) at 65° C for 1-3 days (Maloney et al., 1995; Wirth et al., 1999).Insoluble lysates are precipitated by centrifugation; the collected digest supernatant is then sonicated for 10 min and filtrated through a 0.2 μm polyester filter to isolate the UHMWPE particles. The collected particles are washed with water and sterilized in 70% ethanol, then after final washing, stored in DMEM or saline for later addition to cultures (Maloney et al., 1995; Wirth et al., 1999). UHMWPE debris are retrieved from synovial fluid or wear serum by digesting these samples in 5-10 M sodium hydroxide solution for 12-24 hrs at 65° C (Affatato et al., 2001; Chiu et al., 2009; Minoda et al., 2004; Wolfarth et al., 1997). Serum samples may be lyophilized to dryness before digestion (Chiu et al., 2009). The digest supernatant is sonicated, then ultracentrifuged under a layer of 5% sucrose density gradient at high speed for 3 hrs at 4° C. The sucrose solution is collected and ultracentrifuged under a two-layered isopropanol-water density gradient (0.90, 0.96 g/cm^3) at high speed for 1 hour. The layer containing UHMWPE debris at the interface of the two volumes of isopropanol is collected, filtered through a 0.1 μm polycarbonate filter, and allowed to dry. UHMWPE particles retrieved from patient samples and wear simulator tests are 1.0 μm (0.2 to 1.5 μm) in size according to SEM analysis in numerous reports. UHMWPE particles may be sterilized by gamma irradiation from a cesium-137 source, UV light exposure, 70% ethanol wash, or ethylene oxide treatment. Prior membrane fixation in formalin also destroys endotoxin and microbes. To confirm if the retrieved particles are UHMWPE, micro-Raman spectroscopy is used to generate a spectrum of vibrational frequencies from the particles that are matched with those of a UHMWPE standard reference (Wirth et al., 1999; Wolfarth et al., 1997; Visentin et al., 2004). Energy dispersive x-ray analysis provides spectra of elemental composition and can be used to identify metal (titanium, cobalt chromium) and ceramic (aluminium, zirconium) comtaminants in the UHMWPE particle mixture (Affatado et al., 2001; Wolfarth et al., 1997; Maloney et al., 1995). Studies have shown with SEM that UHMWPE wear debris is mostly spherical or round, elongated, oval, or oblong, with rough, grainy surface containing numerous pits.

Particles should be sterilized and confirmed negative of bacterial endotoxin before addition to culture. Endotoxin induces many of the same biologic reactions as wear particles, including inflammation, cytokine production, and osteoclastogenesis, and potentiates the adverse effects of particles (Bi et al., 2001, 2002; Greenfield et al., 2005). Adherent endotoxin has been detected on commercial titanium particles and actual orthopedic implant materials as a result of the manufacturing process, can also originate from distant infections and accumulate on implants at subclinical levels, and are found at higher levels in patients with inflammatory arthritis such as rheumatoid arthritis (Bi et al., 2001; Nalepka et al., 2006; Greenfield et al., 2008). Endotoxins on particles or in supernantant can be measured using commercial assay kits, such as the Limulus Amoebocyte Lysate Kit from BioWhittaker (Walkersville, MD, USA). Endotoxin, if detected on metal particles, can be removed by five or more alternating cycles of incubation in 25% nitric acid at room temperature, then in 0.1 N sodium hydroxide in 95% ethanol at 30° C, each incubation for 18-20 hrs, with PBS washes in between each step (Ragab et al., 1999).

Osteoblasts may be obtained commercially as tumorigenic cell lines or from primary rodent or human sources. Osteoblast cell lines include MG-63, SaOS-2, U-2OS, HOS, OCT-1, and MLO-Y4, among which MG-63 is most popular. MG-63, SaOS-2, U2OS, and HOS cells are osteosarcoma (osteogenic sarcoma) cells derived from human patients, and show osteoblast traits of polygonal morphology, alkaline phosphatase and osteocalcin expression, collagen matrix deposition, and calcium phosphate mineralization. One study has described MG-63 as immature osteoblasts, and OCT-1 as mature secretory osteoblasts derived from the calvaria, and MYO-L4 as osteocytes derived from the long bones, of transgenic mice that express the SV40 T-antigen oncogene driven by the osteocalcin promoter (Lohmann et al., 2002a; Kato et al., 1997). Lineage-specific cell lines can be readily obtained from transgenic mice in which the SV40 T-antigen is driven by the expression of a lineage-specific gene such as that of osteocalcin, which is expressed only in osteoblasts and osteocytes (Bonewald, 1999; Kato et al., 1997). MG-63, SaOS-2, U2OS, and HOS cells are available commercially from American Type Culture Collection (Manassas, VA, USA); primary osteoblasts are also purchasable from certain commercial sources. Primary osteoblasts are often derived from marrow aspirates of human trabecular bone after hip or knee arthroplasty or iliac crest bone after spine fusion, or from calvaria of neonatal rats. Human trabecular or iliac crest bone or neonatal rat calvarium is first minced into < 1 mm^3 pieces and then plated in DMEM or α-MEM culture medium. Cells migrate out from the minced bone fragments and expand to near confluency in about 2-3 weeks. The minced bone pieces can also be digested in collagenase (1 mg/mL) for 30-60 min or trypsin for ≤ 15 min at 37° C prior to plating, to facilitate release of entrapped cells. The osteoblasts should stain positive for alkaline phosphatase, collagen type I, osteocalcin, bone sialoprotein, and calcium phosphate mineral. Osteoprogenitors and multipotent stem cells with osteochondrogenic potential are subpopulations of heterogeneous marrow stromal cells (MSCs) isolated from the medullary cavities of long bones (Peister et al., 2004; Phinney et al., 1999). MSCs are most commonly used to represent osteoprogenitors in experiments involving osteogenic differentiation, as no marker has yet been discovered that specifically identifies and allows purification of pure osteoprogenitors. Human multipotent stem cells capable of differentiating along osteogenic, chondrogenic, and adipogenic lineages are recognized to be positive for CD markers 27, 44, 90, 105, and 166, and negative for hematopoietic markers such as CD34, 45, and 14. Multipotent stem cells can be isolated by flow cytometry with these antibodies, or may be purchased as pre-purified stocks from commercial sources. MSCs are normally isolated from mice by injecting culture medium through surgically dissected femurs and tibias using a 20-25 gauge needle with syringe, and plated directly into culture (Chiu et al., 2006, 2007; Peister et al., 2004; Phinney et al., 1999). Non-adherent blood cells are removed with subsequent medium exchange. The adherent MSCs, which include osteoprogenitor and multipotent stem cells, can be expanded in culture or used immediately for experimentation. MSCs can be induced to undergo osteogenic differentiation in DMEM or α-MEM containing ascorbic acid or ascorbate-2-phosphate (50 μg/mL), dexamethasone (10 nM), and β-glycerophosphate (10 mM) for 2-3 weeks; a series of studies has also included $1\alpha,25\text{-}(OH)_2D_3$ (vitamin D3 or calcitriol, 10 nM) (Wang et al., 2002, 2003). Human MSCs are isolated from femoral medullary canals of total hip arthroplasty patients and plated/expanded in culture in the same fashion (Wang et al., 2002, 2003). The mouse pre-osteoblast cell line, MC3T3-E1, is commonly used to study osteogenic differentiation and its transcriptional mechanisms. Several subclones of MC3T3-E1 exist with different mineralization potentials and expression patterns of osteocalcin and bone sialoprotein (Wang et al., 1999). Mineralizing subclones 4 and 14, and non-mineralizing subclones 24 and 30, of MC3T3-E1 are available from American Type Culture Collection. All subclones of MC3T3-E1 produce collagenous extracellular matrix, are responsive to ascorbic acid, and express alkaline phosphatase and Runx2/Cbfa1 (Choi et al., 1996; Franceschi et al., 1992, 1994; Quarles et al., 1992; Torii et al., 1996; Xiao et al., 1997, 2002).

Osteoblasts, osteoprogenitors, and MSCs are usually treated with particles in 6-, 12-, or 24-well plates, and occasionally in 96-well plates for proliferation and viability assays. Cells are generally plated at an initial density of 0.5-5.0 x 10^4 cells/cm^2, and then treated with particles after 24 hrs of plating or after reaching 70-80% confluency. hMSCs are usually plated at lower cell densities of 0.5-1.0 x 10^4 cells/cm^2, because of their slow proliferation potential and greater difficulty in expanding these cells to large numbers, compared to osteoblast cell lines which proliferate very robustly. Studies have represented particle doses as weight or volume percentages (relative to culture medium volume), number of particles per cell, number of particles per volume of medium, or mass of particles per well or volume of medium. Units can be interconverted based on knowledge of the average diameter of particles, volume of medium per well, and number of cells per well. PMMA and titanium particles are expressed more often as weight or volume percentages (e.g., 0.1, 0.25, 0.50, 1.0% wt), UHMWPE particles are expressed more often as number of particles per mL of medium

(10^5, 10^6, 10^7, 10^8 particles/mL), and ceramic particles are at times expressed as mass of particles per volume of medium (e.g., 0.1, 1.0, 10.0 mg/mL). Particle doses are also at times expressed as number of particles per cell (e.g., 5, 50, 500, 5000 particles/cell).

7. *In Vivo* experimentation methods

The in vivo response of osteoblasts and osteoprogenitors to orthopaedic wear debris has been studied by our group using two systems: the femoral intramedullary injection model and the bone harvest chamber (BHC). These systems have been used extensively to study tissue reactions to wear debris particles in mouse and rabbit systems, and have been important in helping researchers understand the mechanism of wear particle-induced osteolysis, inflammation, and granulomatosis. The femoral intramedullary injection system allows implant particles suspended in saline or hyaluronan carrier solution to be delivered continuously over a period of weeks into the femoral canal of experimental rodents. The system consists of a mini-osmotic Alzet pump (Durect, Cupertino, CA, USA) that is implanted subcutaneously in the dorsal, interscapular region of the animal. The Alzet pump is connected via tubing passed via a surgically created tunnel in the subcutaneous tissue, to a hollow titanium rod 6 mm, 23 gauge in dimensions. The titanium rod is inserted into the femoral medullary canal through a hole drilled in the intercondylar notch (the groove between the femoral condyles) using needles of increasingly larger diameter (e.g., 27, 25, 23, 21, 19 gauge). The pump holds approximately 250 μL of particle suspension, usually at a concentration of 10^9 to 10^{10} particles/mL, and infuses particles into the femoral canal at a rate of 0.15-0.25 μL/hr over several weeks. The titanium rod localizes particles to the marrow canal and prevents their leakage. After several weeks, the tissue reaction to particles can be evaluated by histology, staining for markers of osteoblasts, such as alkaline phosphatase or osteocalcin, and osteoclasts, such as TRAP (tartrate resistant acid phosphatase) or the vitronectin receptor $\alpha V\beta 3$ to visualize on microscope for cell number and density. Alternatively, particles can be injected as a single bolus in a suspension volume ≤ 10 μL, into the tibial medullary canal through a drilled hole in the proximal tibia, as was done in previous studies. The single bolus injection method, however, is less favorable given that it differs from the clinical scenario in which particles are continuously shed from implants over a long period of time; particles injected this way are also not confined as well to the medullary tissue. Local infusion of particles not only allows the study of resident tissue reactions, but also the migratory patterns of luciferase- and GFP-transfected cells injected intravenously into systemic circulation of the animal. Although the femoral intramedullary injection system theoretically allows the behavior of osteoblasts, osteoprogenitors, and multipotent stem cells to be studied in vivo, in practice, this rests upon identifying single, specific markers for these cells to facilitate histological identification. Alkaline phosphatase is not specific enough to identify osteoblasts or to distinguish them from osteoprogenitors or pre-osteoblasts. Multipotent stem cells are currently not defined by a single marker, but by a large panel of complex surface markers. The in vivo study of osteoblasts, osteoprogenitors, and multipotent stem cells, therefore, rests on the discovery of unique markers that allow for easy and accurate identification of these cells histologically.

The femoral intramedullary injection system involves an arthrotomy of the knee to access the intercondylar notch, which is accomplished via a quadriceps-patellar approach (Zilber et al., 2008). This approach involves a 5-mm incision on the anterior aspect of the knee; the

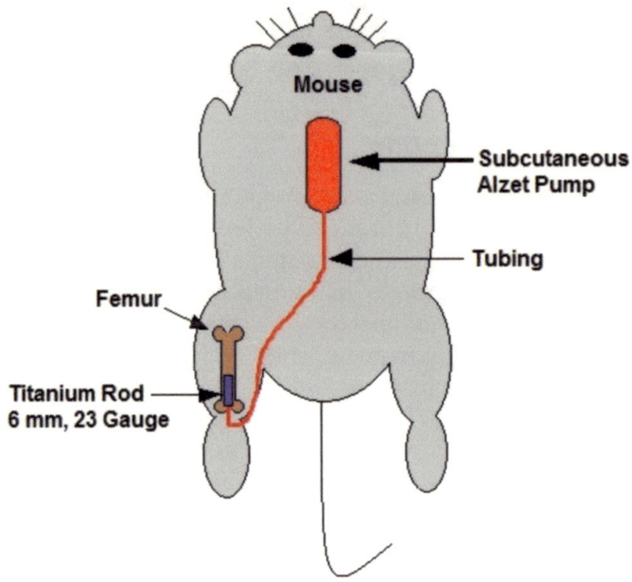

Fig. 3. The femoral intramedullary infusion system (dorsal view of mouse). The model consists of an Alzet mini-osmotic pump that is implanted subcutaneously in the interscapular region of the mouse. The pump is connected via tubing to the titanium rod (6 mm, 23 gauge), which is inserted into the medullary canal of the femur via a hole drilled in the intercondylar notch near the knee joint. The tubing is snugged into a surgically created tunnel in subcutaneous tissue. The pump, which holds about 250 μL of fluid, is used to infuse particle suspensions into the femoral canal at a rate of 0.15-0.25 μL/hour. This model mimics the clinical situation in which bone and marrow tissue are continuously exposed to wear particles produced from implants.

medial patellar ligament is then incised and the patella laterally displaced, which exposes the intercondylar notch for drilling and subsequent insertion of the titanium rod or particle bolus injection. For particle bolus injection, the traditional quadriceps-patellar or the less invasive transpatellar approach can be used (Zilber et al., 2008). In the transpatellar approach, a similar incision is made on the anterolateral side of the knee, the lateral part of the quadriceps is pushed aside, and without cutting the tendons or ligaments or displacing the patella, the intercondylar notch is directly accessed through the patellar tendon for drilling and particle bolus injection. In both approaches, the needle should be drilled 5 mm into the femoral canal to ensure clear passage through the distal femoral growth plate and to prevent leakage. A study has compared the two approaches in mice and shown successful delivery of 10 μL volumes of 10% PMMA particles into the femoral canal, confirmed subsequently by micro-CT imaging (Zilber et al., 2008).

The efficiency of this in vivo particle infusion system has been determined in a series of studies (Ortiz et al., 2008a, 2008b; Ma et al., 2008, 2009a). In this series, the Alzet mini-osmotic pump delivered UHMWPE and polystyrene particles (0.5 ± 0.015 μm) over 4 weeks into an ex vivo collection tube. The pump delivered 10^9 to 10^{11} particles suspended in 200 μL of mouse serum at a rate of 0.25 μL/hr. The efficiency of particle delivery was determined by spectrophotometrically measuring the turbidities of the initial and collected outflow solutions (at 595 nm) and referencing the absorbances against a standard curve of turbidities of known particle concentrations. The efficiency was estimated to be 46% for an original load of 6 x 10^9 polystyrene particles, but it decreased to 23% and then to 15% for approximately each order of magnitude increase in particle number. Efficiency for UHMWPE was approximately one-third for an initial load of 3 x 10^{10} or 1.5 x 10^{11} particles (Ortiz et al., 2008a). Particles were successfully pumped into freshly dissected femurs cultured ex vivo in DMEM F-12 medium, and were visible in the medullary canal upon gross inspection, particularly with blue-dyed polystyrene particles (Ortiz et al., 2008b). The efficiency of particle delivery has also been evaluated in live mice (Ma et al., 2008, 2009a). Blue-dued polystyrene particles were injected successfully into the femoral canal of mice over 4 weeks at an efficiency of 40-50% of the initial 6 x 10^9 particles delivered, and were visible on gross inspection of the dissected femurs (Ma et al., 2009a). UHMWPE particles infused into femurs of mice over 4 weeks led to reduced bone volume and higher numbers of macrophages compared to contralateral control femurs with rod but no particles, as assessed by micro-CT and histology/histomorphometry of femoral cross sections (Ma et al., 2008). These studies established the femoral intramedullary injection model as a successful system for delivering particles in vivo; improvements however, are needed to increase efficiency of particle delivery.

Another series of studies has used the particle injection method to assess in vivo cell responses to titanium particles (Warme et al., 2004; Epstein et al., 2005b; Bragg et al., 2008). In a similar study, UHMWPE particles injected as a single bolus into the femur of C57BL/6 mice (at an average quantity of 3 x 10^9 particles/femur in sodium hyaluronate:PBS carrier solution) also induced intramedullary bone marrow monocytes to increase expression of MCP-1, IL-6, and IL-1β over a 10 week period relative to monocytes from control femurs without particles, as determined by RT-PCR of mRNA from extracted monocytes (Epstein et al., 2005a). In the initial study, 1.39 x 10^8 titanium particles (3.7 ± 1.8 μm) were injected as a single bolus in 10 μL of sodium hyaluronate: PBS carrier solution into the femoral canal, followed by a press-fit 10 mm, 25 gauge stainless steel rod cut from Kirschner wire to prevent particle leakage (Warme et al., 2004). After 26 weeks, femurs were dissected and cultured ex vivo in DMEM-F12 for 72 hrs. ELISA analysis of culture media revealed that femurs infused with particles yielded a 45, 79, and 221% increase in production of IL-6, MCP-1, and M-CSF compared to contralateral femurs not infused with particles, whereas IL-1β and TNF-α levels were not elevated (Warme et al., 2004). Histology of femoral cross sections revealed evidence of endosteal bone scalloping and destruction. In a similar study, the same bolus of titanium particles was injected into femurs of knockout mice lacking IL-1r1, the receptor for IL-1 (B6.129s7-Il1r1, Jackson Laboratories, Bar Harbor, ME, USA) (Epstein et al., 2005b). After 20 weeks, femurs were dissected and placed in organ culture. ELISA analysis of culture medium revealed that the production of MCP-1 by femurs infused with particles in these IL-1r1 knockout mice was no different than contralateral control femurs not infused with particles; the absolute levels of MCP-1 production from these experimental femurs were also significantly lower (6-8 fold lower) than those of wild type mice. However, inflammation and bone loss occurred to similar degrees in both IL-1r1 knockout and wild type mice, which indicated that while lack of the IL-1 receptor limited MCP-1 production, it did not abolish or reduce the overall inflammatory response to particles, due perhaps to activation of alternative inflammatory pathways (Epstein et al., 2005b). A followup study demonstrated histological evidence of inflammation and endosteal erosion characterized by fibrosis, jagged cortical margins, increased porosity, and presence of a periprosthetic membrane in femoral canals of IL-1r1 knockout mice injected with a bolus of titanium particles (Bragg et al., 2008).

The particle injection method has also been employed to study migratory patterns of injected cells, which may theoretically be extended to luciferase- and GFP-labeled marrow stromal or multipotent stem cells, osteoprogenitors, and osteoblasts. A series of studies has tracked the systemic migration of luciferase-transfected reporter macrophages injected into the lateral tail vein of nude mice with previous injection or infusion of particles into the femur (Ren et al., 2008, 2010, 2011). In one study, Simplex P bone cement powder 1-100 μm in diameter (Howmedica Osteonics, Allendale, NJ, USA) consisting of 15% PMMA, 75% methylmethacrylate styrene copolymer, and 10% barium sulfate, as a 10% wt suspension in PBS, was injected as a single bolus of 10 μL into the femoral canal of nude mice, followed 7 days later by injection of luciferase- and GFP-transfected Raw264.7 macrophages (5×10^5 cells in 100 μL HBSS) into their lateral tail vein (Ren et al., 2008). Bioluminescence imaging of mice revealed significantly higher bioluminescent signal in particle-infused femurs at days 6 and 8 post-macrophage injection (4.7 ± 1.6, 7.8 ± 2.9 respectively, ratios of signal of particle-infused femur over contralateral control femur), compared to those of saline-injected controls (1.2 ± 0.2, 1.4 ± 0.5). Histological analysis of femoral cross sections also showed higher numbers of GFP- and MOMA-2-positive macrophages (MOMA-2 is a macrophage marker) in the particle-infused femurs than in control femurs. The imaging and histology results indicated that macrophages from systemic sites migrated to tissues injured by wear debris particles. Similarly, UHMWPE particles (1.0 ± 0.1 μm) injected as a single bolus of 1.2×10^8 particles in 10 μL into femora of nude mice attract luciferase- and GFP-transfected Raw264.7 macrophages to its site of infusion, resulting in significantly larger bioluminescent signals (10.32 ± 7.61 signal ratio) than saline-injected control femurs (signal ratio close to 1) 8 days after macrophage injection. Histological analysis revealed larger number of Raw264.7 macrophages positive for GFP and $\alpha V\beta 3$-positive osteoclasts in particle-infused femurs compared to saline-injected control femurs (Ren et al., 2010). UHMWPE particles continuously infused into femora of nude mice by the Alzet mini-osmotic pump (rather than by single bolus injection), also attracted labeled Raw264.7 macrophages to their site of infusion (Ren et al., 2011). Ten days after macrophage injection, femurs extracted for histology demonstrated increased numbers of GFP-labeled Raw264.7 macrophages, total macrophages (MOMA-2-positive), and vitronectin receptor/TRAP-positive osteoclasts in particle-infused samples than in saline-treated control femurs. Some cells stained positive for both TRAP and MOMA-2, and represent monocytes that have differentiated into osteoclasts. Bioluminescence imaging revealed significantly higher signal ratios in particle-infused femurs (13.95 ± 5.65) compared to saline-treated femurs with signal ratios close to 1. MicroCT scans of femurs infused with particles revealed decreased bone mineral density compared to saline-infused femurs (Ren et al., 2011). Taken together, these results indicate that systemic macrophages migrate to sites of particle infusion in response to particle-induced inflammation. The same model can potentially be applied to study the migratory patterns of systemically infused marrow stromal or multipotent stem cells, osteoprogenitors, and osteoblasts, which may respond to secreted cues of bone injury or osteolysis. The applicability of this model for this purpose rests upon identifying markers that allow appropriate isolation of pure osteogenic cell and progenitor populations for labeling with luciferase or fluorescent proteins.

In vivo cell responses to orthopaedic wear debris can also be evaluated using the bone harvest chamber (BHC). A modified version of the BHC, the drug test chamber (DTC), also allows evaluation of cell responses to infused therapeutic agents and growth factors in vivo under simultaneous exposure to wear particles. Earlier studies on in vivo tissue responses have been conducted by direct surgical implantation of particle boluses (e.g., 60-70 mg of PMMA cement powder) into the medullary tibial canal of rabbits via a drilled hole in the proximal tibia (Goodman et al., 1988, 1991a, 1991b). Though these studies have helped to elucidate the response of tissues to wear debris particles, the introduction of the BHC in the early 1990s has greatly facilitated this research process (Goodman et al., 1994, 1995a, 1995b, 1995c, 1996a, 1996b). The BHC is a titanium device with an inner core containing a 1 x 1 x 5 mm^3 pathway for tissue ingrowth and an outer cylindrical shell with threads for screwing the cylinder into the surrounding bone. The outer shell contains 1 x 1 mm^2 openings on its two ends that are continuous with the pathway in the inner chamber. When implanted into bone, the BHC allows bone ingrowth into its inner core; this bone tissue specimen can be collected at multiple times by removing the inner core, without disrupting the outer shell that has integrated with surrounding bone. In addition, particle suspensions can be placed inside the inner pathway such that ingrown bone reacts to these particulates, allowing the tissue reaction to be studied by histology after retrieval of the tissue sample. The DTC is essentially the BHC setup with an additional Alzet mini-osmotic pump that allows biologics to be infused into the inner core at a regulated rate. This mimics the clinical scenario in which therapeutic drugs are delivered locally to an area of tissue ingrowth. The DTC contains a 10 μL reservoir for holding the infused solution and is linked to the inner core for bone ingrowth. The Alzet pump, which contains around 250 μL of solution, is implanted subcutaneously in the animal and infuses fluid at a rate of 0.25 μL/hr to the DTC reservoir via tubing. From there, the fluid travels to the inner chamber where the tissue is ingrowing and exposed to particles. As fluid builds up in the inner chamber, it is drained via outlet tubing to the skin of the animal. The Alzet pump and its tubing can also be removed and replaced with minimal disturbance to the system. The size of the BHC/DTC permits this device to be used only for rabbits or larger animals. With appropriate markers to identify multipotent stem cells, osteoprogenitors, and osteoblasts, the in vivo behavior of these cells in response to wear particles can potentially be studied using the harvest chamber models.

The BHC has been used in a series of studies to evaluate in vivo tissue responses to wear particles during administration of oral p38 MAP kinase inhibitors in rabbits (Goodman et al., 2007; Ma et al., 2009). p38 MAP kinase mediates various pathways in inflammation, apoptosis, and osteoclast differentiation. In one study, BHCs were implanted and allowed to osseointegrate into the proximal tibial metaphyses of rabbits for 6 weeks. Ingrown tissue was removed and replaced with UHMWPE particles (0.5 ± 0.2 μm) at a concentration of 7.5 x 10^9 particles in 5 μL in 1% sodium hyaluronate carrier solution at one of the 3-week treatment time intervals, with or without oral administration of p38 MAPK inhibitor, with comparison to control BHCs filled with carrier solution only. Tissue ingrowth into the BHC chamber was collected at the end of 3 weeks, and assessed histologically for expression of alkaline phosphatase (osteoblasts) or vitronectin receptor (osteoclasts) (Goodman et al., 2007). Histology tissue sections were also histomorphometrically quantified, using NIH Imaging software, for total tissue area, total bone area, ratio of total bone area over total tissue area, and total area of alkaline phosphatase-positive stains, and counted for the number of vitronectin receptor-positive cells. The oral p38 MAPK inhibitor, expected to inhibit inflammation and bone loss, actually yielded dimnished bone ingrowth and alkaline phosphatase staining, and failed to suppress inflammation or foreign body reactions in the presence of UHMWPE particless (Goodman et al., 2007). A later study testing the effects of the oral p38 MAPK inhibitor SCIO-323, has shown similar results of reduced bone growth with no curtailment of inflammation in particle-treated groups, compared to particle-treated controls not receiving SCIO-323 (Ma et al., 2009). In summary, the BHC experiments have shown that p38 MAPK inhibitors do not improve bone formation in tissues exposed to wear debris particles.

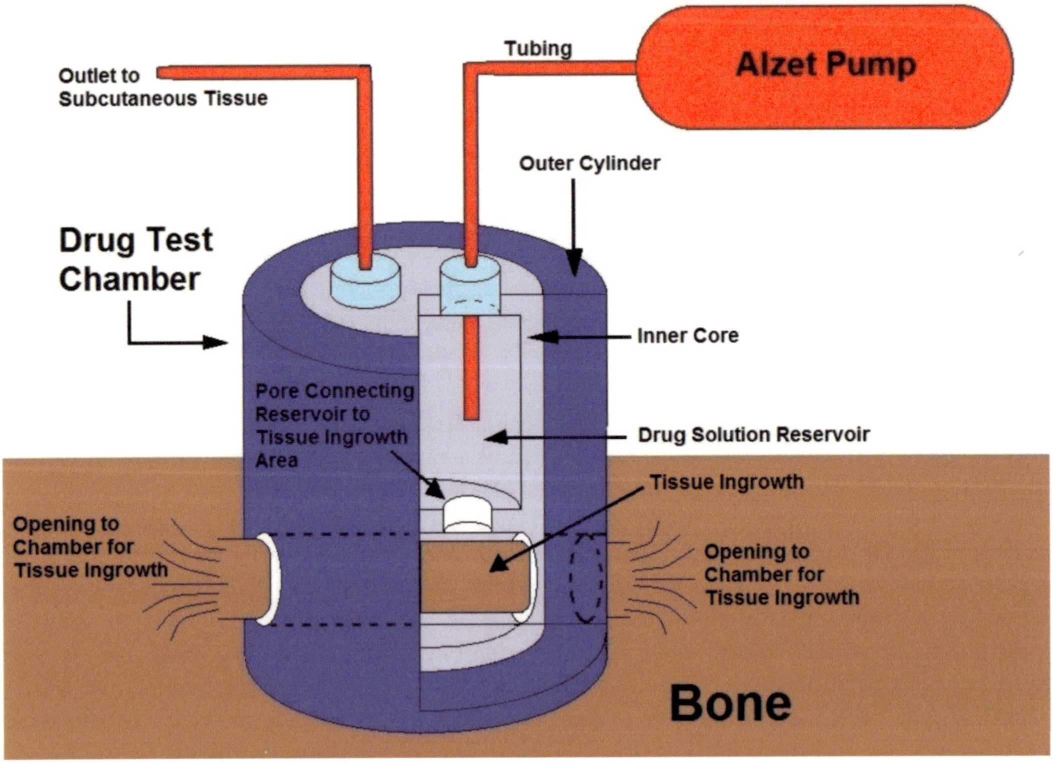

Fig. 4. The drug test chamber (DTC). This system consists of a titanium chamber that permits tissue ingrowth, and an Alzet mini-osmotic pump for infusing biologics into the chamber. The titanium chamber consists of an outer cylinder that allows the device to be screwed into surrounding bone, and an inner core composed of a 10 μL reservoir for holding infused solution and an inner canal/pathway for tissue ingrowth. The inner core is separable from the outer cylinder and allows the ingrown tissue to be collected without disrupting the entire device. The Alzet pump infuses solutions into the reservoir of the inner core, which in turn is connected to the tissue ingrowth canal via an open pore. Fluid outflow is drained via tubing to the subcutaneous tissue.

The DTC has been employed in a series of studies to evaluate in vivo tissue responses to wear particles during local infusion of trophic, osteogenic, or anti-inflammatory factors (Goodman et al., 2003a, 2003b; Ma et al., 2006). In one study, DTC was used to infuse FGF-2, a growth factor that modulates osteoblast proliferation, differentiation, bone formation, and angiogenesis, in the presence of UHMWPE particles in rabbits (Goodman et al., 2003a). FGF-2 was infused at a dose of 50 ng/day over 3 weeks into the DTC, in the presence of a low (5.8×10^{11} particles/mL) or high (1.7×10^{12} particles/mL) concentration of UHMWPE particles (0.5 ± 0.2 μm). After 3 weeks, tissues extracted for histology and histomorphometric analysis revealed that FGF-2 significantly increased bone growth and decreased the number of vitronectin receptor-positive osteoclasts in samples treated with UHWMPE particles, compared to particle-treated samples not infused with FGF-2 (Goodman et al., 2003a). In another study, the DTC was infused with IL-10, an anti-inflammatory cytokine that suppresses Th1 helper cell-mediated inflammation, including expression of IL-1, IL-6, IL-8, TNF-α, and GM-CSF, in the presence of UHMWPE particles in rabbits (Goodman et al., 2003b). IL-10 was infused at increasing doses of 0.1, 1.0, 10.0 and 100.0 ng/mL for 3 weeks at each dose, in the presence or absence of UHMWPE particles (1.7×10^{12} particles/mL) in the DTC. Histology and histomorphometirc analysis revealed that IL-10 infused at 1.0 ng/mL for 3 weeks, significantly increased bone growth up to 48% in the presence of UHMWPE particles, compared to particle-treated samples without IL-10. In the absence of particles, IL-10 had no effect on bone growth relative to controls not treated with IL-10 (Goodman et al., 2003b). In another study, the DTC was infused with OP-1 (also called BMP-7), a growth factor that promotes osteoblast proliferation, differentiation, and mineralization, in the presence of UHMWPE particles in rabbits (Ma et al., 2006). Infusion of OP-1 (110 ng/day) into the DTC for 6 weeks increased bone growth by 38% in the presence of UHMWPE particles, relative to particle-treated samples without OP-1 (Ma et al., 2006).

8. References

[1] Abbas S, Clohisy JC, Abu-Amer Y. (2003). Mitogen-activated protein (MAP) kinases mediate PMMA-induction of osteoclasts. *J Orthop Res*, Vol. 21, No. 6, pp. 1041-1048.

[2] Affatato S, Fernandes B, Tucci A, Esposito L, Toni A. (2001). Isolation and morphological characterization of UHMWPE wear debris generated in vitro. *Biomaterials*, Vol. 22, No. 17, pp. 2325-2331.

[3] Allen MJ, Myer BJ, Millett PJ, Rushton N. (1997). The effects of particulate cobalt, chromium and cobalt–chromium alloy on human osteoblast-like cells in vitro. *J Bone Joint Surg Br*, Vol. 79, No. 3, pp. 475–482.

[4] Andrews RE, Shah KM, Wilkinson JM, Gartland A. (2011). Effects of cobalt and chromium ions at clinically equivalent concentrations after metal-on-metal hip replacement on human osteoblasts and osteoclasts: implications for skeletal health. *Bone*, Vol. 49, No. 4, pp. 717-723.

[5] Atkins GJ, Welldon KJ, Holding CA, Haynes DR, Howie DW, Findlay DM. (2009). The induction of a catabolic phenotype in human primary osteoblasts and osteocytes by polyethylene particles. *Biomaterials*, Vol. 30, No. 22, pp. 3672-3681.

[6] Bi Y, Collier TO, Goldberg VM, Anderson JM, Greenfield EM. (2002). Adherent endotoxin mediates biological responses of titanium particles without stimulating their phagocytosis. *J Orthop Res*, Vol. 20, No. 4, pp. 696-703.

[7] Bi Y, Seabold JM, Kaar SG, Ragab AA, Goldberg VM, Anderson JM, Greenfield EM. (2001). Adherent endotoxin on orthopedic wear particles stimulates cytokine

production and osteoclast differentiation. *J Bone Miner Res*, Vol. 16, No. 11, pp. 2082-2091.

[8] Bonewald LF. (1999). Establishment and characterization of an osteocyte-like cell line, MLO-Y4. *J Bone Miner Metab*, Vol. 17, No. 1, pp. 61-65.

[9] Bragg B, Epstein N, Ma T, Goodman S, Smith RL. (2008). Histomorphometric analysis of the intramedullary bone response to titanium particles in wild-type and IL-1R1 knock-out mice: a preliminary study. *J Biomed Mater Res B Appl Biomater*, Vol. 84, No. 2, pp. 559-570.

[10] Campbell P, Ma S, Yeom B, McKellop H, Schmalzried TP, Amstutz HC. (1995). Isolation of predominantly submicron-sized UHMWPE wear partices from periprosthetic tissues. *J Biomed Mater Res*, Vol. 29, No. 1, pp. 127-131.

[11] Chiu R, Ma T, Smith RL, Goodman SB. (2006). Polymethylmethacrylate particles inhibit osteoblastic differentiation of bone marrow osteoprogenitor cells. *J Biomed Mater Res A*, Vol. 15, No. 4, pp. 850-856.

[12] Chiu R, Ma T, Smith RL, Goodman SB. (2007). Kinetics of polymethylmethacrylate particle-induced inhibition of osteoprogenitor differentiation and proliferation. *J Orthop Res*, Vol. 25, No. 4, pp. 450-457.

[13] Chiu R, Ma T, Smith RL, Goodman SB. (2008). Polymethylmethacrylate particles inhibit osteoblastic differentiation of MC3T3-E1 osteoprogenitor cells. *J Orthop Res*, Vol. 26, No. 7, pp. 932-936.

[14] Chiu R, Ma T, Smith RL, Goodman SB. (2009). Ultrahigh molecular weight polyethylene wear debris inhibits osteoprogenitor proliferation and differentiation in vitro. *J Biomed Mater Res A*, Vol. 89, No. 5, pp. 242-247.

[15] Chiu R, Smith KE, Ma GK, Ma T, Smith RL, Goodman SB. (2010). Polymethylmethacrylate particles impair osteoprogenitor viability and expression of osteogenic transcription factors Runx2, osterix, and Dlx5. *J Orthop Res*, Vol. 28, No. 5, pp. 571-577.

[16] Chiu R, Smith RL, Goodman SB. (2010). Polymethylmethacrylate particles inhibit human mesenchymal stem cell osteogenesis, *Proceedings of Society for Biomaterials*, Seattle, April 2010.

[17] Choi JY, Lee BH, Song KB, Park RW, Kim IS, Sohn KY, Jo JS, Ryoo HM. (1996). Expression patterns of bone-related proteins during osteoblastic differentiation in MC3T3-E1 cells. *J Cell Biochem*, Vol. 61, No. 4, pp. 609-618.

[18] Choi MG, Koh HS, Kleuss D, O'Connor D, Mathur A, Truskey GA, Rubin J, Zhou DX, Sung KL. (2005). Effects of titanium particle size on osteoblast functions in vitro and in vivo. *Proc Natl Acad Sci USA*, Vol. 102, No. 12, pp. 4578-4583.

[19] Ciapetti G, Gonzales-Carrasco JL, Savarino L, Montealegre MA, Pagani S, Baldini N. (2005). Quantitative assessment of the response of osteoblast- and macrophage-like cells to particles of Ni-free Fe-base alloys. *Biomaterials*, Vol. 26, No. 8, pp. 849-859.

[20] Clohisy JC, Yamanak Y, Faccio R, Abu-Amer Y. (2006). Inhibition of IKK activation, through sequestering NEMO, blocks PMMA-induced osteoclastogenesis and calvarial inflammatory osteolysis. *J Orthop Res*, Vol. 24, No. 7, pp. 1358-1365.

[21] Dean DD, Lohmann CH, Sylvia VL, Koster G, Liu Y, Schwartz Z, Boyan BD. (2001). Effect of polymer molecular weight and addition of calcium stearate on response of MG63 osteoblast-like cells to UHMWPE particles. *J Orthop Res*, Vol. 19, No. 2, pp. 179-86.

[22] Dean DD, Schwartz Z, Blanchard CR, Liu Y, Agrawal CM, Lohmann CH, Sylvia VL, Boyan BD. (1999). Ultrahigh molecular weight polyethylene particles have direct effects on proliferation, differentiation, and local factor production of MG63 osteoblast-like cells. *J Orthop Res*, Vol. 17, No. 1, pp. 9-17.

[23] Dean DD, Schwartz Z, Liu Y, Blanchard CR, Agrawal CM, Mabrey JD, Sylvia VL, Lohmann CH, Boyan BD. (1999). The effect of ultra-high molecular weight polyethylene wear debris on MG63 osteosarcoma cells in vitro. *J Bone Joint Surg Am*, Vol. 81, No. 4, pp. 452-461.

[24] DeLaSalle H, Benghuzzi H, Deville R, Tucci M. (2006). The effects of PMMA particle number on MG-63 osteoblast cell function. *Biomed Sci Instrum*, Vol. 42, 48-53.

[25] Epstein NJ, Bragg WE, Ma T, Spanogle, J, Smith RL, Goodman SB. (2005). UHMWPE wear debris upregulates mononuclear cell proinflammatory gene expression in a novel murine model of intramedullary particle disease. *Acta Orthop*, Vol. 76, No. 3, pp. 412-420.

[26] Epstein NJ, Warme BA, Spanogle J, Ma T, Bragg B, Smith RL, Goodman SB. (2005). Interleukin-1 modulates periprosthetic tissue formation in an intramedullary model of particle-induced inflammation. *J Orthop Res*, Vol. 23, No. 3, pp. 501-510.

[27] Fleury C, Petit A, Antoniou J, Zukor DJ, Tabrizian M, Huk OL. (2006). Effect of cobalt and chromium ions on human MG-63 osteoblasts in vitro: morphology, cytotoxicity, and oxidative stress. *Biomaterials*, Vol. 27, No., 18, pp. 3351-3360.

[28] Franceschi RT, Bhanumathi SI, Cui Y. (1994). Effects of ascorbic acid on collagen matrix formation and osteoblast differentiation in murine MC3T3-E1 cells. *J Bone Miner Res*, Vol. 9, No. 6, pp. 843-854.

[29] Franceschi RT, Iyer BS. (1992). Relationship between collagen synthesis and expression of the osteoblast phenotype in MC3T3-E1 cells. *J Bone Miner Res*, Vol. 7, No. 2, pp. 235-246.

[30] Fritz EA, Glant TT, Vermes C, Jacobs JJ, Roebuck KA. (2002). Titanium particles induce the immediate early stress responsive chemokines IL-8 and MCP-1 in osteoblasts. *J Orthop Res*, Vol. 20, No. 3, pp. 490-498.

[31] Fritz EA, Glant TT, Vermes C, Jacobs JJ, Roebuck KA. (2006). Chemokine gene activation in human bone marrow-derived osteoblasts following exposure to particulate wear debris. *J Biomed Mater Res A*, Vol. 77, No. 1, pp. 192-201.

[32] Fritz EA, Jacobs JJ, Glant TT, Roebuck KA. (2005). Chemokine IL-8 induction by particulate wear debris in osteoblasts is mediated by NF-kappaB. *J Orthop Res*, Vol. 23, No. 6, pp. 1249-1257.

[33] Goodman S, Aspenberg P, Song Y, Doshi A, Regula D, Lidgren L. (1995). Effects of particulate high-density polyethylene and titanium alloy on tissue ingrowth into bone harvest chamber in rabbits. *J Appl Biomater*, Vol. 6, No. 1, pp. 27-33.

[34] Goodman S, Aspenberg P, Song Y, Knoblich G, Huie P, Regula D, Lidgren L. (1995). Tissue ingrowth and differentiation in the bone-harvest chamber in the presence of cobalt-chromium-alloy and high-density-polyethylene particles. *J Bone Joint Surg Am*, Vol. 77, No. 7, pp. 1025-1035.

[35] Goodman S, Aspenberg P, Song Y, Regula D, Lidgren L. (1995). Intermittent micromotion and polyethylene particles inhibit bone ingrowth into titanium chambers in rabbits. *J Appl Biomater*, Vol. 6, No. 3, pp. 161-165.

[36] Goodman S, Aspenberg P, Song Y, Regula D, Lidgren L. (1996). Polyethylene and titanium alloy particles reduce bone formation. *Acta Orthop Scand*, Vol. 67, No. 6, pp. 599-605.

[37] Goodman S, Trindade, Ma T, Lee M, Wang N, Ikenou T, Matsuura I, Miyanishi K, Fox N, Regula D, Genovese G, Klein J, Bloch D, Smith RL. (2003). Modulation of bone ingrowth and tissue differentiation by local infusion of interleukin-10 in presence of ultra-high molecular weight polyethylene (UHMWPE) wear particles. *J Biomed Mater Res A*, Vol. 65, No. 1, pp. 43-50.

[38] Goodman SB, Chin RC, Chiou SS, Lee JS. (1991). Suppression of prostaglandin E2 synthesis in the membrane surrounding particulate polymethylmethacrylate in the rabbit tibia. *Clin Orthop Relat Res*, Vol. 271, pp. 300-304.

[39] Goodman SB, Davidson JA, Song Y, Martial N, Fornasier VL. (1996). Histomorphological reaction of bone to different concentrations of phagocytosable particles of high-density polyethylene and Ti-6Al-4V alloy in vivo. *Biomaterials*, Vol. 17, Nol. 20, pp. 1943–1947.

[40] Goodman SB, Fornasier VL, Kei J. (1988). The effects of bulk versus particulate polymethylmethacrylate on bone. *Clin Orthop Relat Res*, Vol. 232, pp. 255-262.

[41] Goodman SB, Fornasier VL, Kei J. (1991). Quantitative comparison of the histological effects of particulate polymethylmethacrylate versus polyethylene in rabbit tibia. *Arch Orthop Trauma Surg*, Vol. 110, No. 3, pp. 123-126.

[42] Goodman SB, Ma T, Spanogle J, Chiu R, Miyanishi K, Oh K, Plouhar P, Wadsworth S, Smith RL. (2007). Effects of a p38 MAP kinase inhibitor on bone ingrowth and tissue differentiation in rabbit chambers. *J Biomed Mater Res A*, Vol. 81, No. 2, pp. 310-316.

[43] Goodman SB, Song Y, Yoo JY, Fox N, Trindade MC, Kajiyama G, Ma T, Regular D, Brown J, Smith RL. (2003). Local infusion of FGF-2 enhances bone ingrowth in rabbit chambers in presence of polyethylene particles. *J Biomed Mater Res A*, Vol. 65, No. 4, pp. 454-461.

[44] Goodman SB. (1994). The effects of micromotion and particulate materials on tissue differentiation: bone chamber studies in rabbits. *Acta Orthop Scand Suppl*, Vol. 258, pp. 1-43.

[45] Granchi D, Amato I, Battistelli L, Ciapetti G, Pagani S, Avnet S, Baldini N, Giunti A. (2005). Molecular basis of osteoclastogenesis induced by osteoblasts exposed to wear particles. *Biomaterials*, Vol. 26, No. 15, pp. 237-239.

[46] Granchi D, Ciapetti G, Amato I, Pagani S, Cenni E, Savarino L, Avnet S, Peris JL, Pallacani A, Baldini N, Giunti A. (2004). The influence of alumina and ultra-high molecular weight polyethylene particles on osteoblast-osteoclast cooperation. *Biomaterials*, Vol. 25, No. 18, pp. 4037-45.

[47] Greenfield EM, Bechtold J, Implant Wear Symposium 2007 Biologic Work Group. (2008). What other biologic and mechanical factors might contribute to osteolysis? *J Am Acad Orthop Surg*, Vol. 16, Suppl 1, pp. S56-62.

[48] Greenfield EM, Bi Y, Ragab AA, Goldberg VM, Nalepka JL, Seabold JM. (2005). Does endotoxin contribute to aseptic loosening of orthopedic implants? *J Biomed Mater Res B Appl Biomater*, Vol. 72, No. 1, pp. 179-185.

[49] Gregory CA, Gunn WG, Peister A, Prockop DJ. (2004). An Alizarin red-based assay of mineralization by adherent cells in culture: comparison with cetylpyridinium chloride extraction. *Anal Biochem*, Vol. 329, No. 1, pp. 77-84.

[50] Heinemann DE, Lohmann C, Siggelkow H, Alves F, Engel I, Koster G. (2000). Human osteoblast-like cells phagocytose metal particles and express the macrophage marker CD68 in vitro. *J Bone Joint Surg Br*, Vol. 82, No. 2, pp. 283-289.

[51] Jeong WK, Park SW, Im GI. (2008). Growth factors reduce the suppression of proliferation and osteogenic differentiation by titanium particles on MSCs. *J Biomed Mater Res A*, Vol. 86, No. 4, pp. 1137-1144.

[52] Kanaji A, Caicedo MS, Virdi AS, Sumner DR, Hallab NJ, Sena K. (2009). Co-Cr-Mo alloy particles induce tumor necrosis factor alpha production in MLO-Y4 osteocytes: a role for osteocytes in particle-induced inflammation. *Bone*, Vol. 45, No. 3, pp. 528-533.

[53] Kann S, Chiu R, Ma T, Goodman SB. (2010). OP-1 (BMP-7) stimulates osteoprogenitor cell differentiation in the presence of polymethylmethacrylate particles. *J Biomed Mater Res A*, Vol. 94, No. 2, pp. 485-488.

[54] Kato Y, Windle JJ, Koop BA, Mundy GR, Bonewald LF. (1997). Establishment of an osteocyte-like cell line, MLO-Y4. *J Bone Miner Res*, Vol. 12, No. 12, pp. 2014-2023.

[55] Komori T. (2006). Regulation of osteoblast differentiation by transcription factors. *J Cell Biochem*, Vol. 99, No. 5, pp. 1233-1239.

[56] Kurtz SM. (2004). *The UHMWPE Handbook: Ultra-High Molecular Weight Polyethylene in Total Joint Replacement*, Academic Press, ISBN 0-12-429851-6, San Diego, United States of America.

[57] Kwon SY, Lin T, Takei H, Ma Q, Wood DJ, O'Connor D, Sung KL. (2001). Alterations in the adhesion behavior of osteoblasts by titanium particle loading: inhibition of cell function and gene expression. *Biorheology*, Vol. 38, No. 2-3, pp. 161-83.

[58] Kwon SY, Takei H, Pioletti DP, Lin T, Ma QJ, Akeson WH, Wood DJ, Sung KL. (2000). Titanium particles inhibit osteoblast adhesion to fibronectin-coated substrates. *J Orthop Res*, Vol. 18, No. 2, pp. 203-211.

[59] Lenz R, Mittelmeier W, Hansmann D, Brem R, Diehl P, Fritsche A, Bader R. (2009). Response of human osteoblasts exposed to wear particles generated at the interface of total hip stems and bone cement. *J Biomed Mater Res A*, Vol. 89, No. 2, pp. 370-378.

[60] Lian JB, Stein GS. (2001). Osteoblast biology. In: *Osteoporosis, 2nd ed.*, Marcus R, Feldman D, Kelsey J. pp. 21-71, Academic Press, ISBN 978-0-12-470862-4, San Diego, United States of America.

[61] Liu F, Zhu Z, Mao Y, Liu M, Tang T, Qiu S. (2009). Inhibition of titanium particle-induced osteoclastogenesis through inactivation of NFATc1 by VIVIT peptide. *Biomaterials*, Vol. 30, No. 9, pp. 1756-1762.

[62] Lohmann CH, Dean DD, Bonewald LF, Schwartz Z, Boyan BD. (2002). Nitric oxide and prostaglandin E2 production in response to ultra-high molecular weight polyethylene particles depends on osteoblast maturation state. *J Bone Joint Surg Am*, Vol. 84, No. 3, pp. 411-419.

[63] Lohmann CH, Dean DD, Koster G, Casasola D, Buchhorn GH, Fink U, Schwartz Z, Boyan BD. (2002). Ceramic and PMMA particles differentially affect osteoblast phenotype. *Biomaterials*, Vol. 23, No. 8, pp. 1855-1863.

[64] Lohmann CH, Schwartz Z, Koster G, Jahn U, Buchhorn GH, MacDougall MJ, Casasola D, Liu Y, Sylvia VL, Dean DD, Boyan BD. (2000). Phagocytosis of wear debris by osteoblasts affects differentiation and local factor production in a manner dependent on particle composition. *Biomaterials*, Vol. 21, No. 6, pp. 551-561.

[65] Ma G, Chiu R, Huang Z, Pearl K, Ma T, Smith RL, Goodman SB. (2010). Polymethylmethacrylate particle exposure causes changes in p38 MAPK and TGF-beta signalling in differentiating MC3T3-E1 cells. *J Biomed Mater Res A*, Vol. 94, No. 1, pp. 234-240.

[66] Ma T, Huang Z, Ren PG, McCally R, Lindsey D, Smith RL, Goodman SB. (2008). An in vivo murine model of continuous intramedullary infusion of particles. *Biomaterials*, Vol. 29, No. 27, pp. 3738-3742.

[67] Ma T, Nelson ER, Mawatari T, Oh KJ, Larsen DM, Smith RL, Goodman SB. (2006). Effects of local infusion of OP-1 on particle-induced and NSAID-induced inhibition of bone ingrowth in vivo. *J Biomed Mater Res A*, Vol. 79, No. 3, pp. 740-746.

[68] Ma T, Ortiz SG, Huang Z, Ren PG, Smith RL, Goodman SB. (2009). In vivo murine model of continuous intramedullary infusion of particles: a preliminary study. *J Biomed Mater Res B Appl Biomater*, Vol. 88, No.1, pp. 250-253.

[69] Ma T, Ren PG, Larsen DM, Suenaga E, Zilber S, Genovese M, Smith RL, Goodman SB. (2009). Efficacy of a p38 mitogen activated protein kinase inhibitor in mitigating an established inflammatory reaction to polyethylene particles in vivo. *J Biomed Mater Res A*, Vol. 89, No. 1, pp. 117-123.

[70] Malaval L, Liu F, Roche P, Aubin JE. (1999). Kinetics of osteoprogenitor proliferation and osteoblast differentiation in vitro. *J Cell Biochem*, Vol. 74, No. 4, pp. 616-627.

[71] Maloney WJ, Smith RL, Schmalzried TP, ChibaJ, Huene D, Rubash H. (1995). Isolation and characterization of wear particles generated in patients who have had failure of a hip arthroplasty without cement. *J Bone Joint Surg Am*, Vol. 77, No. 9, pp. 1301-1310.

[72] Martinez ME, Medina S, del Campo MT, Garcia JA, Rodrigo A, Munuera L. (1998). Effect of polyethylene particles on human osteoblastic cell growth. *Biomaterials*, Vol. 19, No. 1-3, pp. 183-187.

[73] Martinez ME, Medina S, del Campo MT, Sanchez-Cabezudo MJ, Sanchez M, Munuera L. (1998). Effect of polyethylene on osteocalcin, alkaline phosphatase, and procollagen secretion by human osteoblastic cells. *Calcif Tissue Int*, Vol. 62, No. 5, pp. 453-456.

[74] Minoda Y, Kobayashi A, Iwaki H, Miyaguchi M, Kadoya Y, Ohashi H, Takaoka K. (2004). Characteristics of polyethylene wear particles isolated from synovial fluid after mobile-bearing and posterior-stabilized total knee arthroplasties. *J Biomed Mater Res B Appl Biomater*, Vol. 71, No. 1, pp. 1-6.

[75] Nalepka JL, Lee MJ, Kraay MJ, Marcus RE, Goldberg VM, Chen X, Greenfield EM. (2006). Lipopolysaccharide found in aseptic loosening of patients with inflammatory arthritis. *Clin Orthop Relat Res*, Vol. 451, pp. 229-235.

[76] O'Connor DT, Choi MG, Kwon SY, Paul Sung KL. (2004). New insight into the mechanism of hip prosthesis loosening: effect of titanium debris size on osteoblast function. *J Orthop Res*, Vol. 22, No. 2, pp. 229-236.

[77] Okafor CC, Haleem-Smith H, Laqueriere P, Manner PA, Tuan RS. (2006). Particulate endocytosis mediates biological responses of human mesenchymal stem cells to titanium wear debris. *J Orthop Res*, Vol. 24, No. 3, pp. 461-473.

[78] Ortiz SG, Ma T, Epstein NJ, Smith RL, Goodman SB. (2008). Validation and quantification of an in vitro model of continuous infusion of submicron-sized particles. *J Biomed Mater Res B Appl Biomater*, Vol. 84, No. 2, pp. 328-333.

[79] Ortiz SG, Ma T, Regula D, Smith RL, Goodman SB. (2008). Continuous intramedullary polymer particle infusion using a murine femoral explants model. *J Biomed Mater Res B Appl Biomater*, Vol. 87, No. 2, pp. 440-446.

[80] Peister A, Mellad JA, Larson BL, Hall BM, Gibson LF, Prockop DJ. (2004). Adult stem cells from bone marrow (MSCs) isolated from different strains of inbred mice vary in surface epitopes, rates of proliferation, and differentiation potential. *Blood*, Vol. 103, No. 5, pp. 1662-1668.

[81] Peter B, Zambelli PY, Guicheux J, Pioletti DP. (2005). The effect of bisphosphonates and titanium particles on osteoblasts: an in vitro study. *J Bone Joint Surg Br*, Vol. 87, No. 8, pp. 1157-63.

[82] Phinney DG, Kopen G, Isaacson RL, Prockop DJ. (1999). Plastic adherent stromal cells from the bone marrow of commonly used strains of inbred mice: variations in yield, growth, and differentiation. *J Cell Biochem*, Vol. 72, No. 4, pp. 570-585.

[83] Pioletti DP, Leoni L, Genini D, Takei H, Du P, Corbeil J. (2002). Gene expression analysis of osteoblastic cells contacted by orthopedic implant particles. *J Biomed Mater Res*, Vol. 61, No. 3, pp. 408-20.

[84] Piolett DP, Kottelat A. (2004). The influence of wear particles in the expression of osteoclastogenesis factors by osteoblasts. *Biomaterials*, Vol. 25, No. 27, pp. 5803-5808.

[85] Pioletti DP, Takei H, Kwon SY, Wood D, Sung KL. (1999). The cytotoxic effect of titanium particles phagocytosed by osteoblasts. *J Biomed Mater Res*, Vol. 46, No. 3, pp. 399-407.

[86] Quarles LD, Yohay DA, Lever LW, Caton R, Wenstrup RJ. (1992). Distinct proliferative and differentiated stages of murine MC3T3-E1 cells in culture: an in vitro model of osteoblast development. J Bone Miner Res, Vol. 7, No. 6, pp. 683-692.

[87] Queally JM, Devitt BM, Butler JS, Malizia AP, Murray D, Doran PP, O'Bryne JM. (2009). Cobalt ions induce chemokine secretion in primary human osteoblasts. *J Orthop Res*, Vol. 27, No. 7, pp. 855-864.

[88] Ragab AA, Van De Motter R, Lavish SA, Goldberg VM, Ninomiya JT, Carlin CR, Greenfield EM. (1999). Measurement and removal of adherent endotoxin from titanium particles and implant surfaces. *J Orthop Res*, Vol. 17, No. 6, pp. 803-809.

[89] Ramachandran R, Goodman SB, Smith RL. (2006). The effects of titanium and polymethylmethacrylate particles on osteoblast phenotypic stability. *J Biomed Mater Res A*, Vol. 77, No. 3, pp. 512-517.

[90] Ren PG, Huang Z, Ma T, Biswal S, Smith RL, Goodman SB. (2010). Surveillance of systemic trafficking of macrophages induced by UHMWPE particles in nude mice by noninvasive imaging. *J Biomed Mater Res A*, Vol. 94, No. 3, pp. 706-711.

[91] Ren PG, Irani A, Huang Z, Ma T, Biswal S, Goodman SB. (2011). Continuous infusion of UHMWPE particles induces increased bone macrophages and osteolysis. *Clin Orthop Relat Res*, Vol. 469, No. 1, pp. 113-122.

[92] Ren PG, Lee SW, Biswal S, Goodman SB. (2008). Systemic trafficking of macrophages induced by bone cement particles in nude mice. *Biomaterials*, Vol. 29, No. 36, pp. 4760-4765.

[93] Rodrigo AM, Martinez ME, Escudero ML, Ruiz J, Martinez P, Saldana L, Gomez-Garcia L, Fernandez L, Cordero J, Munuera L. (2001). Influence of particle size in the effect of polyethylene on human osteoblastic cells. *Biomaterials*, Vol. 22, No. 8, pp. 755-762.

[94] Rodrigo AM, Martinez ME, Saldana L, Valles G, Martinez P, Gonzales-Carrasco JL, Cordero J, Munuera L. (2002). Effects of polyethylene and alpha-alumina particles on IL-6 expression and secretion in primary cultures of human osteoblastic cells. *Biomaterials*, Vol. 23, No. 3, pp. 901-908.

[95] Roebuck KA, Vermes C, Carpenter LR, Fritz EA, Narayanan R, Glant TT. Down-regulation of procollagen $\alpha 1$[I] messenger RNA by titanium particles correlates with nuclear factor κB (NF-κB) activation and increased Rel A and NF-κB1 binding to collagen promoter. (2001). *J Bone Miner Res*, Vol. 16, No. 3, pp. 501-510.

[96] Sabokbar A, Fujikawa Y, Brett J, Murray DW, Athanasou NA. (1996). Increased osteoclastic differentiation by PMMA particle-associated macrophages. *Acta Orthop Scand*, Vol. 67, No. 6, pp. 593-598.

[97] Sabokbar A, Fujikawa Y, Murray DW, Athanasou NA. (1997). Radio-opaque agents in bone cement increase bone resorption. *J Bone Joint Surg Br*, Vol. 79, No. 1, pp. 129-134.

[98] Sabokbar A, Fujikawa Y, Murray DW, Athanasou NA. (1998). Bisphosphonates in bone cement inhibit PMMA particle induced bone resorption. *Ann Rheum Dis*, Vol. 57, No. 10, pp. 614-618.

[99] Schofer MD, Fuchs-Winkelmann S, Kessler-Thones A, Rudisile MM, Wack C, Paletta JR, Boudriot U. (2008). The role of mesenchymal stem cells in the pathogenesis of Co-Cr-Mo particle induced aseptic loosening: an in vitro study. *Biomed Mater Eng*, Vol. 18, No. 6, pp. 395-403.

[100] Seo SW, Lee D, Cho SK, Kim AD, Minematsu H, Celil Aydemir AB, Geller JA, Macaulay W, Yang J, Young-In Lee F. (2007). ERK signaling regulates macrophages colony-stimulating factor expression by titanium particles in MC3T3-E1 murine calvarial preosteoblastic cells. *Ann N Y Acad Sci*, Vol. 1117, pp. 151-158.

[101] Shida J, Trindade MC, Goodman SB, Schurman DJ, Smith RL. (2000). Induction of interleukin-6 release in human osteoblast-like cells exposed to titanium particles in vitro. *Calcif Tissue Int*, Vol. 67, No. 2, pp. 151-155.

[102] Sommer B, Felix R, Sprecher C, Leunig M, Ganz R, Hofstetter W. (2005). Wear particles and surface topographies are modulators of osteoclastogenesis in vitro. *J Biomed Mater Res A*, Vol. 72, No. 1, pp. 67-76.

[103] Takei H, Pioletti DP, Kwon SY, Sung KL. (2000). Combined effect of titanium particles and TNF-alpha on the production of IL-6 by osteoblast-like cells. *J Biomed Mater Res*, Vol. 52, No. 2, pp. 382-387.

[104] Torii Y, Hitomi K, Tsukagoshi N. (1996). Synergistic effect of BMP-2 and ascorbate on the phenotypic expression of osteoblastic MC3T3-E1 cells. *Mol Cell Biochem*, Vol. 165, No. 1, pp. 25-29.

[105] Tuan RS, Lee FY, Konttinen Y, Wilkinson JM, Smith RL, Implant Wear Symposium 2007 Biologic Work Group. (2008). What are the local and systemic biologic

reactions and mediators to wear debris, and what host factors determine or modulate the biologic response to wear particles? *J Am Acad Orthop Surg*, Vol. 16, Suppl 1, pp. S42-48.

[106] Valles G, Gonzales-Melendi P, Saldana L, Rodriguez M, Munuera L, Vilaboa N. (2008). Rutile and titanium particles differentially affect the production of osteoblastic local factors. *J Biomed Mater Res A*, Vol. 84, No. 2, pp. 324-336.

[107] Vermes C, Chandrasekaran R, Jacobs JJ, Galante JO, Roebuck KA, Glant TT. (2001). The effects of particulate wear debris, cytokines, and growth factors on the functions of MG-63 osteoblasts. *J Bone Joint Surg Am*, Vol. 83, No. 2, pp. 201-211.

[108] Vermes C, Roebuck KA, Chandrasekaran R, Dobai JG, Glante TT. (2000). Particulate wear debris activates protein tyrosine kinases and nuclear factor kappaB, which down-regulates type I collagen synthesis in human osteoblasts. *J Bone Miner Res*, Vol. 15, No. 9, pp. 1756-1765.

[109] Visentin M, Stea S, Squarzoni S, Antonietti B, Reggiani M, Toni A. (2004). A new method for isolation of polyethylene wear debris from tissue and synovial fluid. *Biomaterials*, Vol. 25, No. 24, pp. 5531-5537.

[110] Wang D, Christensen K, Chawla K, Ziao G, Krebsbach PH, Franceschi RT. (1999). Isolation and characterization of MC3T3-E1 preosteoblast subclones with distinct in vitro and in vivo differentiation/mineralization potential. *J Bone Miner Res*, Vol. 14, No. 6, pp. 893-903.

[111] Wang ML, Nesti, LJ, Tuli R, Lazatin J, Danielson KG, Sharkey PF, Tuan RS. (2002). Titanium particles suppress expression of osteoblastic phenotype in human mesenchymal stem cells. *J Orthop Res*, Vol. 20, No. 6, pp. 1175-1184.

[112] Wang ML, Tuli R, Manner PA, Sharkey PF, Hall DJ, Tuan RS. (2003). Direct and indirect induction of apoptosis in human mesenchymal stem cells in response to titanium particles. *J Orthop Res*, Vol. 21, No., 4, pp. 697-707.

[113] Warme BA, Epstein NJ, Trindade MC, Miyanishi K, Ma T, Saket RR, Regular D, Goodman SB, Smith RL. (2004). Proinflammatory mediator expression in a novel murine model of titanium particle-induced intramedullary inflammation. *J Biomed Mater Res B Appl Biomater*, Vol. 71, No. 2, pp. 360-366.

[114] Wirth MA, Agrawal CM, Mabrey JD, Dean DD, Blanchard CR, Miller MA, Rockwood CA Jr. (1999). Isolation and characterization of polyethylene wear debris associated with osteolysis following total shoulder arthroplasty. *J Bone Joint Surg Am*, Vol. 81, No. 1, pp. 29-37.

[115] Wolfarth DL, Han DW, Bushar G, Parks NL. (1997). Separation and characterization of polyethylene wear debris from synovial fluid and tissue samples of revised knee replacements. *J Biomed Mater Res*, Vol. 34, No. 1, pp. 57-61.

[116] Wright T, Goodman SB. (2001). *Implant Wear in Total Joint Replacement*, American Academy of Orthopaedic Surgeons, ISBN 0-89203-261-8, Illinois, United States of America.

[117] Xiao G, Cui Y, Ducy P, Karsenty G, Franceschi RT. (1997). Ascorbic acid-dependent activation of the osteocalcin promoter in MC3T3-E1 preosteoblasts: requirement for collagen matrix synthesis and the presence of an intact OSE2 sequence. *Mol Endocrinol*, Vol. 11, No. 8, pp. 1103-1113.

[118] Xiao G, Gopalakrishnan R, Jiang D, Reith E, Benson MD, Franceschi RT. (2002). Bone morphogenetic proteins, extracellular matrix, and mitogen-activated protein

kinase signalling pathways are required for osteoblast-specific gene expression and differentiation in MC3T3-E1 cells. *J Bone Miner Res*, Vol. 17, No. 1, pp. 101-110.

[119] Yamanaka Y, Abu-Amer W, Foglia D, Otero J, Clohisy JC, Abu-Amer Y. (2008). NFAT2 is an esssential mediator of orthopedic particle-induced osteoclastogenesis. *J Orthop Res*, Vol. 26, No. 12, pp.1577-1584.

[120] Yamanaka Y, Abu-Amer Y, Faccio R, Clohisy JC. (2006). Map kinase c-JUN N-terminal kinase mediates PMMA induction of osteoclasts. *J Orthop Res*, Vol. 24, No. 7, pp. 1349-1357.

[121] Yao J, CS-Szabo G, Jacobs JJ, Kuettner KE, Glant TT. (1997). Suppression of osteoblast function by titanium particles. *J Bone Joint Surg Am*, Vol. 79, No. 1, pp. 107-112.

[122] Zambonin G, Colucci S, Cantatore F, Grano M. (1998). Response of human osteoblasts to polymethylmethacrylate in vitro. Calcif Tissue Int, Vol. 62, No. 4, pp. 362-365.

[123] Zhang H, Ricciardi BF, Yang X, Shi Y, Camacho NP, Bostrom MG. (2008). Polymethylmethacrylate particles stimulate bone resorption of mature osteoclasts in vitro. *Acta Orthop*, Vol. 79, No. 2, pp. 281-288.

[124] Zilber S, Epstein N, Lee S, Larsen M, Ma T, Smith RL, Biswal S, Goodman SB. (2008). Mouse femoral intramedullary injection model: technique and microCT scan validation. *J Biomed Mater Res B Appl Biomater*, Vol. 84, No. 1, pp. 286-290.

[125] Zreigat H, Crotti TN, Howlett CR, Capone M, Markovic B, Haynes DR. (2003). Prosthetic particles modify the expression of bone-related proteins by human osteoblastic cells in vitro. *Biomaterials*, Vol. 24, No. 2, pp. 337-346.

9

Osteogenesis Imperfecta

Roy Morello[1,2] and Paul W. Esposito[3,4]
[1]*Department of Physiology & Biophysics, University of Arkansas for Medical Sciences, Little Rock, AR,*
[2]*Division of Genetics, University of Arkansas for Medical Sciences, Little Rock, AR,*
[3]*Department of Orthopaedic Surgery and Rehabilitation, University of Nebraska Medical Center, The Nebraska Medical Center, Omaha, NE,*
[4]*Department of Orthopaedic Surgery, Childrens Hospital and Medical Center, Omaha, NE, USA*

1. Introduction

Osteogenesis imperfecta (OI) is a congenital, generalized connective tissue disorder characterized by severe osteoporosis and bone fragility. Other features of the disease include dentinogenesis imperfecta, scoliosis, short stature, blue sclerae, hearing loss, and skin and ligament laxity (Cheung and Glorieux, 2008; Rauch and Glorieux, 2004). It is the most commonly inherited connective tissue disorder with a prevalence in the United States of about 25,000-50,000 cases (Martin and Shapiro, 2007). Molecular defects in type I collagen genes, *COL1A1* and *COL1A2*, were first associated with OI in the early 1980's (Chu et al., 1983). Since then, although OI is most commonly an autosomal dominant disease, it became evident that in certain pedigrees with recurrence of OI in children of unaffected parents, other mechanisms of inheritance were at play. While germline mosaicism for a type I collagen mutation was demonstrated in some rare cases (Cohn et al., 1990; Edwards et al., 1992), in others where no collagen primary sequence defects were evident, the existence of recessively inherited forms of OI had to be postulated. It is known that 10-15% of all OI cases are not caused by type I collagen mutations and some of these can be distinguished from others based on specific bone histological features (Glorieux et al., 2002), clinical features (Glorieux et al., 2000), or because they are linked to a genetic region not containing type I collagen genes (Labuda et al., 2002). It took about a quarter of a century to identify the first gene responsible for some cases of recessive OI, i.e. *CRTAP* (encoding Cartilage-associated protein) (Morello et al., 2006). This initial discovery led the way to the identification of several novel genes whose mutations cause recessive forms of OI. It has rapidly become evident that while dominant forms of OI are caused by mutations in type I collagen genes, recessive forms of OI are almost always caused by mutations in genes encoding for proteins involved in the type I collagen synthetic pathway and often residing in the rough endoplasmic reticulum (rER). Thus, all direct and indirect collagen interactors, either in the rER or Golgi apparatus or involved in intracellular collagen trafficking, have become new candidates for recessive or atypical forms of OI. This chapter will provide the reader with an update on the latest developments in the OI field, including description of new genes causing OI, mechanisms of disease and novel therapeutic approaches.

2. Classification of OI, clinical features and differential diagnosis

Osteogenesis imperfecta was classified several years ago into four types based on clinical, radiological and genetic features (Sillence, 1988; Sillence et al., 1979). Type II OI is the perinatal lethal form followed by types III, IV and I, in decreasing order of severity with type I OI being the mildest form. The mode of inheritance is not unique to each type with at least types II (further sub-classified into IIA, IIB and IIC) and III that could be inherited in a dominant or recessive fashion. More recently, out of the more heterogeneous group of type IV patients, novel types V, VI and VII OI were described based on unique clinical and/or histological features and linkage to loci where no type I collagen genes were mapped (Glorieux et al., 2000; Glorieux et al., 2002; Labuda et al., 2002).

The nosology of OI has been a subject of discussion and revision in light of recent discoveries of novel genes causing recessive forms of the disease. Plotkin (Plotkin, 2004) proposed to classify as OI all those cases in which a mutation in either *COL1A1* or *COL1A2* can be identified. Cases resulting from mutations in other genes would be classified as syndromes resembling OI. Others have proposed to adopt a revised Sillence classification of OI type I through VI but removing types VII and VIII which are due to mutations in *CRTAP* and *LEPRE1*, respectively, but have clinical and radiological features indistinguishable from types II-IV (Van Dijk et al., 2010). A more genetically oriented classification has also being proposed (Forlino et al., 2011). Here the classical Sillence OI types I-IV are maintained (all due to either *COL1A1* or *COL1A2* defects), followed by the previously described types V, VI and VII, and then in increasing order new types of OI (the latest is number XI) where each new type (from types V-XI) is due to a mutation in a different gene (**Table 1**). Conversely, the 2010 Revision of the Nosology and Classification of Genetic Skeletal Disorders (Warman et al., 2011) has agreed to retain the Sillence classification as the universally accepted way to classify the degree of OI severity but to free it from any direct molecular reference.

Because the original Sillence classification has been in use for over 30 years and instantly refers to the clinical severity of the disease, it is likely that physicians will continue to use it at least until the underlying genetic mutation of a patient has been clearly determined. The strictly genetic classification could be quite useful though as it is indeed possible that different genetic etiology and hence mechanism of disease may require a different therapeutic approach. This is beginning to emerge for instance in patients with *SERPINF1* mutations who have not shown beneficial effects from bisphosphonate treatment (Homan et al., 2011).

Although there remains a great deal of difficulty making a definitive diagnosis in many of the children, recognition that there are recessive forms of osteogenesis imperfecta has clarified a historically confusing differential diagnosis. Utilization of these modified classifications also assists in identifying individuals without the classic types I – IV from normal children with nonaccidental trauma and other unrelated metabolic bone diseases.

OI type	Inheritance	Clinical features	Gene defect	Protein
I	AD	Mild	*COL1A1 (null alleles)*	a1(I)
II	AD	Lethal	*COL1A1 or COL1A2*	a1(I) or a2(I)
III	AD	Severe, deforming	*COL1A1 or COL1A2*	a1(I) or a2(I)
IV	AD	Moderate	*COL1A1 or COL1A2*	a1(I) or a2(I)
V	AD	Hypertrophic callus, dense metaphyseal band, calcification of radio-ulnar interosseus membrane	*Unknown*	Unknown
VI	AR	Severe: mineralization defect, 'fish scale' bone lamellae, slightly elevated AP	*SERPINF1*	PEDF
VII	AR	Very severe to lethal, rhyzomelia	*CRTAP*	CRTAP
VIII	AR	Severe to lethal, rhyzomelia	*LEPRE1*	P3H1
IX	AR	Moderate to severe	*PPIB*	CYPB
X	AR	Severe	*SERPINH1*	HSP47
XI	AR	Moderate to severe with joint contractures (Bruck syndrome 1?)	*FKBP10*	FKBP10
NC	AR	Moderate to severe with joint contractures and pterygia, Bruck syndrome 2	*PLOD2*	LH2
NC	AR	Ocular form of OI, osteoporosis pseudoglioma syndrome	*LRP5 (null alleles)*	LRP5
NC	AR	Moderate to severe	*SP7*	OSX (Osterix)

Table 1. Genetic classification of OI (AD = autosomal dominant; AR = autosomal recessive; NC = not classified)

Type I: These individuals typically do not have major bone deformity and have a significant variability in terms of number of fractures, even within the same family. Fractures typically begin when the children start to ambulate. Plain radiographs often are normal in appearance. These individuals may have blue sclera and hearing loss, although this may not occur before the second or third decade. Dentinogenesis imperfecta is not typically a major component of Type I. There may be subtle dental findings. There are no long-term studies to determine if the collagen defect might lead to later dental problems. Growth and stature are typically mildly decreased in type I OI (Forlino et al., 2011; Sillence et al., 1979).

Type II: Type II is historically described as perinatally lethal, typically from pulmonary failure related to the severe involvement of the chest cavity with small volume, deformity, and recurrent rib fractures. There may also be some involvement of the intrinsic collagen of the lung parenchyma (Forlino et al., 2011; Sillence et al., 1979).

These children are frequently diagnosed in prenatal ultrasounds with short, severely bowed long bones with multiple fractures. Radiographically, at the time of birth, they have severe bowing of the long bones, multiple fractures in different stages of healing, poorly defined cortices, and crumpling or wrinkling of the bones in an accordion-type fashion. There is poor tubulation with wide medullary canals. There is typically severe wedging deformity of the vertebrae. The skull is usually quite soft and large (Forlino et al., 2011; Sillence et al., 1979). Some of these children, including some treated with bisphosphonates, have survived for several years.

Type III: These patients are also frequently diagnosed on prenatal ultrasound. They also have relative shortening of the long bones, significant bowing, and multiple prenatal and postnatal fractures. These children continue to have fractures even with gentle handling. This is the most severe non-lethal form. They may have a very typical triangular facies, blue sclerae, dentinogenesis imperfecta, vertebral fractures, and frequently scoliosis. Without treatment with bisphosphonates, this OI type frequently demonstrates classic "popcorn epiphyses" of the long bones and patients have significant short stature (Forlino et al., 2011; Sillence et al., 1979).

Type IV: Traditionally, this classification has included children with phenotypes that did not fit into Sillence type I or III. These children typically have multiple fractures, varying degrees of deformity, as well as a great deal of variation in terms of color of the sclera, cranial settling, dentinogenesis imperfecta, and stature. With the recognition of recessive forms, many of these children previously classified as having type IV are now recognized as having one of these other, less common forms (Forlino et al., 2011; Sillence et al., 1979).

Type V: These individuals have increasing bone fragility and a moderately severe phenotype of OI. They also have calcification of the interosseous membrane which can be noted in the first year of life. This causes a significant decrease in pronation and supination. The radial head dislocates anteriorly, and long bone fracture can result in a very hypertrophic callus. There can be a radio-dense band at the end of the metaphysis. There is a unique mesh-like pattern of lamination histologically under polarizing light. (Arundel et al., 2011; Glorieux et al., 2000).

The clinical features of the recessive types of OI are described in section 4 (Molecular genetics of dominant and recessive OI).

3. Management and treatment

A team approach is vital to care for children with OI because many of them have not only recurrent fractures and severe bowing deformities, but also lax joints and connective tissue-associated problems. Long-term, individuals may develop other significant health issues, including cardiac, pulmonary, and joint problems. Unfortunately, to this point there is no good long-term data to determine what types of problems individuals with OI develop, their frequency, and appropriate treatment, or whether present medical management will improve long-term function. There is also very likely a significant difference in long-term function and the rate of deterioration that is dependent upon the specific genetic defect, but this has not been studied.

Bisphosphonates have been utilized extensively over the past decade in the treatment of osteogenesis imperfecta and other disorders with brittle bones and have been shown to clearly increase cortical thickness (Arikoski et al., 2004; Rauch and Glorieux, 2006). They improve comfort and function (Land et al., 2006a) but they do not lead pre-existing bony deformity and bowing to remodel (Astrom et al., 2007; Forin et al., 2005; Land et al., 2006a; Plotkin et al., 2006) (**Figure 1**). Decreases in fracture rates have been difficult to document.

Centers that treat large numbers of these children however have anecdotally noted a marked increase in activity level and ambulation, even in children with severe type III OI. Present indications for treatment with bisphosphonates in children with the more severe forms of OI include marked bowing, which is interfering with comfort and function, and recurrent fractures (de Graaff et al., 2011; Forin et al., 2005; Glorieux, 2007; Glorieux et al., 1998; Plotkin et al., 2006; Rauch and Glorieux, 2006).

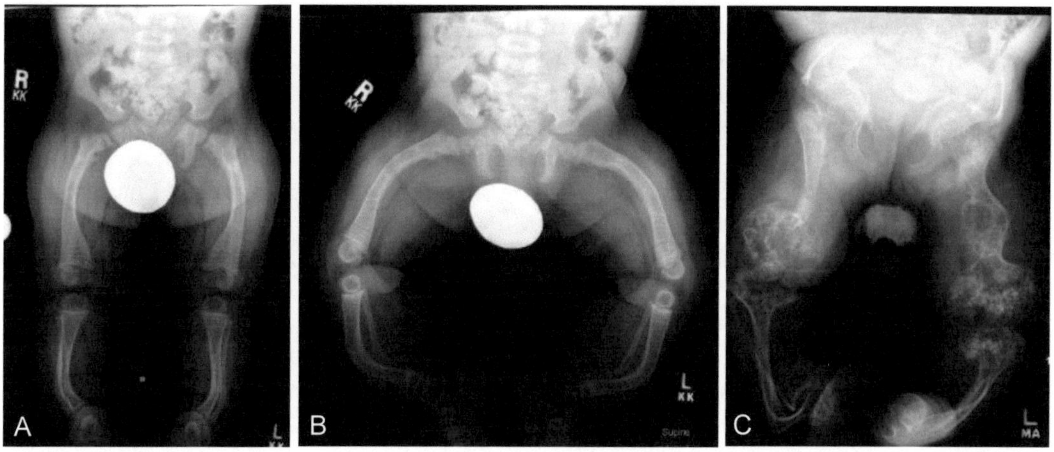

Fig. 1. A, B: 15-month old with type III OI. Note the relatively normal physis, and reasonable bone development following treatment with pamidronate since infancy. However, the significant bowing will not remodel, and as these children begin to pull up to stand they will predictably fracture at the apex of the bow. C: untreated 17 year old also with type III demonstrating popcorn epiphysis and signs of recurrent fractures.

The greatest improvement in areal bone density occurs in the first year of treatment. Pamidronate has been studied the most extensively, and has been shown to improve vertebral height and development in children with compressed vertebral bodies (Land et al., 2006b). Infants and young children with more severe OI with bowing and recurrent fractures have been safely treated with pamidronate (Astrom et al., 2007; Land et al., 2006a; Plotkin et al., 2006)· The DEXA scan is the most frequent test utilized to help determine the relative severity of the OI, and the Z-score has ben utilized to monitor the response to treatment. However, there is not data suggesting that the goal of treatment is to develop a bone density in the normal range. At the present time, the clinical parameters of improved comfort, decreased fracture rate, and progression of normal developmental milestones offers the best clinical assessment of effective treatment. Zoledronic acid is a more potent bisphosphonate, which requires only one intra-venous treatment per year. It is presently being studied, but this data and results are not yet available (Shapiro and Sponsellor, 2009).

Initial treatment protocols with pamidronate were for a set number of years depending on the treating center. However, it has been noted that if the treatment is discontinued in a growing child, the bone that is developing at the proximal and distal end of the long bones is not treated. This gives rise to a stress riser between the treated bone of the shaft and the relatively soft bone at either end of the long bones (Breslau-Siderius et al., 1998; Rauch et al., 2006)· Theoretically, this is a concern with the longer acting agents, which may be given only once per year (Rauch et al., 2007; Rauch et al., 2006; Ward et al., 2007). The ideal treatment protocol is not universally agreed upon and it is recognized that other forms of treatment in the future will improve the lives of these individuals (Devogelaer and Coppin, 2006; Glorieux, 2007; Glorieux et al., 1998; Plotkin et al., 2006; Rauch and Glorieux, 2006).

There are a number of recent review papers dealing with the evaluation and treatment of osteogenesis imperfecta. These papers very nicely demonstrate the impact of the team approach, early medical management with bisphosphonates combined with prudent surgical management, address the questions that remain to be answered, and address the differences in approach between centers (Esposito and Plotkin, 2008; Forlino et al., 2011; Shapiro and Sponsellor, 2009).

It is less clear when to treat children with type I OI. Many centers recommend that treatment with bisphosphates be withheld unless the children are having recurrent fractures. Whether or not the bone density as measured on DEXA results as an isolated parameter has a role in determining treatment in this patient population with type I OI is unclear. Bone density has been correlated with disease severity, and may be predictive of long-term function (Plotkin et al., 2006).

The role of bisphosphonate treatment with non-union fractures is also unclear. Non-unions have been noted in 15% of children with osteogenesis imperfecta even prior to treatment with bisphosphonates (Agarwal and Joseph, 2005). There is one report of delay in healing following osteotomies but not fractures (Pizones et al., 2005). Non-unions have been reported post surgically (Cho et al., 2011). There are other reports that patients receiving bisphosphonates did not have issues with bone healing. El Sobky et al reported that children treated with pamidronate prior to surgery and afterwards function better than children treated with surgery alone (el-Sobky et al., 2006). In our experience with a large OI clinic population, when pamidronate is discontinued, some of the children have increased bone pain, which decreases after treatment is restored, and an increase in fracture rate, although this is not reported definitively in the literature.

Bisphosphonate treatment has clearly been shown to improve vertebral height even after significant wedge compression deformity of the vertebrae (Land et al., 2006b). However, there is no report of whether this treatment changes the incidence or severity of scoliosis. One recent spine x-ray review of a large osteogenesis imperfecta clinic population showed a significant increase in spondylolysis and spondylolisthesis above the incidence reported in otherwise normal children. The vast majority of these children had type III and type IV OI, and were ambulatory following treatment with bisphosphonates (Hatz et al., 2011). The long term implications are unclear.

3.1 Surgical treatment

Preoperative assessment and planning are critical to successful surgical outcomes in these individuals. The indications for surgical realignment include recurrent fractures and severe deformities in children with severe osteogenesis imperfecta who are making attempts to stand. Children with type I may also benefit from telescoping percutaneous intramedullary nailing to avoid the necessity of spica casting. Children with severe OI who sustained fractures in areas of pre-existing deformity very consistently have had increase in the deformity from muscle pull even though they are casted. This leads to a repetitive cycle of fracture and progressive deformity. The children with significant bowing who are beginning to stand will predictably fracture. This cycle of recurrent fracture very clearly interferes with their psychomotor development. There is rarely an indication for operative treatment prior to the children attempting to stand as most of the fractures are low energy and can be splinted for a brief period of time. Age is not necessarily a major factor in determining when to perform the surgery but may have an impact on the type of fixation utilized (Fassier et al., 2006; Fassier and Glorieux, 2003).Lower extremities are typically more severely involved than the upper extremities and interfere with psychomotor development more significantly than upper extremity deformities early in life. However, there are some children who benefit from upper extremity surgery, especially of the humerus, because of the use of arms for weight bearing to a much greater extent than their peers in the normal population (Amako et al., 2004; Gargan et al., 1996; Montpetit et al., 2003; Sulko and Radlo, 2005).

3.2 Principles of surgery

The goal of surgery in a child who is attempting to bear weight or has recurrent fractures, which interfere with his or her ability to ambulate comfortably even in a wheelchair, is to obtain anatomic mechanical alignment while load sharing with the bone and intramedullary device. Surgery should not be performed for deformity until bone density has been optimized medically. Fractures may require operative treatment prior to medical treatment if a child presents with a disabling injury and the surgeon's assessment is that the bone structure is adequate to allow for fixation. Ideally, this device will telescope and grow with the child. The principles include minimizing injury to the soft tissue envelope of the bone and to the adjacent joints. The most frequently utilized device is the Fassier-Duval nail, as this has been shown to be a safe and effective means of treatment and may increase the time to revision surgery (Esposito, 2010; Fassier et al., 2006; Turman et al., 2006). This device also decreases the need for arthrotomies. However, other intramedullary devices continue to be used with good results (Boutaud and Laville, 2004; Cho et al., 2007; Cho et al., 2011; Joseph et al., 2005; Luhmann et al., 1998). Treatment of younger children and toddlers may require earlier revision because the length of the rods are short initially because of the size and length of the child's one. However, the toddler years are a vital time of growth and development in the ability to stand, transfer, and ambulate. This technique also allows for the treatment of multiple bones simultaneously without the necessity of prolonged spica casting.

Osteotomies can be performed in the majority of children through a small incision percutaneously. This minimizes the injury to the soft tissue envelope and allows for some inherent rotational stability. The Fassier Duval technique also decreases the need for arthrotomies (Boutaud and Laville, 2004; Cho et al., 2007; Esposito, 2010; Fassier et al., 2006; Fassier and Glorieux, 2003; Joseph et al., 2005; Luhmann et al., 1998; Turman et al., 2006). Although most frequently utilized to correct femoral and tibial deformities, it is quite effective in the humerus (Figure 2A, B). There are specific deformities such as true coxa vara, which must be differientiated from the more common apparent coxa vara caused by anterolateral bowing of the proximal femoral diaphysis, which now can be effectively treated (Fassier and Glorieux, 2003). Femoral neck fractures can also be treated but the diaphysis must be protected with an intramedullary nail (Fassier and Glorieux, 2003; Tsang and Adedapo, 2011) (Figure 2C). True coxa vara can develop post surgical rodding but can also be seen to develop after trivial trauma or without known trauma.

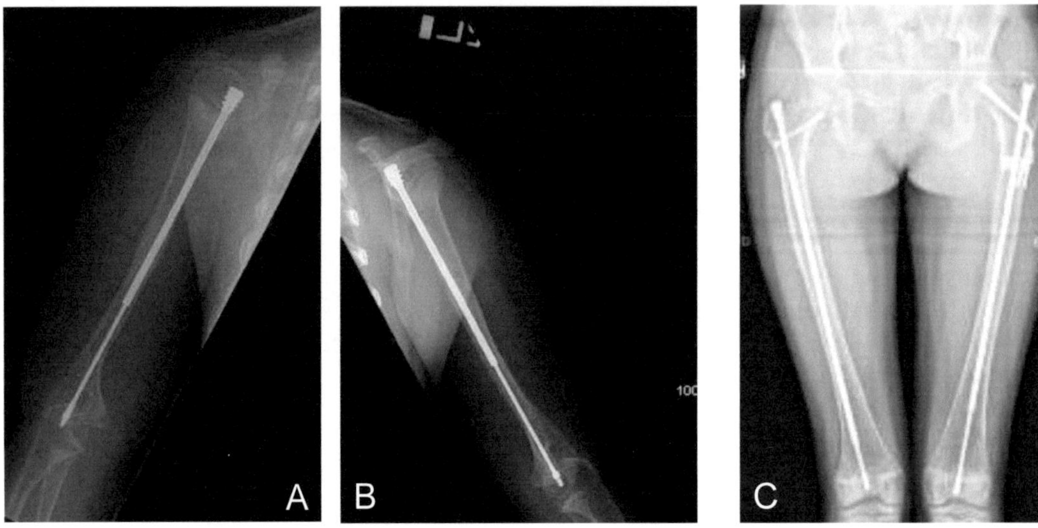

Fig. 2. A, B: 5-year old child with type III OI - 2 years post-op bilateral humeral osteotomies for recurrent fractures and severe bowing that were interfering with weight bearing function. C: 12 year old female with type I OI with sub-trochanteric fracture on the left and femoral neck fracture on the right side. The Fassier Duval percutaneous technique is not only useful in younger children with corrective osteotomies, but is very useful in dealing with adolescents with fractures. These children typically have small canals and need protection until at least skeletal maturity regardless of the age at initial surgery.

3.3 Pitfalls

Rigid devices should be avoided as some of the children will develop resorption of bone around the device because of this rigidity and stress shielding. Plates and screws not combined with an intramedullary device are stress risers and very clearly and predictably will develop bowing and fracture at the ends of the plates (Enright and Noonan, 2006).

Careful evaluation for associated problems such as cranial settling on the cervical spine must be undertaken (Forlino et al., 2011)· Maintaining gentle longitudinal traction and supporting the neck greatly assists the anesthesiologist during intubation process and may prevent neurologic or bony spinal injury.

The majority of these children tend to have an elevated temperature because of their underlying metabolism. However, malignant hyperthermia is not associated with osteogenesis imperfecta. With the percutaneous techniques, significant bleeding is rarely encountered. However, when multiple bones are treated at one surgical setting, cumulative bleeding may necessitate transfusion.

The entire operative team must be educated in the care and handling of these children. It is not mandatory in all of the children to utilize an arterial line, monitor blood pressure, if they have been treated with bisphosphonates and had a good response to that treatment. Setting the blood pressure cuff to neonatal pressures only in children with reasonable bone density and structure can allow for safe monitoring. This is especially true if the cuff is placed over a bone that has previously had an intramedullary nail placed. Obviously in a child with severe bone weakness and deformity, an arterial line may be indicated.

Post operative pain can be a difficult problem, with spasm necessitating treatment such as diazepam. Recent experience in one of our centers with epidural technique has shown that this can be done safely and has made a significant improvement in comfort and has enhanced post operative rehabilitation. Post operative casting or splinting is necessary only for a brief period of time if the surgeon determines that it is necessary to control rotation or to provide comfort. In some series and in our ongoing experience, splinting for 3-4 weeks is adequate. Protected weight-bearing can then begin, minimizing muscle atrophy, joint stiffness and osteoporosis from immobilization. Correcting as many deformities as necessary at one episode may decrease the number of fractures and total time of immobilization for these children.

4. Molecular genetics of dominant and recessive OI

Osteogenesis imperfecta is commonly an autosomal dominant disease; however, about 10-15% of all OI cases are due to a recessively inherited mutation in a non-collagen coding gene.

4.1 Dominant OI

Dominant forms of osteogenesis imperfecta are always associated with mutations in the *COL1A1* or *COL1A2* gene encoding the a1(I) or a2(I) chain of type I collagen, respectively. *COL1A1* mutations causing a reduced synthesis of type I collagen via haploinsufficiency are referred to as 'quantitative mutations' and usually result from nonsense substitutions or frameshifts that cause a premature termination codon and subsequent degradation of the transcript by the nonsense-mediated RNA degradation mechanism. These mutations typically result in mild forms of OI (i.e. type I OI) where each cell produces less collagen but of normal quality and structure. Patients with these mutations have short to normal stature, little to no deformities, bluish sclerae and increased susceptibility to fractures (Forlino et al., 2011; Rauch and Glorieux, 2004). In contrast, missense mutations in the a1(I) or a2(I) chain, especially glycine (Gly) substitutions in the Gly-X-Y repeat along the triple helical domain, as well as splice mutations causing in-frame deletions or exon skipping are usually referred to as 'qualitative or structural mutations' and cause lethal (OI type II), severe (type III), or moderate (type IV) disease. These mutations significantly impact the normal structure and assembly of the procollagen heterotrimer and may trigger a cascade of deleterious events at both the intracellular level, including abnormal collagen post-translational modification, folding, trafficking and ER-stress, and extracellular level, including reduced collagen in the matrix, abnormal mineralization and altered matrix-to-cell signaling. Although well over 1000 different dominant mutations in *COL1A1* or *COL1A2* have been described, it has been quite difficult to establish a genotype-phenotype correlation among the many different structural mutations and that could explain the spectrum of clinical severity ranging from moderate to lethal (Byers et al., 1991). Some general rules though have held true. 1) Because the trimer assembly and the winding of the triple helical domain proceed in a zipper-like manner from the C- terminus to the N-terminus, mutations closer to the C-terminus cause a more severe phenotype. 2) A greater proportion of lethal mutations affect the a1(I) versus the a2(I) chain. 3) One third of all Gly substitutions in the triple helical domain are lethal, especially when Gly is replaced by a charged or a branched side chain amino acid. 4) Two and eight lethal regions in the helical domain of a1(I) and a2(I), respectively, have been identified and align with major ligand binding sites such as those for integrins, matrix metalloproteinases and various matrix molecules including proteoglycans (for a review see (Marini et al., 2007)).

In conclusion, it is also important to remember that some rare mutations in either *COL1A1* or *COL1A2* can cause a form of Ehlers-Danlos syndrome (EDS) (reviewed in (Beighton et al., 1998)).

4.2 Recessive OI due to mutations of Leprecan family members

The recently identified family of proteins called Leprecans includes five members: cartilage-associated protein (CRTAP), synaptonemal complex 65 (SC65 or No55), prolyl 3-hydroxylase 1 (P3H1 or Leprecan, encoded by the *LEPRE1* gene), prolyl 3-hydroxylase 2 (P3H2, encoded by the *LEPREL1* gene), and prolyl 3-hydroxylase 3 (P3H3, encoded by the *LEPREL2* gene). Initial studies showed that *Crtap* loss of function in mice causes an osteochondrodysplasia characterized by short stature, kyphosis, shortening of the first segment of the limb (i.e. rhizomelia), and severe osteopenia (Morello et al., 2006). The osteoclast counts and function were normal with absence of a hyper-resorptive phenotype. However, bone histomorphometry showed functional osteoblast defects with reduced mineral apposition rate (MAR) hence, decreased bone formation rate (BFR). Osteoid surfaces and volumes were reduced and mineralization showed a shorter lag time. Transmission electron microscopy studies of mouse skin fibroblasts showed that type I collagen fibrils formed in the extracellular matrix although they had, on average, a significantly increased diameter. Although CRTAP has no enzymatic activity, it can bind to P3H1 in the rough endoplasmic reticulum (rER) and somehow facilitate its activity. Biochemically, the *Crtap-/-* mouse phenotype is associated with lack of conversion of Pro^{986} into the 3-hydroxy-proline normally found at that position in the triple helical domain of a1(I), a1(II) and a2(V) chains (Baldridge et al., 2010; Morello et al., 2006). Severely decreased *CRTAP* expression due to a hypomorphic mutation with residual expression of normal protein is associated with "rhizomelic" recessive osteogenesis imperfecta type VII, described by Ward et al. (Ward et al., 2002) in a unique First Nations Community pedigree of Northern Quebec. Instead, complete absence of CRTAP (mostly due to loss of function mutations) causes lethal to severe recessive OI in humans (Barnes et al., 2006; Morello et al., 2006). Although initially classified as type IIB-III, also these cases are tentatively classified as **type VII OI**. Because Crtap can form a trimeric complex (so called prolyl 3-hydroxylation complex) together with prolyl 3-hydroxylase 1 (P3h1, encoded by *LEPRE1*) and cyclophilin B (CypB, encoded by *PPIB*) (Morello et al., 2006) in the rER, the genes encoding these interactors became new candidates for causing recessive OI. Mutations in *LEPRE1* were then identified in probands affected with recessive OI (tentatively classified as **type VIII OI**) and negative for mutations in *COL1A1*, *COL1A2* or *CRTAP* (Cabral et al., 2007). It has been estimated that *CRTAP* and *LEPRE1* mutations contribute to about 5 to 7% of all severe recessive OI cases (Barnes et al., 2010). This number may be higher in certain populations or geographic regions. In fact, recurrent pathogenetic *LEPRE1* alleles have been described in populations of West African origin (Cabral et al., 2007) or Ireland (Irish Travelers) (Baldridge et al., 2008). Clinically, newborns with either *CRTAP* or *LEPRE1* mutations are indistinguishable and characterized by multiple healing fractures, short tubular femurs due to lack of modeling, and extreme low bone mineralization (Baldridge et al., 2008; Marini et al., 2010; Willaert et al., 2009). Their sclerae are usually white. P3H1 is the enzyme responsible for the conversion of proline into 3-hydroxy-proline (3-Hyp) (Vranka et al.,

2004) and decreased/lack of this modification at Pro^{986} in the triple helical domain of type I collagen also characterizes these patients (Cabral et al., 2007). More recently, it was demonstrated that in tissues as well as fibroblast cultures, loss of CRTAP protein was associated with loss of P3H1 protein and loss of P3H1 was associated with loss of CRTAP (Baldridge et al., 2010; Chang et al., 2009; van Dijk et al., 2009). This evidence indicated that CRTAP is required for P3H1 stabilization and activity in vivo and vice versa, suggesting a common pathogenetic mechanism and thus providing an explanation for the very similar clinical findings in probands with mutations in these two genes. The generation of *Lepre1* null mice was recently reported and the phenotype is highly similar to that of *Crtap-/-* mice (Vranka et al., 2010).

Further characterization of the phenotype of *Crtap-/-* mice demonstrated primary subtle defects in the lung and kidney with increased cell proliferation and also skin laxity with reduced thickness, stiffness, and overall strength (Baldridge et al., 2010). This is consistent with a generalized connective tissue disease, but it may also indicate the existence of a primary defect in the OI lung; respiratory distress and failure have been documented in OI patients with *CRTAP* or *LEPRE1* mutations (Baldridge et al., 2008).

4.3 Recessive OI due to mutations of peptidyl-prolyl cis-trans isomerases

At least three structurally distinct families of proteins have been linked by their ability to catalyze the bond preceding a proline residue between its *cis* and *trans* forms: the Cyclophilins (cyclosporine A binding proteins), the FKBPs (FK506-binding proteins), and the Parvulins (Gothel and Marahiel, 1999). The peptidyl-prolyl cis-trans isomerases (PPIase), also known as immunophilins, were initially identified as the intracellular receptors of the immunosuppressive drugs cyclosporine A and FK506/rapamycin (Gothel and Marahiel, 1999). They are widely distributed in all eukaryotes, prokaryotes and archaea and are present in all major cell compartments indicating that their function is required in several cellular processes. The cis-trans isomerization of peptidyl-prolyl bonds that they catalyze is a protein conformational change occurring during protein folding and thought to be rate limiting for type I collagen which contains about 20% proline residues (Gothel and Marahiel, 1999). Unlike most Cyclophilins which are predicted to localize either in the nuclear or cytosolic compartment, Cyclophilin B is localized in the ER (Pemberton and Kay, 2005) or secreted extracellularly (Yao et al., 2005). Because of its interaction with Crtap and P3h1 to form the prolyl 3-hydroxylation complex in the ER, Cyclophilin B became the next logical candidate potentially implicated in recessive forms of OI. Mutations in *Ppib* (encoding CypB) were first identified in hereditary equine regional dermal asthenia (HERDA) (Tryon et al., 2007), a recessive condition affecting Quarter Horses with features resembling those of Ehlers Danlos and Epidermolysis Bullosa syndromes. However, more recently *PPIB* mutations were also associated with recessive OI in three distinct families (Barnes et al., 2010; van Dijk et al., 2009). It is important to note that lack of PPIB causes shorter, undertubulated, bowed and fractured long bones but without rhizomelia. The degree of severity seems variable and is, perhaps, dependent upon the location of the mutations. One report described 4 probands with severe type IIB/III OI and frameshift mutations in either exon 4 or 5 (van Dijk et al., 2009), while another report described two siblings with a moderately severe OI who were able to reach independent ambulation. They had a mutation in the first coding triplet modifying the initial methionine into arginine with apparent lack of protein (Barnes et al., 2010). These patients are sometimes classified as having **type IX OI**.

A controversy also exists regarding the modification status of type I collagen chains in probands' fibroblasts with *PPIB* mutations. Those affected with severe OI were shown to have over-modification of type I collagen chains and a significantly reduced level of Pro^{986} 3-hydroxylation (but higher than those observed in patients with mutations in either *CRTAP* or *LEPRE1*) (van Dijk et al., 2009) while those with moderate OI showed normal levels of collagen modification and prolyl 3-hydroxylation (Barnes et al., 2010). The description of additional families with *PPIB* mutations will help to clarify this important aspect. Absence of Cyclophilin B only moderately affected expression levels of either CRTAP or P3H1 protein, indicating its higher degree of independence from the prolyl 3-hydroxylation complex (van Dijk et al., 2009). Due to the fact that the whole 3-hydroxylation complex was previously shown to possess, besides prolyl 3-hydroxylase and peptidyl-prolyl isomerase activity, a collagen chaperone function (Ishikawa et al., 2009), it is still unclear what independent contributions these activities have to the phenotype of OI when they are impaired. Mice deficient in Cyclophilin B have been shown to have severe recessive OI phenotype with collagen over-modification, absence of Pro^{986} 3-hydroxylation, and also reduced levels of P3h1 (Choi et al., 2009).

Mutations in a second immunophilin molecule, called FKBP65/FKBP10 (encoded by the *FKBP10* gene), have been initially detected in a few Turkish families and a Mexican-American family (Alanay et al., 2010). FKBP65 resides in the rough ER and is a protein known to interact with nascent matrix molecules, including tropoelastin and type I collagen, and have a molecular chaperone activity (Ishikawa et al., 2008; Patterson et al., 2005). Patients with mutations in *FKBP10* were described as having a progressive severe form of OI. Born with normal length and weight, they had an early history of long bone fractures leading to progressive deformities of the limbs and eventually were wheelchair bound. Progressive kyphoscoliosis with flattening and wedging of the vertebral bodies is a distinctive feature of this recessive form of OI with absence of dentinogenesis imperfecta or hearing loss (Alanay et al., 2010). The procollagen chains synthesized by these patients' fibroblasts were not over-modified and prolyl 3-hydroxylation of Pro^{986} was normal, suggesting a downstream defect in the collagen synthetic pathway compared to this earlier modification. Further analyses showed a delayed secretion of type I collagen chains with dilation of the rER and evidence of abnormal intracellular collagen trafficking (Alanay et al., 2010). A second report described additional mutations in *FKBP10* in patients affected with a recessive form of OI who also had contractures of the large joints, thus reminiscent of Bruck syndrome (Kelley et al., 2011). *FKBP10* maps on chromosome 17q21 and further investigations are required to understand if *FKBP10* is indeed the causative gene for Bruck syndrome type I (recessive OI with large joint contractures -MIM ID#259450) whose critical region, however, had been originally mapped to 17p12 (Bank et al., 1999). These patients are sometimes classified as having **type XI OI**.

4.4 Recessive OI due to mutations of Serpin family members

The Serpins (serine protease inhibitors) constitute a very large and broadly distributed superfamily of protease inhibitors which can be further subdivided into 16 clades (Law et al., 2006). They are thought to be important regulators of enzymes involved in proteolytic cascades and their role in human disease has clearly emerged (Roussel et al., 2011). Although grouped under the same superfamily due to sequence homology and common protein structure, two distinct groups can be identified: the first comprises the predominant family of protease inhibitors in mammals and is involved in the modulation of extracellular matrix remodeling, inflammation, and blood clotting (van Gent et al., 2003); the second includes a number of proteins without protease inhibitor activity and with a diverse array of functions, including molecular chaperones. Within the 36 identified human serpins, both HSP47 (heat-shock protein 47 or serpin peptidase inhibitor, clade H, member 1 encoded by the *SERPINH1* gene) and PEDF (pigment epithelium derived factor or serpin peptidase inhibitor, clade F, member 1 encoded by the *SERPINF1* gene) belong to this second group of proteins and have been linked to recessive OI.

At present, one single proband with severe recessive OI was found to have a homozygous missense mutation in the *SERPINH1* gene, encoding the collagen chaperone molecule HSP47 (Christiansen et al., 2010). Mutations in the *Serpinh1* gene had been described earlier in a dog breed affected with OI (Drogemuller et al., 2009) while *Serpinh1*-null mice die in utero with multiple collagens defects (Nagai et al., 2000). The proband was born with typical OI features with generalized osteopenia, thin ribs with healing fractures, blue sclerae, dentinogenesis imperfecta, platyspondyly, short limbs with bowed femora, joint laxity, and relative macrocephaly. Additional complications included respiratory distress, pyloric stenosis, renal stones, hypotonia; he died at the age of 3 years and 6 months due to sudden respiratory failure (Christiansen et al., 2010). Similar to what was described with mutations in *FKBP10*, type I procollagen chains were not over-modified and were normally prolyl 3-hydroxylated. However, they were noticed to accumulate in the Golgi apparatus and to be more susceptible to protease digestion, indicating a compromised helical structure. It appears that HSP47 may play a monitoring function for proper triple helical structure assembly and, like FKBP65, acts downstream of the prolyl 3-hydroxylation complex (Christiansen et al., 2010). This was tentatively classified as **type X OI**.

Recently mutations in *SERPINF1*, encoding the pigment epithelium derived factor (PEDF) have been identified in a few cases of recessive OI some of which were originally classified as **OI type VI** (Becker et al., 2011; Glorieux et al., 2002; Homan et al., 2011). Clinically these patients are born of normal weight and length, without fractures, limb deformities or joint laxity, with gray-white sclerae and normal facial features. Biochemically, they are characterized by a slight elevation in serum alkaline phosphatase and bone turn-over and by the absence of circulating levels of PEDF. They can begin to fracture early (before the first year of life) and progress to experience several other fractures which result in bone deformities and usually lack or loss of ambulation. The progressive worsening of the symptoms suggests a post-natal early onset of the skeletal phenotype; importantly, at the histological level, iliac bone biopsies show a large amount of un-mineralized osteoid on their cancellous bone due to a mineralization defect and a 'fish-scale' pattern of bone deposition instead of normal bone lamellation (Glorieux et al., 2002; Homan et al., 2011). All patients identified were homozygous for either nonsense mutations or frameshift mutations leading to a premature termination codon and likely to nonsense-mediated RNA decay, resulting in null alleles. Of note, PEDF-deficient mice were described earlier and showed increased stromal vessels and epithelial cell hyperplasia in both the prostate and pancreas (Doll et al., 2003). PEDF has been described as a multi-functional protein with roles as a potent inhibitor of angiogenesis, neurotrophic factor and collagen-interacting molecule among others (Dawson et al., 1999; Filleur et al., 2009; Meyer et al., 2002). It is a protein circulating in serum and the pathogenetic mechanisms leading to forms of recessive OI are currently unclear. This adds an exciting puzzle to solve about its multiple functions.

4.5 Recessive OI due to mutations of other genes

A second locus responsible for recessive OI with joint contractures (Bruck syndrome type II -MIM ID #609220) had been previously identified and mapped at 3q23-q24 (van der Slot et al., 2003). Probands had a combination of OI and arthrogryposis, showing osteoporosis, long bone deformities, scoliosis and congenital joint contractures (Breslau-Siderius et al., 1998; Ha-Vinh et al., 2004). Mutations in the *PLOD2* gene, encoding the lysyl-hydroxylase 2 enzyme which is a collagen telopeptide lysyl hydroxylase, were identified in 2003 (van der Slot et al., 2003).

The ocular form of OI is a recessive condition causing very low bone mass with fractures and severe eye defects that can lead to early blindness. These include hyperplasia of the vitreous, corneal opacity, secondary glaucoma, and the formation of retrolental masses resembling a retinoblastoma (Beighton et al., 1985; De Paepe et al., 1993). It was later recognized as the osteoporosis pseudoglioma syndrome (OPPG) (Beighton, 1986; Brude, 1986; Frontali and Dallapiccola, 1986; Superti-Furga et al., 1986). The OPPG locus was linked to the long arm of chromosome 11 (Gong et al., 1996) and the gene responsible for the disease was later identified as the LDL-receptor related protein 5 or LRP5 (Gong et al., 2001). LRP5 is an important regulator of bone mass accrual during growth and a co-receptor in the canonical Wnt pathway: null mutations cause OPPG while heterozygous carriers have also low bone mass (Gong et al., 2001). In addition, several missense mutations in the LRP5 gene have been associated with other conditions such as recessive and dominant familial exudative vitreoretinopathy 4 (Jiao et al., 2004; Toomes et al., 2004), and high bone mass phenotypes (Boyden et al., 2002; Little et al., 2002; Van Wesenbeeck et al., 2003).

	SERPINF1	*CRTAP*	*LEPRE1*	*PPIB*	*SERPINH1*	*FKBP10*	*PLOD2*
Dentinogenesis Imperfecta		+/-			+		
Rhizomelia		+	+				
Coxa vara	+	+				+	
Femur undertubulation		+	+	+			
Popcorn epiphyses	+	+/-	+/-				
Scoliosis	+	+	+	+	+	+	+
Platyspondyly			+				
Vertebral wedging						+	
Ligamentous laxity		+	+	+	+	+	
Joint contractures						+	+
Wormian bones		+	+			+	+
White/Grey/Blue sclerae	W/B/G	W/G	W/G/B	W/B	B	W/G/B	W/G/B
Proptosis		+		+			
Respirat. distress		+	+		+		
Pterygia						+	+
Skin blisters					+	+	
Elev. alkal. phosp.	+						

Table 2. Tentative table for the differential diagnosis of recessive OI forms (+/- may or may not be present).

Finally, in a unique patient diagnosed with OI a homozygous single base pair deletion causing a frameshift and a premature termination codon in the gene *SP7/OSX* encoding the transcription factor Osterix was described (Lapunzina et al.). The mutation eliminates the last of three zinc-finger DNA binding domains at the C-terminus of Osterix, likely affecting its transactivation function. In mice, Osterix is an essential transcription factor for proper osteoblast lineage differentiation and directly or indirectly activates the expression of a host of osteoblast genes beyond type I collagen. As a result, considering the importance of Osterix for murine skeletal development and homeostasis (Nakashima et al., 2002; Zhou et al., 2010), this finding was rather surprising because the predicted human phenotype would have been possibly even more dramatic than seen in the described proband. However, the molecular consequences and the mechanism behind the emergence of an OI phenotype due to *OSX* mutations are completely unknown, and the description of additional patients with OSX mutations will facilitate an understanding of the inherent pathogenetic process.
A list of clinical features identified in different forms of recessive OI is presented in **Table 2.**

5. Mouse models of OI

Different mouse models showing many of the clinical features of OI have been identified or generated in the past years. The phenotype severity of each model has been compared to the severity of human OI as classified by Sillence (Sillence et al., 1979).

5.1 Mouse models due to alterations of type I collagen genes

One of the most commonly utilized OI mouse models is the oim mouse (osteogenesis imperfecta murine) (Chipman et al., 1993). This is a naturally occurring strain of mice with a spontaneous nucleotide deletion in the *Col1a2* gene that results in a frameshift and the alteration of the a2(I) procollagen C-propeptide. The phenotype is recessively inherited and homozygous mutant mice have osteopenia, small body size, limb deformity and skeletal fractures; it mimics a moderate to severe human OI and thus considered a model for OI type III. Interestingly, tissues of homozygous mutant mice accumulate a1(I) homotrimers.
The Mov13 mouse was instead generated by the germline insertion of Moloney murine leukemia virus (MMLV) into intron 1 of *Col1a1* (Breindl et al., 1984; Jaenisch et al., 1983; Schnieke et al., 1983). The retroviral insertion blocks the initiation of transcription and inactivates the *Col1a1* allele (Hartung et al., 1986). The insertion is lethal at midgestation in homozygous mice (comparable to a type II OI though causing earlier lethality) while heterozygous mice are viable and constitute a model for the mild type I OI with increased skeletal fragility but also interesting adaptations that lead to improved cortical mechanical properties (Bonadio et al., 1993).
The use of Cre-lox recombination technology made it possible to obtain the first knock-in mouse model for OI. An allele harboring a G to T transversion (nt 1546) and causing an a1(I) Gly^{349} to Cys substitution that was initially identified in a type IV OI patient was generated (Forlino et al., 1999). Heterozygous mice with this mutation, named Brittle IV (BrtlIV), express a tissue-specific balanced ratio of normal and mutant allele, have a dominant phenotype and moderately severe skeletal phenotype comparable to a human type IV OI; hence they represent a suitable model for the study of the pathophysiology of OI. They showed bone deformity, osteopenia, fragility and disorganized trabecular structure with phenotypic variability that goes from perinatal lethality to long term survival (Forlino et al.,

1999). The phenotypic variability was shown to be dependent on the differential expression of both extracellular and intracellular proteins (Forlino et al., 2007). Also the BrtlIV mouse model undergoes post-pubertal adaptations that increase femoral strength and stiffness perhaps by improvement of bone matrix material properties (Kozloff et al., 2004). Interestingly, homozygous BrtlIV mice carrying the single base pair substitution on both *Col1a1* alleles have a near normal phenotype without fractures or altered bone mineral density (Forlino and al., 2005). The mechanism behind this phenomenon is currently poorly understood.

Other mice bearing point mutations in the *Col1a1* gene were generated. These, for instance, include transgenic mice with specific substitution of Gly^{859} into either Cys or Arg and resulting in a dominant lethal phenotype (Stacey et al., 1988). Mice with an ENU-mutagenesis induced frameshift mutation in the C-terminal domain of *Col1a1* (named Aga2 from abnormal gait 2). The phenotype of these mice was dominant with decreased bone mass, fractures, early lethality, increased bone turnover and intracellular accumulation of abnormal procollagen chains that triggered an endoplasmic reticulum-associated stress response and osteoblast apoptosis (Lisse et al., 2008). Or transgenic mice carrying a mini-gene version of the human *COL1A1* gene and reproducing a lethal in-frame deletion identified in an OI patient (Khillan et al., 1991; Pereira et al., 1993).

5.2 Mouse models due to alterations of other genes

The fragilitas ossium (fro/fro) mouse is a model for recessively inherited OI and was generated by treatment of mice with a chemical mutagen (Guenet et al., 1981). A high percentage of mutant pups die in the perinatal period with radiographic findings similar to a severe recessive OI type II. The surviving mice have progressive deformity but reduced fracture frequency (Sillence et al., 1993). The underlying mutation is a deletion in the sphingomyelin phosphodiesterase 3 (*Smpd3*) gene (Aubin et al., 2005) which was recently shown to be a positive regulator of mineralization in *in vitro* osteoblast cultures (Khavandgar et al., 2011).

Mice carrying genetically engineered mutations in *Crtap*, *Leprel* and *Ppib* genes encoding the components of the rER heterotrimeric prolyl 3-hydroxylation complex (namely cartilage-associated protein, prolyl 3-hydroxylase 1 and cyclophilin B, respectively) have been generated (Choi et al., 2009; Morello et al., 2006; Vranka et al., 2010). Their phenotype is very similar with severe osteopenia, kyphosis, skin laxity, abnormal collagen fibrils at the ultrastructural level and lack of collagen prolyl 3-hydroxylation (see more details on the phenotypes of these mice in the paragraph on Molecular Genetics of OI). They represent useful models for the study of recessively inherited OI and great tools for understanding its pathophysiology.

6. Pathogenesis and disease mechanisms in OI

As discussed above, *COL1A1* null alleles cause dominant OI through a mechanism of haploinsufficiency whereby about half normal type I collagen trimers are secreted in the extracellular matrix causing a decreased bone mass and an osteoporotic phenotype (Willing et al., 1992). Contrary to homozygous *COL1A1* null mutations that are most likely incompatible with life as seen in the Mov13 mice, patients with homozygous *COL1A2* null mutations have a phenotype more similar to EDS (Malfait et al., 2006; Nicholls et al., 2001;

Schwarze et al., 2004). They synthesize a(I)$_3$ homotrimers which were shown to be overmodified, to alter the triple helical structure and to resist collagenases digestion (Deak et al., 1985; Han et al., 2010; Kuznetsova et al., 2001).

Collagen structural mutations instead often have a profound impact on procollagen chains register and assembly and may slow down the winding of the triple helix resulting in over-modification of additional proline and lysine residues by ER resident enzymes (i.e. prolyl- and lysyl-hydroxylases). In addition, an increase in hydroxylysines can generate an abnormal glycosylation and intra/inter-molecular crosslink pattern in the collagen fibril (Kivirikko and Pihlajaniemi, 1998). The deceleration of collagen synthesis results in slower secretion and accumulation of misfolded procollagen chains in the ER. Indeed OI can be considered a conformational disease where stable misfolded procollagen chains assume a dominant negative effect. Importantly, depending on the location and the effect of the individual mutation the cellular response is different. Those mutations (e.g. those in the C-terminal propeptide) that interfere with chains association trigger an unfolded protein response (UPR) and target the misfolded polypeptides to proteosomes via the ER-associated degradation pathway (Chessler et al., 1993; Ishida et al., 2009; Lisse et al., 2008). Whereas mutations localized in the triple helix cause only regional misfolding, do not activate the UPR but rather autophagy and the autophagic elimination of these stable collagen aggregates (Bateman et al., 2009; Ishida et al., 2009; Makareeva et al., 2011). The overall cellular consequences of the activation of either pathway are likely to have a significant chronic effect on multiple osteoblast functions (Rutkowski et al., 2006; Tsang et al., 2010).

At the extracellular level, there is an alteration in the quality and quantity of secreted collagen. This causes an imbalance in the stoichiometry of matrix components (Fedarko et al., 1995) and altered interactions between collagen and non-collagenous proteins and between collagen and substrate adhesion molecules (e.g. integrins) (Marini et al., 2007). The changes in the matrix and its components affect the mineralization process and, irrespective of the type I collagen mutation, cause a shift towards increased mineralization density (Bateman et al., 2009; Camacho et al., 1996; Roschger et al., 2008a; Roschger et al., 2008b).

Based on recent findings, it has become clear that recessive OI can be caused by mutations in genes encoding collagen modifier molecules such as prolyl- or lysyl-hydroxylases, prolyl isomerases, collagen specific chaperones, and also 'adapter proteins' such as CRTAP. Loss of function of the prolyl 3-hydroxylation complex caused by mutations in *CRTAP, LEPRE1,* or *PPIB* causes early post-translational defects in the procollagen synthesis, slowing down the triple helical winding with over-modification of prolyl and lysyl residues. With one exception (Barnes et al., 2010), the OI phenotype resulting from loss of function of these genes is almost invariably lethal to severe and comparable to a type II/III OI according to the original Sillence classification. Mutations in either *FKBP10* or *SERPINH1* do not cause procollagen chain over-modification and do not interfere with prolyl 3-hydroxylation, but somehow they affect collagen transport between the rER and Golgi. Thus, their effect on procollagen appears to be downstream of the prolyl 3-hydroxylation complex, but the resulting OI phenotype is still quite severe and similar to a type III/IV OI. Mutations in both *PLOD2* (Bruck syndrome type II) and *FKBP10* genes also cause joint contractures suggesting, perhaps, a potential interaction between their encoded proteins. It is still unknown how *SP7/OSX* mutations cause OI other than the simple consideration that type I collagen is a target of *OSX* and, therefore, may be down-regulated with impaired OSX function.

With a few exceptions, the effects that mutations in genes causing recessive OI have on bone quality and bone matrix mineralization is still unclear. While in all cases there is severe osteopenia, mouse models for *Crtap*, *Lepre1* and *Ppib* lack of function have overmodified collagen lacking 3-Hyp at Pro^{986}, increased diameter of collagen fibrils, and decreased irregular deposition of ECM (Choi et al., 2009; Morello et al., 2006; Vranka et al., 2010). Fibroblasts from a patient with null *CRTAP* mutation were recently shown to depose less collagen in the matrix (Valli et al., 2011). Quantitative backscattered electron imaging studies on *Crtap*-null as well as OI-VII bones to determine bone mineralization density distribution have shown a higher calcium content of the bone matrix (Fratzl-Zelman et al., 2010); these results are similar to what has been observed in classical OI due to mutations in type I collagen genes (Boyde et al., 1999; Roschger et al., 2008a). In addition, those studies suggested altered mineralization kinetics resulting in an elevated tissue mineralization density (Fratzl-Zelman et al., 2010). Taken together these data suggest that any alteration in collagen structure or its post-translational modification may result in abnormal protein and mineral stoichiometry and likely abnormal mineralization kinetics.
However, among the different recessive forms of OI, OI VI (due to mutations in *SERPINF1*) shows a unique mineralization defect with persistence of non-mineralized osteoid on the cancellous bone and indicating a different pathogenetic mechanism (Homan et al., 2011).

7. Conclusion

Mutations affecting a specific collagen chain have a primary impact on tissues with higher expression of that chain (e.g. bone for *COL1A1* or *COL1A2*, blood vessels for *COL3A1*, skin for *COL7A1*, etc…), and cause milder connective tissue abnormalities in tissues which express lower levels. These are usually dominant mutations. Instead, mutations affecting collagen modifying proteins in the rER or Golgi, or those involved in collagen intracellular transport, usually cause recessive conditions; clinically these can be even more severe than the former because they have an impact on multiple collagen chains based on the collagen chain substrate specificity of the modification being affected. Importantly, the biological relevance of that modification will emerge in the most severely affected tissue(s). Hence, the clinical signs of mutations in genes encoding either one of the collagen chains or one of the collagen modifying proteins often share many similarities and contribute to generate the disease spectrum that goes from Osteogenesis Imperfecta to Bruck to Ehlers Danlos to Epidermolysis Bullosa syndromes (see **Table 2**). A careful assessment of the proband's clinical features may provide essential hints toward the underlying molecular defect (e.g. joint contractures in case of *PLOD2* or *FKBP10* mutations), the correct diagnosis and the proper therapy and follow-up.
Additional cases of recessive OI are waiting further elucidation to uncover the yet unidentified culprit genes. With the discovery of new genes involved in skeletal dysplasias, and specifically OI, our understanding of the underlying pathogenetic processes will continue to improve as well as our ability to devise and then test new therapeutic approaches.
At the present time, the ability to care for these individuals, by combining the benefits of early bisphosphonate treatment with appropriate surgical techniques, has greatly enhanced the comfort and function of these children. Minimizing the soft tissue trauma associated with surgery and avoiding long-term and recurrent episodes of immobilization is also a

major advance in recent years. Questions clearly remain with regard to the long-term implications of the medical and surgical treatments, as well as how to transition treatment as the children mature. Clearly, this is an interim approach and the advances in the genetic and molecular understanding of these disorders will lead to more appropriate and effective treatment of the underlying disease.

8. Acknowledgements

The authors would like to thank Dr. Michael Jennings (University of Arkansas for Medical Sciences, Little Rock, AR) and Linda Kraut (University of Nebraska, Omaha, NE) for editorial assistance. This work was supported in part by the Arkansas Biosciences Institute, the major research component of the Arkansas Tobacco Settlement Proceeds Act of 2000 (RM). Additional research support was obtained from the William R. Patrick Foundation (PWE).

9. References

Agarwal, V., and Joseph, B. (2005). Non-union in osteogenesis imperfecta. Journal of pediatric orthopaedics Part B / European Paediatric Orthopaedic Society, Pediatric Orthopaedic Society of North America *14*, 451-455.

Alanay, Y., Avaygan, H., Camacho, N., Utine, G.E., Boduroglu, K., Aktas, D., Alikasifoglu, M., Tuncbilek, E., Orhan, D., Bakar, F.T., *et al.* (2010). Mutations in the gene encoding the RER protein FKBP65 cause autosomal-recessive osteogenesis imperfecta. American journal of human genetics *86*, 551-559.

Amako, M., Fassier, F., Hamdy, R.C., Aarabi, M., Montpetit, K., and Glorieux, F.H. (2004). Functional analysis of upper limb deformities in osteogenesis imperfecta. J Pediatr Orthop *24*, 689-694.

Arikoski, P., Silverwood, B., Tillmann, V., and Bishop, N.J. (2004). Intravenous pamidronate treatment in children with moderate to severe osteogenesis imperfecta: assessment of indices of dual-energy X-ray absorptiometry and bone metabolic markers during the first year of therapy. Bone *34*, 539-546.

Arundel, P., Offiah, A., and Bishop, N.J. (2011). Evolution of the radiographic appearance of the metaphyses over the first year of life in type V osteogenesis imperfecta: clues to pathogenesis. Journal of bone and mineral research : the official journal of the American Society for Bone and Mineral Research *26*, 894-898.

Astrom, E., Jorulf, H., and Soderhall, S. (2007). Intravenous pamidronate treatment of infants with severe osteogenesis imperfecta. Arch Dis Child *92*, 332-338.

Aubin, I., Adams, C.P., Opsahl, S., Septier, D., Bishop, C.E., Auge, N., Salvayre, R., Negre-Salvayre, A., Goldberg, M., Guenet, J.L., *et al.* (2005). A deletion in the gene encoding sphingomyelin phosphodiesterase 3 (Smpd3) results in osteogenesis and dentinogenesis imperfecta in the mouse. Nature genetics *37*, 803-805.

Baldridge, D., Lennington, J., Weis, M., Homan, E.P., Jiang, M.M., Munivez, E., Keene, D.R., Hogue, W.R., Pyott, S., Byers, P.H., *et al.* (2010). Generalized connective tissue disease in Crtap-/- mouse. PloS one *5*, e10560.

Baldridge, D., Schwarze, U., Morello, R., Lennington, J., Bertin, T.K., Pace, J.M., Pepin, M.G., Weis, M., Eyre, D.R., Walsh, J., *et al.* (2008). CRTAP and LEPRE1 mutations in recessive osteogenesis imperfecta. Human mutation *29*, 1435-1442.

Bank, R.A., Robins, S.P., Wijmenga, C., Breslau-Siderius, L.J., Bardoel, A.F., van der Sluijs, H.A., Pruijs, H.E., and TeKoppele, J.M. (1999). Defective collagen crosslinking in bone, but not in ligament or cartilage, in Bruck syndrome: indications for a bone-specific telopeptide lysyl hydroxylase on chromosome 17. Proc Natl Acad Sci U S A *96*, 1054-1058.

Barnes, A.M., Carter, E.M., Cabral, W.A., Weis, M., Chang, W., Makareeva, E., Leikin, S., Rotimi, C.N., Eyre, D.R., Raggio, C.L., *et al.* (2010). Lack of cyclophilin B in osteogenesis imperfecta with normal collagen folding. The New England journal of medicine *362*, 521-528.

Barnes, A.M., Chang, W., Morello, R., Cabral, W.A., Weis, M., Eyre, D.R., Leikin, S., Makareeva, E., Kuznetsova, N., Uveges, T.E., *et al.* (2006). Deficiency of cartilage-associated protein in recessive lethal osteogenesis imperfecta. The New England journal of medicine *355*, 2757-2764.

Bateman, J.F., Boot-Handford, R.P., and Lamande, S.R. (2009). Genetic diseases of connective tissues: cellular and extracellular effects of ECM mutations. Nat Rev Genet *10*, 173-183.

Becker, J., Semler, O., Gilissen, C., Li, Y., Bolz, H.J., Giunta, C., Bergmann, C., Rohrbach, M., Koerber, F., Zimmermann, K., *et al.* (2011). Exome sequencing identifies truncating mutations in human SERPINF1 in autosomal-recessive osteogenesis imperfecta. American journal of human genetics *88*, 362-371.

Beighton, P. (1986). Osteoporosis-pseudoglioma syndrome. Clin Genet *29*, 263.

Beighton, P., De Paepe, A., Steinmann, B., Tsipouras, P., and Wenstrup, R.J. (1998). Ehlers-Danlos syndromes: revised nosology, Villefranche, 1997. Ehlers-Danlos National Foundation (USA) and Ehlers-Danlos Support Group (UK). American journal of medical genetics *77*, 31-37.

Beighton, P., Winship, I., and Behari, D. (1985). The ocular form of osteogenesis imperfecta: a new autosomal recessive syndrome. Clin Genet *28*, 69-75.

Bonadio, J., Jepsen, K.J., Mansoura, M.K., Jaenisch, R., Kuhn, J.L., and Goldstein, S.A. (1993). A murine skeletal adaptation that significantly increases cortical bone mechanical properties. Implications for human skeletal fragility. The Journal of clinical investigation *92*, 1697-1705.

Boutaud, B., and Laville, J.M. (2004). [Elastic sliding central medullary nailing with osteogenesis imperfecta. Fourteen cases at eight years follow-up]. Rev Chir Orthop Reparatrice Appar Mot *90*, 304-311.

Boyde, A., Travers, R., Glorieux, F.H., and Jones, S.J. (1999). The mineralization density of iliac crest bone from children with osteogenesis imperfecta. Calcified tissue international *64*, 185-190.

Boyden, L.M., Mao, J., Belsky, J., Mitzner, L., Farhi, A., Mitnick, M.A., Wu, D., Insogna, K., and Lifton, R.P. (2002). High bone density due to a mutation in LDL-receptor-related protein 5. The New England journal of medicine *346*, 1513-1521.

Breindl, M., Harbers, K., and Jaenisch, R. (1984). Retrovirus-induced lethal mutation in collagen I gene of mice is associated with an altered chromatin structure. Cell *38*, 9-16.

Breslau-Siderius, E.J., Engelbert, R.H., Pals, G., and van der Sluijs, J.A. (1998). Bruck syndrome: a rare combination of bone fragility and multiple congenital joint contractures. Journal of pediatric orthopaedics *7*, 35-38.

Brude, E. (1986). Ocular osteogenesis imperfecta. Clin Genet *29*, 187.

Byers, P.H., Wallis, G.A., and Willing, M.C. (1991). Osteogenesis imperfecta: translation of mutation to phenotype. Journal of medical genetics *28*, 433-442.

Cabral, W.A., Chang, W., Barnes, A.M., Weis, M., Scott, M.A., Leikin, S., Makareeva, E., Kuznetsova, N.V., Rosenbaum, K.N., Tifft, C.J., *et al.* (2007). Prolyl 3-hydroxylase 1 deficiency causes a recessive metabolic bone disorder resembling lethal/severe osteogenesis imperfecta. Nat Genet *39*, 359-365.

Camacho, N.P., Landis, W.J., and Boskey, A.L. (1996). Mineral changes in a mouse model of osteogenesis imperfecta detected by Fourier transform infrared microscopy. Connect Tissue Res *35*, 259-265.

Chang, W., Barnes, A.M., Cabral, W.A., Bodurtha, J.N., and Marini, J.C. (2009). Prolyl 3-Hydroxylase 1 and CRTAP are Mutually Stabilizing in the Endoplasmic Reticulum Collagen Prolyl 3-Hydroxylation Complex. Human molecular genetics.

Chessler, S.D., Wallis, G.A., and Byers, P.H. (1993). Mutations in the carboxyl-terminal propeptide of the pro alpha 1(I) chain of type I collagen result in defective chain association and produce lethal osteogenesis imperfecta. The Journal of biological chemistry *268*, 18218-18225.

Cheung, M.S., and Glorieux, F.H. (2008). Osteogenesis Imperfecta: update on presentation and management. Rev Endocr Metab Disord *9*, 153-160.

Chipman, S.D., Sweet, H.O., McBride, D.J., Jr., Davisson, M.T., Marks, S.C., Jr., Shuldiner, A.R., Wenstrup, R.J., Rowe, D.W., and Shapiro, J.R. (1993). Defective pro alpha 2(I) collagen synthesis in a recessive mutation in mice: a model of human osteogenesis imperfecta. Proceedings of the National Academy of Sciences of the United States of America *90*, 1701-1705.

Cho, T.J., Choi, I.H., Chung, C.Y., Yoo, W.J., Lee, K.S., and Lee, D.Y. (2007). Interlocking telescopic rod for patients with osteogenesis imperfecta. The Journal of bone and joint surgery American volume *89*, 1028-1035.

Cho, T.J., Kim, J.B., Lee, J.W., Lee, K., Park, M.S., Yoo, W.J., Chung, C.Y., and Choi, I.H. (2011). Fracture in long bones stabilised by telescopic intramedullary rods in patients with osteogenesis imperfecta. J Bone Joint Surg Br *93*, 634-638.

Choi, J.W., Sutor, S.L., Lindquist, L., Evans, G.L., Madden, B.J., Bergen, H.R., 3rd, Hefferan, T.E., Yaszemski, M.J., and Bram, R.J. (2009). Severe osteogenesis imperfecta in cyclophilin B-deficient mice. PLoS genetics *5*, e1000750.

Christiansen, H.E., Schwarze, U., Pyott, S.M., AlSwaid, A., Al Balwi, M., Alrasheed, S., Pepin, M.G., Weis, M.A., Eyre, D.R., and Byers, P.H. (2010). Homozygosity for a missense mutation in SERPINH1, which encodes the collagen chaperone protein HSP47, results in severe recessive osteogenesis imperfecta. American journal of human genetics *86*, 389-398.

Chu, M.L., Williams, C.J., Pepe, G., Hirsch, J.L., Prockop, D.J., and Ramirez, F. (1983). Internal deletion in a collagen gene in a perinatal lethal form of osteogenesis imperfecta. Nature *304*, 78-80.

Cohn, D.H., Starman, B.J., Blumberg, B., and Byers, P.H. (1990). Recurrence of lethal osteogenesis imperfecta due to parental mosaicism for a dominant mutation in a human type I collagen gene (COL1A1). American journal of human genetics *46*, 591-601.

Dawson, D.W., Volpert, O.V., Gillis, P., Crawford, S.E., Xu, H., Benedict, W., and Bouck, N.P. (1999). Pigment epithelium-derived factor: a potent inhibitor of angiogenesis. Science *285*, 245-248.

de Graaff, F., Verra, W., Pruijs, J.E., and Sakkers, R.J. (2011). Decrease in outpatient department visits and operative interventions due to bisphosphonates in children with osteogenesis imperfecta. J Child Orthop *5*, 121-125.

De Paepe, A., Leroy, J.G., Nuytinck, L., Meire, F., and Capoen, J. (1993). Osteoporosis-pseudoglioma syndrome. American journal of medical genetics *45*, 30-37.

Deak, S.B., van der Rest, M., and Prockop, D.J. (1985). Altered helical structure of a homotrimer of alpha 1(I)chains synthesized by fibroblasts from a variant of osteogenesis imperfecta. Coll Relat Res *5*, 305-313.

Devogelaer, J.P., and Coppin, C. (2006). Osteogenesis imperfecta : current treatment options and future prospects. Treat Endocrinol *5*, 229-242.

Doll, J.A., Stellmach, V.M., Bouck, N.P., Bergh, A.R., Lee, C., Abramson, L.P., Cornwell, M.L., Pins, M.R., Borensztajn, J., and Crawford, S.E. (2003). Pigment epithelium-derived factor regulates the vasculature and mass of the prostate and pancreas. Nat Med *9*, 774-780.

Drogemuller, C., Becker, D., Brunner, A., Haase, B., Kircher, P., Seeliger, F., Fehr, M., Baumann, U., Lindblad-Toh, K., and Leeb, T. (2009). A missense mutation in the SERPINH1 gene in Dachshunds with osteogenesis imperfecta. PLoS genetics *5*, e1000579.

Edwards, M.J., Wenstrup, R.J., Byers, P.H., and Cohn, D.H. (1992). Recurrence of lethal osteogenesis imperfecta due to parental mosaicism for a mutation in the COL1A2 gene of type I collagen. The mosaic parent exhibits phenotypic features of a mild form of the disease. Human mutation *1*, 47-54.

el-Sobky, M.A., Hanna, A.A., Basha, N.E., Tarraf, Y.N., and Said, M.H. (2006). Surgery versus surgery plus pamidronate in the management of osteogenesis imperfecta patients: a comparative study. Journal of pediatric orthopaedics Part B / European Paediatric Orthopaedic Society, Pediatric Orthopaedic Society of North America *15*, 222-228.

Enright, W.J., and Noonan, K.J. (2006). Bone plating in patients with type III osteogenesis imperfecta: results and complications. Iowa Orthop J *26*, 37-40.

Esposito, P., and Plotkin, H. (2008). Surgical treatment of osteogenesis imperfecta: current concepts. Current opinion in pediatrics *20*, 52-57.

Esposito, P.W. (2010). Multiple Percutaneous Osteotomies and Fassier-Duval Telescoping Nailing of Long Bone in Osteogenesis Imperfecta. In Operative Techniques in Orthopedic Surgery, S. Wiesel, ed. (Philadelphia, PA, Wolters Kluwer/Lippincott Williams & Wilkins), pp. 1284-1294.

Fassier, F., Esposito, P., Sponseller, P.D., and al., e. (2006). Multicenter radiological assessment of the Fassier-Duval femoral rodding. In Pediatric Orthopaedic Society of North America (San Diego, CA).

Fassier, F., and Glorieux, D.F. (2003). Osteogenesis Imperfecta. In Surgical Techniques in Orthopaedics and Traumatology (Elsevier).

Fedarko, N.S., Robey, P.G., and Vetter, U.K. (1995). Extracellular matrix stoichiometry in osteoblasts from patients with osteogenesis imperfecta. Journal of bone and mineral research : the official journal of the American Society for Bone and Mineral Research *10*, 1122-1129.

Filleur, S., Nelius, T., de Riese, W., and Kennedy, R.C. (2009). Characterization of PEDF: a multi-functional serpin family protein. Journal of cellular biochemistry *106*, 769-775.

Forin, V., Arabi, A., Guigonis, V., Filipe, G., Bensman, A., and Roux, C. (2005). Benefits of pamidronate in children with osteogenesis imperfecta: an open prospective study. Joint Bone Spine *72*, 313-318.

Forlino, A., and al., e. (2005). Maturation or homozygosity modulates OI phenotype in BRTL mouse. In 9th International Meeting on Osteogenesis Imperfecta (Annapolis, MD).

Forlino, A., Cabral, W.A., Barnes, A.M., and Marini, J.C. (2011). New perspectives on osteogenesis imperfecta. Nat Rev Endocrinol *7*, 540-557.

Forlino, A., Porter, F.D., Lee, E.J., Westphal, H., and Marini, J.C. (1999). Use of the Cre/lox recombination system to develop a non-lethal knock-in murine model for osteogenesis imperfecta with an alpha1(I) G349C substitution. Variability in phenotype in BrtlIV mice. The Journal of biological chemistry *274*, 37923-37931.

Forlino, A., Tani, C., Rossi, A., Lupi, A., Campari, E., Gualeni, B., Bianchi, L., Armini, A., Cetta, G., Bini, L., *et al.* (2007). Differential expression of both extracellular and intracellular proteins is involved in the lethal or nonlethal phenotypic variation of BrtlIV, a murine model for osteogenesis imperfecta. Proteomics *7*, 1877-1891.

Fratzl-Zelman, N., Morello, R., Lee, B., Rauch, F., Glorieux, F.H., Misof, B.M., Klaushofer, K., and Roschger, P. (2010). CRTAP deficiency leads to abnormally high bone matrix mineralization in a murine model and in children with osteogenesis imperfecta type VII. Bone *46*, 820-826.

Frontali, M., and Dallapiccola, B. (1986). Osteoporosis-pseudoglioma syndrome and the ocular form of osteogenesis imperfecta. Clin Genet *29*, 262.

Gargan, M.F., Wisbeach, A., and Fixsen, J.A. (1996). Humeral rodding in osteogenesis imperfecta. J Pediatr Orthop *16*, 719-722.

Glorieux, F.H. (2007). Experience with bisphosphonates in osteogenesis imperfecta. Pediatrics *119 Suppl 2*, S163-165.

Glorieux, F.H., Bishop, N.J., Plotkin, H., Chabot, G., Lanoue, G., and Travers, R. (1998). Cyclic administration of pamidronate in children with severe osteogenesis imperfecta. The New England journal of medicine *339*, 947-952.

Glorieux, F.H., Rauch, F., Plotkin, H., Ward, L., Travers, R., Roughley, P., Lalic, L., Glorieux, D.F., Fassier, F., and Bishop, N.J. (2000). Type V osteogenesis imperfecta: a new form of brittle bone disease. J Bone Miner Res *15*, 1650-1658.

Glorieux, F.H., Ward, L.M., Rauch, F., Lalic, L., Roughley, P.J., and Travers, R. (2002). Osteogenesis imperfecta type VI: a form of brittle bone disease with a mineralization defect. J Bone Miner Res *17*, 30-38.

Gong, Y., Slee, R.B., Fukai, N., Rawadi, G., Roman-Roman, S., Reginato, A.M., Wang, H., Cundy, T., Glorieux, F.H., Lev, D., *et al.* (2001). LDL receptor-related protein 5 (LRP5) affects bone accrual and eye development. Cell *107*, 513-523.

Gong, Y., Vikkula, M., Boon, L., Liu, J., Beighton, P., Ramesar, R., Peltonen, L., Somer, H., Hirose, T., Dallapiccola, B., *et al.* (1996). Osteoporosis-pseudoglioma syndrome, a disorder affecting skeletal strength and vision, is assigned to chromosome region 11q12-13. American journal of human genetics *59*, 146-151.

Gothel, S.F., and Marahiel, M.A. (1999). Peptidyl-prolyl cis-trans isomerases, a superfamily of ubiquitous folding catalysts. Cell Mol Life Sci *55*, 423-436.

Guenet, J.L., Stanescu, R., Maroteaux, P., and Stanescu, V. (1981). Fragilitas ossium: a new autosomal recessive mutation in the mouse. J Hered *72*, 440-441.

Ha-Vinh, R., Alanay, Y., Bank, R.A., Campos-Xavier, A.B., Zankl, A., Superti-Furga, A., and Bonafe, L. (2004). Phenotypic and molecular characterization of Bruck syndrome (osteogenesis imperfecta with contractures of the large joints) caused by a recessive mutation in PLOD2. American journal of medical genetics *131*, 115-120.

Han, S., Makareeva, E., Kuznetsova, N.V., DeRidder, A.M., Sutter, M.B., Losert, W., Phillips, C.L., Visse, R., Nagase, H., and Leikin, S. (2010). Molecular mechanism of type I collagen homotrimer resistance to mammalian collagenases. The Journal of biological chemistry *285*, 22276-22281.

Hartung, S., Jaenisch, R., and Breindl, M. (1986). Retrovirus insertion inactivates mouse alpha 1(I) collagen gene by blocking initiation of transcription. Nature *320*, 365-367.

Hatz, D., Esposito, P.W., Schroeder, B., Burke, B., Lutz, R., and Hasley, B.P. (2011). The incidence of spondylolysis and spondylolisthesis in children with osteogenesis imperfecta. J Pediatr Orthop *31*, 655-660.

Homan, E.P., Rauch, F., Grafe, I., Lietman, C., Doll, J.A., Dawson, B., Bertin, T., Napierala, D., Morello, R., Gibbs, R., *et al.* (2011). Mutations in SERPINF1 cause Osteogenesis imperfecta Type VI. Journal of bone and mineral research : the official journal of the American Society for Bone and Mineral Research.

Ishida, Y., Yamamoto, A., Kitamura, A., Lamande, S.R., Yoshimori, T., Bateman, J.F., Kubota, H., and Nagata, K. (2009). Autophagic elimination of misfolded procollagen aggregates in the endoplasmic reticulum as a means of cell protection. Molecular biology of the cell *20*, 2744-2754.

Ishikawa, Y., Vranka, J., Wirz, J., Nagata, K., and Bachinger, H.P. (2008). The rough endoplasmic reticulum-resident FK506-binding protein FKBP65 is a molecular chaperone that interacts with collagens. J Biol Chem *283*, 31584-31590.

Ishikawa, Y., Wirz, J., Vranka, J.A., Nagata, K., and Bachinger, H.P. (2009). Biochemical characterization of the prolyl 3-hydroxylase 1.cartilage-associated protein.cyclophilin B complex. J Biol Chem *284*, 17641-17647.

Jaenisch, R., Harbers, K., Schnieke, A., Lohler, J., Chumakov, I., Jahner, D., Grotkopp, D., and Hoffmann, E. (1983). Germline integration of moloney murine leukemia virus at the Mov13 locus leads to recessive lethal mutation and early embryonic death. Cell *32*, 209-216.

Jiao, X., Ventruto, V., Trese, M.T., Shastry, B.S., and Hejtmancik, J.F. (2004). Autosomal recessive familial exudative vitreoretinopathy is associated with mutations in LRP5. American journal of human genetics *75*, 878-884.

Joseph, B., Rebello, G., and B, C.K. (2005). The choice of intramedullary devices for the femur and the tibia in osteogenesis imperfecta. Journal of pediatric orthopaedics Part B / European Paediatric Orthopaedic Society, Pediatric Orthopaedic Society of North America *14*, 311-319.

Kelley, B.P., Malfait, F., Bonafe, L., Baldridge, D., Homan, E., Symoens, S., Willaert, A., Elcioglu, N., Van Maldergem, L., Verellen-Dumoulin, C., *et al.* (2011). Mutations in FKBP10 cause recessive osteogenesis imperfecta and type 1 bruck syndrome. J Bone Miner Res.

Khavandgar, Z., Poirier, C., Clarke, C.J., Li, J., Wang, N., McKee, M.D., Hannun, Y.A., and Murshed, M. (2011). A cell-autonomous requirement for neutral sphingomyelinase 2 in bone mineralization. The Journal of cell biology *194*, 277-289.

Khillan, J.S., Olsen, A.S., Kontusaari, S., Sokolov, B., and Prockop, D.J. (1991). Transgenic mice that express a mini-gene version of the human gene for type I procollagen (COL1A1) develop a phenotype resembling a lethal form of osteogenesis imperfecta. The Journal of biological chemistry *266*, 23373-23379.

Kivirikko, K.I., and Pihlajaniemi, T. (1998). Collagen hydroxylases and the protein disulfide isomerase subunit of prolyl 4-hydroxylases. Adv Enzymol Relat Areas Mol Biol *72*, 325-398.

Kozloff, K.M., Carden, A., Bergwitz, C., Forlino, A., Uveges, T.E., Morris, M.D., Marini, J.C., and Goldstein, S.A. (2004). Brittle IV mouse model for osteogenesis imperfecta IV demonstrates postpubertal adaptations to improve whole bone strength. Journal of bone and mineral research : the official journal of the American Society for Bone and Mineral Research *19*, 614-622.

Kuznetsova, N., McBride, D.J., Jr., and Leikin, S. (2001). Osteogenesis imperfecta murine: interaction between type I collagen homotrimers. J Mol Biol *309*, 807-815.

Labuda, M., Morissette, J., Ward, L.M., Rauch, F., Lalic, L., Roughley, P.J., and Glorieux, F.H. (2002). Osteogenesis imperfecta type VII maps to the short arm of chromosome 3. Bone *31*, 19-25.

Land, C., Rauch, F., Montpetit, K., Ruck-Gibis, J., and Glorieux, F.H. (2006a). Effect of intravenous pamidronate therapy on functional abilities and level of ambulation in children with osteogenesis imperfecta. J Pediatr *148*, 456-460.

Land, C., Rauch, F., Munns, C.F., Sahebjam, S., and Glorieux, F.H. (2006b). Vertebral morphometry in children and adolescents with osteogenesis imperfecta: effect of intravenous pamidronate treatment. Bone *39*, 901-906.

Lapunzina, P., Aglan, M., Temtamy, S., Caparros-Martin, J.A., Valencia, M., Leton, R., Martinez-Glez, V., Elhossini, R., Amr, K., Vilaboa, N., *et al.* Identification of a frameshift mutation in Osterix in a patient with recessive osteogenesis imperfecta. American journal of human genetics *87*, 110-114.

Law, R.H., Zhang, Q., McGowan, S., Buckle, A.M., Silverman, G.A., Wong, W., Rosado, C.J., Langendorf, C.G., Pike, R.N., Bird, P.I., *et al.* (2006). An overview of the serpin superfamily. Genome biology *7*, 216.

Lisse, T.S., Thiele, F., Fuchs, H., Hans, W., Przemeck, G.K., Abe, K., Rathkolb, B., Quintanilla-Martinez, L., Hoelzlwimmer, G., Helfrich, M., *et al.* (2008). ER stress-mediated apoptosis in a new mouse model of osteogenesis imperfecta. PLoS genetics *4*, e7.

Little, R.D., Carulli, J.P., Del Mastro, R.G., Dupuis, J., Osborne, M., Folz, C., Manning, S.P., Swain, P.M., Zhao, S.C., Eustace, B., *et al.* (2002). A mutation in the LDL receptor-related protein 5 gene results in the autosomal dominant high-bone-mass trait. American journal of human genetics *70*, 11-19.

Luhmann, S.J., Sheridan, J.J., Capelli, A.M., and Schoenecker, P.L. (1998). Management of lower-extremity deformities in osteogenesis imperfecta with extensible intramedullary rod technique: a 20-year experience. J Pediatr Orthop *18*, 88-94.

Makareeva, E., Aviles, N.A., and Leikin, S. (2011). Chaperoning osteogenesis: new protein-folding disease paradigms. Trends Cell Biol *21*, 168-176.

Malfait, F., Symoens, S., Coucke, P., Nunes, L., De Almeida, S., and De Paepe, A. (2006). Total absence of the alpha2(I) chain of collagen type I causes a rare form of Ehlers-Danlos syndrome with hypermobility and propensity to cardiac valvular problems. Journal of medical genetics *43*, e36.

Marini, J.C., Cabral, W.A., and Barnes, A.M. (2010). Null mutations in LEPRE1 and CRTAP cause severe recessive osteogenesis imperfecta. Cell and tissue research *339*, 59-70.

Marini, J.C., Forlino, A., Cabral, W.A., Barnes, A.M., San Antonio, J.D., Milgrom, S., Hyland, J.C., Korkko, J., Prockop, D.J., De Paepe, A., *et al.* (2007). Consortium for osteogenesis imperfecta mutations in the helical domain of type I collagen: regions rich in lethal mutations align with collagen binding sites for integrins and proteoglycans. Human mutation *28*, 209-221.

Martin, E., and Shapiro, J.R. (2007). Osteogenesis imperfecta:epidemiology and pathophysiology. Current osteoporosis reports *5*, 91-97.

Meyer, C., Notari, L., and Becerra, S.P. (2002). Mapping the type I collagen-binding site on pigment epithelium-derived factor. Implications for its antiangiogenic activity. The Journal of biological chemistry *277*, 45400-45407.

Montpetit, K., Plotkin, H., Rauch, F., Bilodeau, N., Cloutier, S., Rabzel, M., and Glorieux, F.H. (2003). Rapid increase in grip force after start of pamidronate therapy in children and adolescents with severe osteogenesis imperfecta. Pediatrics *111*, e601-603.

Morello, R., Bertin, T.K., Chen, Y., Hicks, J., Tonachini, L., Monticone, M., Castagnola, P., Rauch, F., Glorieux, F.H., Vranka, J., *et al.* (2006). CRTAP is required for prolyl 3-hydroxylation and mutations cause recessive osteogenesis imperfecta. Cell *127*, 291-304.

Nagai, N., Hosokawa, M., Itohara, S., Adachi, E., Matsushita, T., Hosokawa, N., and Nagata, K. (2000). Embryonic lethality of molecular chaperone hsp47 knockout mice is associated with defects in collagen biosynthesis. The Journal of cell biology *150*, 1499-1506.

Nakashima, K., Zhou, X., Kunkel, G., Zhang, Z., Deng, J.M., Behringer, R.R., and de Crombrugghe, B. (2002). The novel zinc finger-containing transcription factor osterix is required for osteoblast differentiation and bone formation. Cell *108*, 17-29.

Nicholls, A.C., Valler, D., Wallis, S., and Pope, F.M. (2001). Homozygosity for a splice site mutation of the COL1A2 gene yields a non-functional pro(alpha)2(I) chain and an EDS/OI clinical phenotype. Journal of medical genetics *38*, 132-136.

Patterson, C.E., Abrams, W.R., Wolter, N.E., Rosenbloom, J., and Davis, E.C. (2005). Developmental regulation and coordinate reexpression of FKBP65 with extracellular matrix proteins after lung injury suggest a specialized function for this endoplasmic reticulum immunophilin. Cell stress & chaperones *10*, 285-295.

Pemberton, T.J., and Kay, J.E. (2005). Identification and comparative analysis of the peptidyl-prolyl cis/trans isomerase repertoires of H. sapiens, D. melanogaster, C. elegans, S. cerevisiae and Sz. pombe. Comparative and functional genomics *6*, 277-300.

Pereira, R., Khillan, J.S., Helminen, H.J., Hume, E.L., and Prockop, D.J. (1993). Transgenic mice expressing a partially deleted gene for type I procollagen (COL1A1). A breeding line with a phenotype of spontaneous fractures and decreased bone collagen and mineral. The Journal of clinical investigation *91*, 709-716.

Pizones, J., Plotkin, H., Parra-Garcia, J.I., Alvarez, P., Gutierrez, P., Bueno, A., and Fernandez-Arroyo, A. (2005). Bone healing in children with osteogenesis imperfecta treated with bisphosphonates. J Pediatr Orthop *25*, 332-335.

Plotkin, H. (2004). Syndromes with congenital brittle bones. BMC Pediatr *4*, 16.

Plotkin, H., Coughlin, S., Kreikemeier, R., Luksan, M., and Esposito, P. (2006). Low Doses of Pamidronate for Children with Osteogenesis Imperfecta (OI). Paper presented at: Proceedings of the 28th Annual Meeting of the American Society for Bone and Mineral Research (Philadelphia, PA, JBMR).

Rauch, F., Cornibert, S., Cheung, M., and Glorieux, F.H. (2007). Long-bone changes after pamidronate discontinuation in children and adolescents with osteogenesis imperfecta. Bone *40*, 821-827.

Rauch, F., and Glorieux, F.H. (2004). Osteogenesis imperfecta. Lancet *363*, 1377-1385.

Rauch, F., and Glorieux, F.H. (2006). Treatment of children with osteogenesis imperfecta. Current osteoporosis reports *4*, 159-164.

Rauch, F., Munns, C., Land, C., and Glorieux, F.H. (2006). Pamidronate in children and adolescents with osteogenesis imperfecta: effect of treatment discontinuation. The Journal of clinical endocrinology and metabolism *91*, 1268-1274.

Roschger, P., Fratzl-Zelman, N., Misof, B.M., Glorieux, F.H., Klaushofer, K., and Rauch, F. (2008a). Evidence that abnormal high bone mineralization in growing children with osteogenesis imperfecta is not associated with specific collagen mutations. Calcified tissue international *82*, 263-270.

Roschger, P., Paschalis, E.P., Fratzl, P., and Klaushofer, K. (2008b). Bone mineralization density distribution in health and disease. Bone *42*, 456-466.

Roussel, B.D., Irving, J.A., Ekeowa, U.I., Belorgey, D., Haq, I., Ordonez, A., Kruppa, A.J., Duvoix, A., Rashid, S.T., Crowther, D.C., *et al.* (2011). Unravelling the twists and turns of the serpinopathies. The FEBS journal *278*, 3859-3867.

Rutkowski, D.T., Arnold, S.M., Miller, C.N., Wu, J., Li, J., Gunnison, K.M., Mori, K., Sadighi Akha, A.A., Raden, D., and Kaufman, R.J. (2006). Adaptation to ER stress is mediated by differential stabilities of pro-survival and pro-apoptotic mRNAs and proteins. PLoS Biol *4*, e374.

Schnieke, A., Harbers, K., and Jaenisch, R. (1983). Embryonic lethal mutation in mice induced by retrovirus insertion into the alpha 1(I) collagen gene. Nature *304*, 315-320.

Schwarze, U., Hata, R., McKusick, V.A., Shinkai, H., Hoyme, H.E., Pyeritz, R.E., and Byers, P.H. (2004). Rare autosomal recessive cardiac valvular form of Ehlers-Danlos syndrome results from mutations in the COL1A2 gene that activate the nonsense-mediated RNA decay pathway. American journal of human genetics *74*, 917-930.

Shapiro, J.R., and Sponsellor, P.D. (2009). Osteogenesis imperfecta: questions and answers. Current opinion in pediatrics *21*, 709-716.

Sillence, D.O. (1988). Osteogenesis imperfecta nosology and genetics. Ann N Y Acad Sci *543*, 1-15.

Sillence, D.O., Ritchie, H.E., Dibbayawan, T., Eteson, D., and Brown, K. (1993). Fragilitas ossium (fro/fro) in the mouse: a model for a recessively inherited type of osteogenesis imperfecta. American journal of medical genetics *45*, 276-283.

Sillence, D.O., Senn, A., and Danks, D.M. (1979). Genetic heterogeneity in osteogenesis imperfecta. Journal of medical genetics *16*, 101-116.

Stacey, A., Bateman, J., Choi, T., Mascara, T., Cole, W., and Jaenisch, R. (1988). Perinatal lethal osteogenesis imperfecta in transgenic mice bearing an engineered mutant pro-alpha 1(I) collagen gene. Nature *332*, 131-136.

Sulko, J., and Radlo, W. (2005). [Operative management of long-bone of the upper limb in children with osteogenesis imperfecta]. Chir Narzadow Ruchu Ortop Pol *70*, 195-199.

Superti-Furga, A., Steinmann, B., and Perfumo, F. (1986). Osteoporosis-pseudoglioma or osteogenesis imperfecta? Clin Genet *29*, 184-185.

Toomes, C., Bottomley, H.M., Jackson, R.M., Towns, K.V., Scott, S., Mackey, D.A., Craig, J.E., Jiang, L., Yang, Z., Trembath, R., *et al.* (2004). Mutations in LRP5 or FZD4 underlie the common familial exudative vitreoretinopathy locus on chromosome 11q. American journal of human genetics *74*, 721-730.

Tryon, R.C., White, S.D., and Bannasch, D.L. (2007). Homozygosity mapping approach identifies a missense mutation in equine cyclophilin B (PPIB) associated with HERDA in the American Quarter Horse. Genomics *90*, 93-102.

Tsang, K.S., and Adedapo, A. (2011). Cannulated screw fixation of fracture neck of femur in children with osteogenesis imperfecta. Journal of pediatric orthopaedics Part B / European Paediatric Orthopaedic Society, Pediatric Orthopaedic Society of North America *20*, 287-290.

Tsang, K.Y., Chan, D., Bateman, J.F., and Cheah, K.S. (2010). In vivo cellular adaptation to ER stress: survival strategies with double-edged consequences. Journal of cell science *123*, 2145-2154.

Turman, K., Esposito, P., Plotkin, H., and al., e. (2006). Initial results with Fassier-Duval telescoping rods in osteogenesis imperfecta. In Pediatric Orthopaedic Society of North America (San Diego, CA).

Valli, M., Barnes, A.M., Gallanti, A., Cabral, W.A., Viglio, S., Weis, M., Makareeva, E., Eyre, D., Leikin, S., Antoniazzi, F., *et al.* (2011). Deficiency of CRTAP in Non-lethal Recessive Osteogenesis Imperfecta Reduces Collagen Deposition into Matrix. Clin Genet.

van der Slot, A.J., Zuurmond, A.M., Bardoel, A.F., Wijmenga, C., Pruijs, H.E., Sillence, D.O., Brinckmann, J., Abraham, D.J., Black, C.M., Verzijl, N., *et al.* (2003). Identification of PLOD2 as telopeptide lysyl hydroxylase, an important enzyme in fibrosis. J Biol Chem *278*, 40967-40972.

van Dijk, F.S., Nesbitt, I.M., Zwikstra, E.H., Nikkels, P.G., Piersma, S.R., Fratantoni, S.A., Jimenez, C.R., Huizer, M., Morsman, A.C., Cobben, J.M., *et al.* (2009). PPIB mutations cause severe osteogenesis imperfecta. American journal of human genetics *85*, 521-527.

Van Dijk, F.S., Pals, G., Van Rijn, R.R., Nikkels, P.G., and Cobben, J.M. (2010). Classification of Osteogenesis Imperfecta revisited. European journal of medical genetics *53*, 1-5.

van Gent, D., Sharp, P., Morgan, K., and Kalsheker, N. (2003). Serpins: structure, function and molecular evolution. Int J Biochem Cell Biol *35*, 1536-1547.

Van Wesenbeeck, L., Cleiren, E., Gram, J., Beals, R.K., Benichou, O., Scopelliti, D., Key, L., Renton, T., Bartels, C., Gong, Y., *et al.* (2003). Six novel missense mutations in the LDL receptor-related protein 5 (LRP5) gene in different conditions with an increased bone density. American journal of human genetics *72*, 763-771.

Vranka, J.A., Pokidysheva, E., Hayashi, L., Zientek, K., Mizuno, K., Ishikawa, Y., Maddox, K., Tufa, S., Keene, D.R., Klein, R., *et al.* (2010). Prolyl 3-hydroxylase 1 null mice display abnormalities in fibrillar collagen-rich tissues such as tendons, skin and bones. J Biol Chem.

Vranka, J.A., Sakai, L.Y., and Bachinger, H.P. (2004). Prolyl 3-hydroxylase 1: Enzyme characterization and identification of a novel family of enzymes. J Biol Chem.

Ward, K.A., Adams, J.E., Freemont, T.J., and Mughal, M.Z. (2007). Can bisphosphonate treatment be stopped in a growing child with skeletal fragility? Osteoporosis international : a journal established as result of cooperation between the European Foundation for Osteoporosis and the National Osteoporosis Foundation of the USA *18*, 1137-1140.

Ward, L.M., Rauch, F., Travers, R., Chabot, G., Azouz, E.M., Lalic, L., Roughley, P.J., and Glorieux, F.H. (2002). Osteogenesis imperfecta type VII: an autosomal recessive form of brittle bone disease. Bone *31*, 12-18.

Warman, M.L., Cormier-Daire, V., Hall, C., Krakow, D., Lachman, R., LeMerrer, M., Mortier, G., Mundlos, S., Nishimura, G., Rimoin, D.L., *et al.* (2011). Nosology and classification of genetic skeletal disorders: 2010 revision. American journal of medical genetics Part A *155A*, 943-968.

Willaert, A., Malfait, F., Symoens, S., Gevaert, K., Kayserili, H., Megarbane, A., Mortier, G., Leroy, J.G., Coucke, P.J., and De Paepe, A. (2009). Recessive osteogenesis imperfecta caused by LEPRE1 mutations: clinical documentation and identification of the splice form responsible for prolyl 3-hydroxylation. Journal of medical genetics *46*, 233-241.

Willing, M.C., Pruchno, C.J., Atkinson, M., and Byers, P.H. (1992). Osteogenesis imperfecta type I is commonly due to a COL1A1 null allele of type I collagen. American journal of human genetics *51*, 508-515.

Yao, Q., Li, M., Yang, H., Chai, H., Fisher, W., and Chen, C. (2005). Roles of cyclophilins in cancers and other organ systems. World journal of surgery *29*, 276-280.

Zhou, X., Zhang, Z., Feng, J.Q., Dusevich, V.M., Sinha, K., Zhang, H., Darnay, B.G., and de Crombrugghe, B. (2010). Multiple functions of Osterix are required for bone growth and homeostasis in postnatal mice. Proc Natl Acad Sci U S A *107*, 12919-12924.

10

The Retinoblastoma Protein in Osteogenesis and Osteosarcoma Formation

Pedro G. Santiago-Cardona
Ponce School of Medicine and Health Sciences, Ponce, Puerto Rico

1. Introduction

The retinoblastoma tumor suppressor as a cell cycle regulator, a brief overview

The retinoblastoma tumor suppressor protein (pRb) is a 928 amino acids nuclear phosphoprotein that functions predominantly as a transcriptional regulator (Knudsen and Knudsen, 2006). It possesses a weak, non-specific DNA binding capacity, therefore, its role as a transcriptional regulator requires that it forms part of protein complexes in which its binding partners provide the capacity to interact with *cis* regulatory elements in the promoters of particular target genes. Evidence supporting its predominantly tumor suppressive function rapidly accumulated since its discovery. First, its deletion in humans was found to be an important causative agent in the genesis of malignant tumors of the retina, or retinoblastomas (Cavenee et al., 1983; Friend et al., 1986; Godbout et al., 1983; Lee et al., 1987), hence its name. This was followed by studies with oncogenic viruses such as some strains of the Human Papilloma Virus (HPV), Adenovirus, and the Simian Vacuolating Virus 40 (SV40). These viruses were found to engender an oncogenic programme in their host cells in which virus-encoded oncoproteins inactivate pRb and other important host tumor suppressors (Ludlow et al., 1989). These studies reinforced the conception of pRb as a tumor suppressor by directly showing that abrogation of pRb function is a necessary step in the chain of events resulting in oncogenic transformation. Further research efforts were aimed at elucidating the precise cellular and molecular mechanisms by which pRb exerts its tumor suppressive function. The generation of the first mice in which the gene encoding pRb, *RB1*, was genetically deleted was very informative in regards to pRb function. These studies showed that mice deficient for pRb in a homozygous manner are non-viable and show a host of defects in neurogenesis and hematopoiesis. These homozygous mutants showed an increased pool of immature nucleated erythrocyte progenitors, together with ectopic mitoses in the nervous system. On the other hand, heterozygous mice, while viable, were prone to develop pituitary and thyroid tumors, strictly dependent on the loss of wild type allele of the *RB1* gene (Lee et al., 1992). These early studies suggested that pRb may be essential for the irreversible cell cycle arrest that is now considered to be a precondition of the fully differentiated post-mitotic state. Therefore, absence of pRb loss could result in an enrichment of proliferative cells with a restricted capacity to withdraw from the cell cycle and subsequently engage in a differentiation programme. These studies led to the early suspicion that these pools of undifferentiated progenitor cells, impaired in their ability to differentiate, could provide a fertile ground for the emergence of tumor forming cells, a suspicion that later studies confirmed. Today, pRb´s tumor suppressive function is widely regarded to depend on a great measure on its capacity to act as a cell cycle repressor, specifically, on its capacity to engender the irreversible cell cycle arrest that is now considered a pre-condition to achieve a fully differentiated state.

pRb´s function as a cell cycle repressor revolves around its capacity to bind and functionally repress the activity of its best characterized binding partners, the E2F transcription factors. These transcription factors, together with their heterodimeric partner DP, trigger the expression of several genes whose products are required for cell cycle progression. Known E2F/DP target genes include proteins involved in DNA synthesis and cell cycle progression such as Thymidine Kinase, Dihydrofolate Reductase (DHFR), DNA Polα, and Types E and A cyclins Cyclins (Knudsen and Knudsen, 2006; Lipinski and Jack, 1999). E2F transcription factors promote cell cycle-related transcription by recruiting pre-initiation complexes consisting of TFIIA and TFIID to E2F-responsive promoters (Nguyen and McCance, 2005; Ross et al., 1999; Zheng and Lee, 2001). As mentioned above, pRb is a phosphoprotein, and it is well established that its function is adversely affected by phosphorylation. In non-dividing cells, pRb is hypophosphorylated and therefore maximally activated, i.e., able to interact with E2F and block its activity (Buchkovich et al., 1989; Cobrinik, 2005; Dyson, 1998; Knudsen and Knudsen, 2006; Knudsen and Wang, 1996). pRb binding to E2F abolishes E2F´s transactivating capacity by recruiting transcriptional repressor complexes to promoters containing E2F binding sites. For example, pRb is known to recruit histone deacetylase (HDAC) enzymes to E2F bound promoters. These HDACs remove acetyl groups from histone proteins, thus strengthening their interactions with DNA thus provoking a local remodelling and condensation of chromatin to make it more compact and therefore less accessible to transcription factors (Lipinski and Jacks, 1999; Steveaux and Dyson, 2002; Zheng and Lee, 2001). pRb also represses transcription directly through direct contact with the basal transcription machinery without the requirement of HDAC activity (Ross and Dynlacht, 1999; Zheng and Lee, 2001).

Under the influence of mitogenic signals acting on a cell, pRb´s capacity to block E2F-dependent transcriptional activity is abolished when it is hyperphosphorylated by heterodimeric complexes containing a Cyclin regulatory component bound to a Cyclin-dependent protein kinase (Cdk). The Cdk component of these complexes gains its catalytic activity only when bound by its cyclin regulatory partner. At least three different Cyclin/Cdk complexes have been shown to phosphorylate pRb during cell cycle progression, each complex phosphorylating pRb in a specific phase of the cell cycle, and each phosphorylation rendering pRb progressively less capable of binding to and inactivating E2F (Harbour and Dean, 2000). Upon cell stimulation by mitogenic growth factors acting via receptor tyrosine kinases and the Ras/MAPK pathway, the mitogen dependent-accumulation of D-type Cyclins drives the formation of complexes between D-type cyclins and Cdk4 and Cdk6 catalytic partners, which phosphorylate pRb in early G1. This relieves the repressive effect of pRb on E2F, the later now being free to command cell cycle-related gene expression. pRb phosphorylation is propagated beyond G1 when E2Fs induce the expression of Cyclins E and A, which in complex with Cdk2 collaborate with CyclinD/Cdk4-6 complexes to sustain phosphorylation during the late G1 and S phases, respectively (Harbour and Dean, 2000; Sheer and Roberts, 1999; Zheng and Lee, 2001). In summary, the concerted actions of these Cyclin/Cdk complexes ensure pRb hyperphosphorylation and inactivation through the complete cell cycle, allowing the cells to proceed unhampered by pRb function through all phases of the cycle. In this scenario, E2F is free to trigger proliferation-related gene expression thus promoting entry into the S-phase and further progression through of cell cycle (Harbour and Dean, 2000; Zheng and Lee, 2001).

Upon completion of mitosis, and provided that anti-mitogenic signals are enriched in the extracellular milleu, pRb is hypophosphorylated and returned to its active, E2F repressive state (Dyson, 1998). This is engendered due the induction by anti-mitogenic signals of the expression of protein phosphatase 1 (PP1), which de-phosphorylates pRb. Further pRb phosphorylation is prevented when these anti-mitogenic signals induce the activities of Smad proteins, which then relocate to the nucleus upon activation and promote the expression of Cyclin-dependent kinase inhibitors (CKIs) such as p15, p16, p21 and p27. As implied by their name, these CKIs repress the actions of the Cyclin/Cdk complexes responsible for pRb phosphorylation. Thus, the concerted actions of PP1 and CKIs restore pRb to its hypo-phosphorylated, fully functional state (Durfee et al., 1993; Ludlow et al., 1993; Nguyen and McCance, 2005).

It is noteworthy that the paramount biological importance of pRb as a master controller of the cell cycle transcends mammals and is highlighted by the fact that conserved pRb homologues have been identified and shown to play crucial roles in cell cycle control and differentiation in *Drosophila* (Du et al., 1996) and *C. elegans* (Lu and Horvitz, 1998). In both of these organisms pRb performs similar roles in cell cycle regulation and differentiation.

2. pRb inactivation in human cancers: All roads lead to Rome

From the previous description of pRb's mechanism of action, pRb abrogation is expected to lead to a major breakdown in cell cycle control with consequent unrestricted proliferation. A corollary of this statement is that a functional pRb pathway represents a major roadblock to oncogenic transformation. Consistent with this, it is now well established that either pRb itself or proteins that funnel their anti-mitogenic activities through pRb are lost or mutationally inactivated in the vast majority of human tumors (Hanahan and Weinberg, 2011; Nguyen and McCance, 2005). Therefore, it is not an overstatement to say that the pRb pathway is inactivated in most, if not all, human tumors. This observation strongly supports the tumor suppressive nature of pRb, while hinting at the strong selective pressures faced by incipient cancer cells to inactivate pRb.

Given the close relationship between pRb and E2F in cell cycle control, it is not surprising then that some human tumors are comprised by transformed cells bearing mutant *RB1* alleles coding for pRb proteins that are defective in their capacity to block E2F action. This is observed with high frequency in retinoblastomas, osteosarcomas, bladder carcinomas and small-cell lung carcinomas, where the *RB1* gene itself is a usual target of mutational hits (Horowitz et al., 1990). However, given the strong selective pressure for pRb inactivation faced by transformed cells, even tumors comprised of cells with wild type *RB1* alleles usually harbor mutations in genes coding for other pRb pathway components. Excessive expression of Cdk4 or Cyclin D by gene amplication or chromosomal translocation is related to several cancer types. For example, amplification of Cyclin D1 genes have been found in breast, thyroid, head and neck tumors as well as in mantle cell lymphomas, while Cdk4 overexpression or Cdk4 mutations that render it insensitive to CKI inhibition have been found in melanomas and glioblastomas (Liu et al., 2004; Sherr and McCormick, 2002; Vooijs and Berns, 1999). Other cancer types such as non-small cell lung carcinomas, melanomas, pancreatic carcinomas and T cell lymphomas show mutational inactivation of the CKI p16 (Kaye, 2002). Melanomas are notable for the high frequency with which they bear mutations in the gene coding for the p53 tumor suppressor, a transcription factor that is a potent inducer of the CKI p21, as well as mutations in the p16 gene (Hussussian et al., 1994). Finally, mutations in the *APC* gene, occurring with high frequency in colorectal carcinomas, lead to unrestricted activation of the Wnt signalling pathway, with consequent up-regulation of Cyclin D genes (López-Kostner, 2010). It can be clearly appreciated that all of the mutational scenarios described above result in abrogation of pRb function, even in the ones in which there is a wild type pRb status. In other words, in most human cancers, pRb itself is missing or defective, or it is inactivated due to hyperphosphorylation. Independently of the mode of pRb inactivation, the end result is always unchecked E2F activity. As can be discerned in the examples above, the mechanism of pRb inactivation during tumorigenesis is clearly tissue specific. Nevertheless, independently of the tissue of origin, the acquisition of a fully transformed phenotype is strongly dependent on the acquisition of mechanisms to circumvent pRb activity.

From what was discussed above, it is more than evident that pRb abrogation signifies a major contribution to carcinogenic transformation by removing the primary obstacle to over-proliferation. However, it is widely regarded that oncogenic transformation is rarely, if ever, the end result of mutations in one or just a few genes. On the contrary, it has been established that a minimum of at the very least 6 mutations in critical genes in the same cell are required to drive cells into full malignancy (Hanahan and Weinberg; 2000). It is well known that other aspects of cellular homeostasis, in addition to cell cycle control, must be dysregulated to achieve a fully malignant phenotype. For example, for the development malignat tumors to occur, unrestricted proliferation must be accompanied by other traits such as evasion of apoptosis, increased angiogenic capacity, loss of intercellular contacts, increased proclivity for migratory activity, and production of extracellular matrix degrading enzymes, among others (Hanahan and Weinberg, 2000). Although pRb loss is apparently more relevant for the early stages of hyperplastic proliferation, it is clear that pRb loss at such a stage can enrich the incipient tumor tissue with proliferative cells in which additional mutant alleles are likely to arise due to DNA replication errors during their prolonged and unrestricted proliferation. These mutant alleles can accumulate and propagate in rapidly dividing pRb-deficient cells and they can cooperate with pRb deficiency to drive full oncogenic transformation. It is important to note that pRb has also been assigned a very important role as guardian of the genome (Zheng and Lee, 2001). Therefore, pRb loss has the dual effect of enhancing proliferative capacity while leading to a state of genomic instability. Therefore, pRb null cells are known not only by their capacity to proliferate unrestrictedly, but also by being prone to acquire genetic alterations ranging from point mutations to gross genetic rearrangements. This in turn can result in inactivation of other tumor suppressors and/or in constitutive activation of oncogenes. Thus pRb contributes to early carcinogenesis by allowing the emergence of a pool of rapidly dividing cells that serves as a fertile ground for the acquisition of further genetic changes that will later contribute to the more advanced stages of malignant transformation, and that together with pRb loss confer cells a selective advantage over normal cells.

3. Additional roles for pRb beyond cell cycle control

It was expected that a powerful tumor suppressor such as pRb, whose inactivation has been so intricately linked to the molecular etiology of most human cancers, would become a focus of intense research in cancer biology. Research on pRb has indeed been intensive for over two decades now, and as a result of this, pRb is now appreciated as a complex multifunctional protein with a wider relevance to cellular homeostasis. As a reflection of this, a wide repertoire of pRb-interacting proteins, in addition to E2F transcription factors, has been identified, each of them mediating a particular function, and all of them together reflecting the complex multifunctional nature of this protein. The list of pRb functions has grown over the years and currently includes, among others, roles in stem cell maintenance, senescence, tissue differentiation, morphogenesis and regeneration, modulation of hormone response, genomic integrity, chromosome segregation, cell-to-cell adhesion and global genomic fluidity. In depth-discussion of each of these additional functions is beyond the scope of this chapter and has been reviewed or reported elsewhere (Braig and Schmitt, 2006; Campisi, 2001; Liu et al., 2004; Lundberg et al., 2000; Narita et al., 2003; Sosa-García et al., 2010; Wynford-Thomas, 1999; Xu et al., 1997; Zheng and Lee, 2001). Further underscoring pRb's tremendous biological importance, pRb is now known to be required for the proper formation of the cellular architecture of the placenta. Using a combination of tetraploid aggregation and conditional *RB1* genetic knock-out strategies Wu et al. (2003) were able to identify an important contribution of pRb to extraembryonic cell lineages required for embryonic development and viability. Interestingly, in these studies, most of the neurological and erythoid abnormalities originally described in pRb-null mice were virtually absent in pRb-deficient embryos when these were rescued with a wild type placenta. A defective placenta in the absence of pRb function can significantly contribute to the embryonic lethality of pRb abrogation during development.

3.1 A role for pRb in tissue differentiation

pRb's role as a cell cycle repressor is intricately linked to its role as an inducer of differentiation. This is consistent with the notion that cell differentiation is a post-mitotic state that is achieved only after a cell undergoes an irreversible withdrawal from the cell cycle. Therefore, pRb can be considered as an integrator between permanent cell cycle arrest and the initiation of cellular programmes that culminate in differentiation. pRb's function in this context can be said to consist in ensuring that a cell does not initiate differentiation before arresting its proliferation. As will be discussed below, this is turn predicts that a breakdown of pRb function can result in the accumulation in tissues of proliferating progenitor cells with tumorigenic potential. The phenotype of the pRb knock-out mice described above supports this notion. pRb's contribution to differentiation is complex and at many levels. pRb function confers differentiating cells with the capacity to irreversibly exit the cell cycle while coordinating this exit with the initiation of differentiation. pRb also protects developing tissues from apoptosis, induces and sustains cell type specific-gene expression, and maintains the differentiated post-mitotic state (Lipinski and Jacks, 1999). It is known that in addition to E2F-bound pRb, free unphosphorylated pRb accumulates after cells reach a post-mitotic state and it is this free active pRb that is responsible for driving and sustaining the various aspects of differentiation (Lipinski and Jacks, 1999).

pRb has been intimately linked to the differentiation of several cell types such as cerebellar granule cells, adipocytes, keratinocytes, myoblasts and osteoblasts (Classon et al., 2000;

Landsberg et al., 2003; Liu et al., 2004; Marino et al., 2003). pRb's participation in myogenic, adipogenic and osteogenic differentiation has been particularly well-studied. As will be discussed in details below, pRb's role in differentiation is a dual one, on the one hand promoting terminal cell cycle arrest, an on the other hand, enhancing the activity of tissue-specific transcription factors that in turn trigger the expression of tissue specific differentiation. It is important to note that in both cell cycle repression and in tissue differentiation, pRb functions predominantly as a transcriptional regulator by a mechanism that essentially consists in binding to, and regulating the transactivating capacity of the main transcription factors involved in these processes. However, pRb's effect on transcription is context-dependent, being repressive in cell cycle control while being activating in regards to cellular differentiation. Specifically, while pRb represses the activity of E2Fs transcription factors during cell cycle regulation, it enhances the activity of the transcription factors that drive tissue-specific gene expression during differentiation. Therefore, pRb's capacity to induce terminal cell cycle arrest is tightly coordinated to its capacity to drive cells into differentiation pathways, both roles being evoked in a complementary manner. This is fully consistent with the notion that cell proliferation and differentiation are mutually exclusive processes, and places pRb in the position of an overseer of the mechanisms that prevent the onset of premature differentiation before precursor cells are fully arrested. In terms of protection of tissues undergoing morphogenesis from undue apoptosis, pRb's role seems to be dependent on its capacity to bind and repress E2F1, which is unique among E2F transcription factors for being the only member capable of inducing apoptosis (DeGregori et al., 1997).

As mentioned above, pRb's participation in myogenic, osteogenic and adipogenic differentiation has been particularly well studied. pRb's involvement in myogenic and adipogenic differentiation will be briefly discussed here, while pRb's role in osteogenic differentiation will be the topic of section 5 of this chapter. In regards to myogenic differentiation, it is now well established that it depends on pRb function for the expression of muscle-specific markers (Gu et al., 1993). pRb abrogation severely impairs myogenic differentiation. In addition, pRb-deficient myoblasts cannot maintain a post-mitotic state following differentiation, being susceptible to mitogenic-re-stimulation (Novitch et al., 1999). This again points to a role for pRb in promoting and sustaining the post-mitotic state associated with differentiation. On the other hand, pRb significantly upregulates the expression of MyoD, a myogenic transcription factor, while increasing its transactivating capacity. In this way pRb contributes to the expression of late muscle differentiation markers such as MHC, MCK and MEF2 (Gu et al., 1993; Novitch et al., 1999). A direct pRb-MyoD interaction has been demonstrated *in vitro* (Gu et al., 1993), although there is still controversy as to the possible relevance of this interaction *in vivo* (Nguyen and McCance, 2005). Furthermore, the specific mechanism accounting for the pRb-dependent upregulation of MyoD still awaits clarification. Several scenarios have been proposed to explain pRb's involvement in myogenic differentiation. In addition to directly activating MyoD transcriptional activity, pRb may sequester inhibitors of muscle specific transcription such as HBP-1, leading to a pRb-mediated de-repression of MyoD activity (Nguyen and McCance, 2005; Zheng and Lee, 2001). Therefore, although the details of the mechanisms by which pRb impinges upon myogenic differentiation are still the subject of research, pRb's importance for myogenic differentiation is widely accepted, whether its role consists in directly transcriptionally activating MyoD expression and function, or in removing a block hampering MyoD expression.

In relation to adipogenic differentiation, pRb has also been shown to bind and increase the transactivation capacities of CCAAT/enhancer binding proteins (C/EBPs), which are the central transcription factors driving adipocyte differentiation (Zheng and Lee, 2001). NF-IL6, another transcription factor member of the C/EBP family which is important for leukocyte differentiation, was also shown to be activated by pRb (Chen et al., 1996). pRb is also known to be involved in promoting erythrocyte and neuron differentiation by abrogating the function of differentiation blockers such as Id2 (Zheng and Lee, 2001). Taken together, the findings obtained from studies in differentiation reveal a common mechanism by which pRb regulates differentiation. pRb does so by interacting with transcription factors associated with differentiation, enhancing the activity of those that promote tissue-specific gene expression while blocking the activity of those that hamper such gene expression.

It is noteworthy that the distinct developmental abnormalities observed in the pRb-null mice, i.e., defects in erythropoiesis, lens, skeleton and muscle differentiation, can be explained in light of pRb's functions in differentiation as just described. Defective tissues in these pRb-null mice were predominantly characterized by an enrichment of poorly differentiated progenitor cells, again pointing to an inability to exit the cell cycle in preparation for differentiation. The embryonic lethality can be explained at least in part by the widespread differentiation defects observed in these animals, together with the defects in the placenta described above.

4. Cellular and molecular mechanisms of osteogenic differentiation

The role of pRb in osteogenic differentiation has been well studied and established. Before discussing pRb's participation in this process, an in-depth discussion of the molecular mechanisms associated with osteogenic differentiation is in order.

4.1 Overview of osteogenic differentiation and skeletal morphogenesis

Osteogenic differentiation is a central component of developmental skeletogenesis. Furthermore, it goes beyond embryogensis and continues afterwards as an ongoing process through adult life, intimately linked to bone remodelling. Bone remodelling in post-natal life serves first in the growth phase and later in adult life to replace aging tissue and repair injuries (Day et al., 2005). This necessitates osteoblast proliferation and differentiation through the entire life of an organism in order to continuously supply bone-forming cells and thus maintain bone homeostasis (Mbalaviele et al., 2005). Bone and cartilage are major tissues in the vertebrate skeletal system, which is primarily composed of three cell types: osteoblasts, chondrocytes, and osteoclasts (Day et al., 2005). In bone homeostasis, osteoblasts participate in the synthesis, deposition and mineralization of the matrix that will form the bone, while osteoclasts resorb this mineralized matrix allowing this rigid tissue to remodel (Ducy, 2000).

Bone marrow mesenchymal stem cells are the source of osteoprogenitor cells in adult life. Bone marrow contains a complex and heterogeneous mixture of pluripotent stem cells that can differentiate not only into osteoblasts, but also into fibroblasts, adipocytes, myocytes, hematopoietic cells, and endothelial cells under the induction by systemic or local factors (Marie, 2002). In the developing skeleton, osteoblasts and chondrocytes both differentiate from a common mesenchymal progenitor *in situ*, whereas osteoclasts are of hematopoietic origin and brought in later by invading blood vessels (Day et al., 2005).

Embryonic skeletogenesis *in situ* starts with the condensation of undiffentiated mesenchymal cells. These condensations, also called anlagen, occur in structures and locations that prefigure each future skeletal element (Ducy, 2000; Hall and Miyake, 2002). Depending on the anatomic location, skeletogenesis can occur by two distinct mechanisms: intramembranous and endochondral ossification (Day et al., 2005). Intramembranous ossification occurs by the direct transformation of mesenchymal cell within condensates into osteoblasts, and is limited to bones of the cranial vault, some facial bones, and part of the mandible and clavicle (Day et al., 2005). On the other hand, the axial and appendicular skeletal elements, i.e., bones that participate in joints and bear weight such as long bones, the spine and ribs, form by endochondral ossification. In this mechanism, the condensed embryonic mesenchyme first transforms into a cartilage template of the future bone while osteoblasts differentiate and mature in the periphery of the cartilage (perichondrium) to form bone collars. The whole template is later remodelled and ossified to produce the mature bone when a collagen type I-rich extracellular matrix (ECM) becomes mineralized by the action of mature osteoblasts (Day et al., 2005; Ducy, 2000).

Osteogenic differentiation is a major driving force of skeletogenesis by providing a constant pool of differentiated osteoblasts, which will form the bone structure by synthesizing, depositing and mineralizing the bone matrix. *In vitro* studies of osteogenic differentiation have supplemented *in vivo* studies and have contributed significantly to the elucidation of the details of this process. Osteogenic differentiation is a complex multi-step process that can be roughly divided into two major stages. The first stage involves the commitment of bone marrow stem cells to the osteogenic lineage, a commitment that imposes a restriction to their pluripotency. This leads to the production of a pool of osteoprogenitor cells that eventually convert to pre-osteoblasts or immature osteoblasts, that will then differentiate into fully mature osteoblasts upon receiving the appropriate stimuli. While osteoprogenitor cells still retain some level of plasticity in their differentiation potential, pre-osteoblast are irreversibly committed to differentiate into osteoblasts. In the second stage, irreversibly committed pre-osteoblasts fully differentiate into mature osteoblasts with bone-producing capabilities. This second stage entails a series of intermediate steps along the osteoblast lineage, each characterized by the expression of specific differentiation-stage-specific markers. Based on the expression patterns of differentiation markers studied in osteoblasts cultured in differentiation inducing medium, most of the steps along the differentiation pathway have been elucidated. Based on the outcomes of in vitro studies (Aubin, 1999; Marie, 2002; Marom, 2004), the second stage can be further subdivided into four main periods as follows. First, pre-confluent proliferation supports expansion of the pre-osteoblasts, which are also active in the biosynthesis of the type I collagen that predominates in bone ECM. This period results in the formation of a confluent monolayer of pre-osteoblasts anchored to a collagen type I ECM. At this time, and in addition to type I collagen, genes related to proliferation (e.g., c-myc, c-fos and c-jun) and cell cycle progression (e.g., histones and cyclins) are expressed together with genes encoding cell adhesion-related molecules (e.g., fibronectin, cadherins, integrins). This period culminates with the establishment of confluent monolayers of post-mitotic pre-osteoblasts that have undergone the contact-dependent growth arrest normally experienced at high cellular densities. In the second period, a second wave of post-confluent proliferation ensues, but only in a very limited population of pre-osteoblasts that become irreversibly committed to enter the full differentiation programme. This post-confluent proliferation allows clonal expansion to increase the mass of future bone forming cells. It occurs at multiple foci scattered through the monolayer of growth-arrested pre-osteoblasts and supports their multilayering to develop bone-forming nodules. Eventually cells within each nodule become growth arrested and start expressing markers of osteoblast differentiation. This step is characterized by the expression of genes that support organization, maturation, and mineralization of the bone ECM (Aubin, 1999; Marie, 2002). This is a post-proliferative gene expression pattern restricted to subgroup of cells within the nodule and serves predominantly to render the ECM competent for mineralization, a process that is essential for the complete expression of the mature osteoblast phenotype. The genes predominantly expressed at this time include genes coding for Alkaline Phosphatase (AP), a cell surface glycoprotein early marker involved in ECM mineralization and in the synthesis and deposition of type I collagen and other non-collagenous bone matrix proteins (Marom et al., 2004). The third period is completely post-mitotic and involves gene expression related to subsequent and more advanced stages of differentiation, specifically related to the ordered deposition of hydroxyapatite, which is the predominant bone mineral. The main characteristic of this period is the appearance of a mineralized bone ECM with which fully mature osteoblasts interact. Osteopontin, Bone Sialoprotein (BSP) and Osteocalcin, which are late markers of full osteoblast differentiation, exhibit maximal expression at this time when maturation of osteoblasts and mineralization of bone tissue reach their peaks (Aubin, 1999; Marie, 2002; Marom, 2004). Osteoponting and BSP are secreted proteins, they bind cell surface integrin receptors, and regulate mineralization (Marom, 2004). Osteocalcin is a matrix protein that regulates osteoclast activity (Marom, 2004), which must be later balanced with osteoblast function to sustain proper bone remodelling and homeostasis. *In vivo*, mature osteoblasts that are actively forming the bone matrix have cuboidal shapes, they line the forming bone, and form extensive cell-to-cell contacts. Once the bone matrix has been deposited, most of these cuboidal osteoblasts become flattened, and a fraction of them loose cell-to-cell adhesion and become embedded within the matrix to become osteocytes (Marie, 2002). Finally, the fourth period is not directly involved in the initial osteogenic differentiation related to skeletogenesis, but is more related to editing and remodelling of the bone ECM. Consistent with editing and remodelling, this period is characterized by increased expression of not only collagen type I, but also of collagenase enzyme. This period is also characterized by apoptosis of osteoblasts and a compensatory proliferative activity that replenishes the osteoblasts lost to apoptosis. As discussed above, there is a reciprocal and functionally coupled relationship between proliferation and differentiation, since full differentiation and maturation of osteoblasts in the third period needs to be preceded by their terminal withdrawal from the cell cycle. The first three periods described above are visually represented in Figure 1.

4.2 Runx2 as a master switch of osteogenic differentiation and bone formation

The events described above are notable for the progressive expression of markers associated with each differentiation step and culminating with the expression of genes that are typical of the fully differentiated osteoblast such as Osteocalcin, Bione Sialoprotein and Osteopontin. The main players in this sequential pattern of differentiation specific gene expression are usually tissue-specific transcription factors that temporally regulate the expression of these markers. In the process of osteogenic differentiation, the predominant, and so far considered the most important, tissue-specific transcription factor identified is the

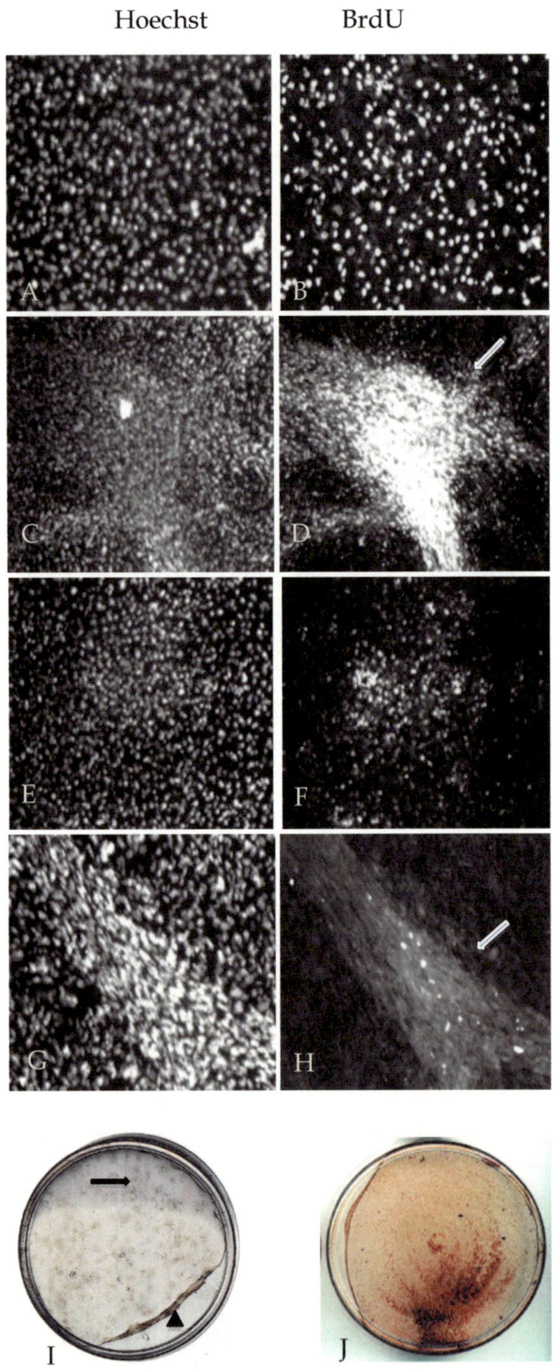

Fig. 1. Main events associated with osteogenic differentiation. The calvaria osteoblast cell line MC3T3-E1 can be induced to differentiate *in vitro* in the presence of ascorbic acid and β-glycerophospahate. This system has been very useful to study the main events and the

transcriptional changes associated to osteogenic differentiation. Panels A, C, E, G and I show total nuclei stained with Hoechst nuclear stain, while panels B, D, F, H and J show nuclei of proliferating cells immunostained for BrdU. Pre-confluent pre-osteoblasts show robust proliferation until high-density cultures are reached (A, B), in which eventually cells undergo contact-dependent growth arrest to produce a confluent cell monolayer. In this stage cells predominantly express collagen type I and genes involved in cell proliferation. At 7 days after confluence (dac), a second wave of proliferation ensues to allow clonal expansion of pre-osteoblast that are irreversibly committed to produce mature osteoblasts (C, D). This clonal expansion results in the formation of multi-layered bone-forming nodules (arrow in D) analogous to the anlagen formed *in vivo*. Notice that cell proliferation is restricted to the bone-forming nodule while cells at the periphery of the nodule are growth arrested, as determined by their lack of incorporated BrdU. At this stage collagen type I continues to be produced robustly, while Alkaline Phosphatase expression is initiated in preparation for the mineralization of the collagen I matrix. At 14 dac, cell proliferation starts to decrease within the bone-forming nodules (E, F), in preparation for the mineralization of the matrix. At 21 dac (G, H), proliferation has completely stopped within the bone-forming nodules (arrow in H). At this time point the bone-forming nodules are apparent to the unaided eye due to their refractive properties and can be seen as mineral- and matrix-dense areas (arrow in I) interspersed through the cell monolayer, which in turn is embedded in a dense collagen type I matrix, seen peeling-off the culture plate in I and J (arrowheads). At this time point markers of late differentiation such as Osteocalcin, Osteopontin and Bone Sialiprotein are being expressed, while mineralization of the bone matrix can bee seen by staining the cultures with alizarin red, which stains bone mineral.

Runt-related transcription factor 2 (Runx2), formerly known as Core Binding Factor α1, or Cbfa1. Runx2 is the earliest molecular marker of the osteoblastic lineage, its expression is both necessary and sufficient to induce osteoblast differentiation (Bialek et al., 2004; Ducy, 2000; Komori, 2002). Evidence pointing to the pivotal role of Runx2 in the regulation of osteogenesis has accumulated to the extent that Runx2 is now considered the main intrinsic regulator of osteogenic differentiation. Runx2 was first identified as the nuclear protein binding to an osteoblast-specific cis-acting element activating the expression of Osteocalcin, the most osteoblast-specific gene. Sequences analyses followed by DNA binding assays located putative Runx2 binding sites in the promoters of other major osteoblast specific genes such as Bone Sialoprotein, Osteopontin and the α1 type I collagen gene (Ducy, 2000). Further confirming the regulatory effect of Runx2 over these genes, *in vitro* studies showed that addition of Runx2 anti-sense oligonucleotides to cultured osteoblasts specifically decreased their expressions (Banerjee, et al., 1997; Ducy, 2000). More importantly, forced expression of Runx2 in non-osteoblastic cells such as primary fibroblasts can activate the expression of Osteocalcin and Bone Sialoprotein in them (Ducy, 2000). The accumulated evidence suggests that Runx2 expression is a key event in the commitment of multipotent mesenchymal stem cells to the osteogenic lineage (Komori, 2002). In addition to participating in the early commitment stage, Runx2 function is also apparently necessary at the later stages of osteogenic differentiation since it is also required for the induction of alkaline phosphatase activity, expression of bone matrix protein genes, and mineralization of that matrix to form bone structures (Banerjee et al., 1997; Ducy, 2000; Komori, 2002; Otto et al., 1997).

The importance of Runx2 for osteogenic differentiation was also established *in vivo*. In mouse embryogenesis, by 12.5 days post-coitum (dpc) every anlage expresses high levels of Runx2. Runx2 is expressed in every future osteoblast, independently of its embryonic origin and regardless of the future mode of ossification, whether intramembranous or perichondrial (Ducy, 2000). Two groups independently deleted the Runx2 gene in mice using homologous recombination (Komori et al., 1997; Otto et al., 1997). Consistent with an important role in osteogenesis, the Runx2 homozygously deficient mice, although normally patterned and of nearly normal size, have skeletons that are entirely cartilaginous. Histologically, these animals lack osteoblasts and their skeletons show a complete lack of bone tissue. Those mice were able to construct a nearly complete cartilage model of the skeleton, but having lost all bone matrix production, failed to mineralize the cartilage scaffold. Further analysis of Runx2 deficient mice revealed that osteogenic differentiation was arrested in the absence of Runx2, demonstrating both that Runx2 is important to that process and that there is no other parallel pathway that can replace its absence (Ducy, 2000). At the molecular level, *in situ* hybridization studies established that there is no expression of differentiation markers expressed exclusively in osteoblasts such as Osteopontin Bone Sialoprotein and Osteocalcin (Komori et al., 1997; Otto et al., 1997), indicative of the absence of mature osteoblasts in these mice. Further supporting a role for Runx2 in bone formation, the heterozygous mice showed a phenotype strongly suggestive of the syndrome known as cleidocranial dysplasia, which arises in humans as a consequence of Runx2 haploid insufficiency and is characterized by generalized bone defects including a ridged skull and lack of clavicles (Otto et al., 1997). Additional evidence has consistently documented a role for Runx2 in the maintenance of the osteoblast differentiated state. For example, Runx2 was shown to regulate the rate of bone mineral deposition by differentiated osteoblasts. Consistent with this, Runx2 expression is sustained post-natally in mice and in fully differentiated osteoblasts (Ducy, 2000). As stated above, Runx2 is an inducer of the expression of Osteocalcin, a gene that is an exclusive trait of fully differentiated osteoblasts (Aubin, 1999; Ducy, 2000). Taken together, the data summarized above suggest that Runx2 modulates commitment of pluripotent stem cells to an osteogenic lineage, while being also a major force driving cells into the osteogenic differentiation. Once osteoblasts reach their maturity, Runx2 regulates their functions and sustains their differentiated state. Clearly then, Runx2 acts as a master regulator of osteoblast differentiation and bone synthesis acting in several stages of the process.

It is important to note that Runx2, although considered a master regulator of the osteogenic differentiation, it is by no means the only osteoblast specific transcription factor related to osteogenic differentiation. In fact, Runx2 is known to act in close concert with another osteoblast specific transcription factor known as Osterix (Osx). In fact, Runx2´s function in the initial commitment to the osteoblast lineage strongly depends on having Osx acting downstream of Runx2. Inactivation of Osx, even in the presence of a fully functional Runx2, results in the formation of ectopic chondrocytes at the expense of osteoblasts (Day et al., 2005). These studies indicate that the initial Runx2-induced commitment to the osteoblastic lineage needs Osx activity to be sustained, and that in the absence of Osx this commitment is fragile, with cells retaining a certain degree of plasticity (Day et al., 2005). These results further indicate that the concerted action of Runx2 and Osx is required not only for determination of one cell type, but also for suppressing the genetic and molecular programs leading to another cell type. Consistent with this, expression of Runx2 in an osteochondral progenitor cell line inhibited chondrocyte differentiation (Lengner et al., 2005).

The mechanisms related to the regulation of Runx2 function have been the subject of intensive research, and there are data suggesting that the regulation of Runx2 function itself may be complex. In light of Runx2´s powerful osteogenic effect, it is puzzling that in mice development, Runx2 expression precedes the appearance of osteoblasts by at least 4 days. Runx2 expression is detected in lateral plate mesoderm as early as E10 during mouse development (Bialek et al., 2004), yet expression of molecular markers of differentiated osteoblasts cannot be detected before E13 at the earliest, and in most skeletal elements, replacement of the cartilaginous template by bone does not occur before E15 (Bianco, et al., 1991). It is puzzling then how such a powerful inducer of osteogenesis can be present in the embryo for a time window of approximately 4 days without exerting its powerful osteogenic effect. Some observations have suggested answers to this puzzle. It has been observed that Twist 1 and 2, which are basic helix-loop-helix (bHLH) containing transcription factors, are expressed in Runx2-expressing cells throughout the skeleton during early development, and osteoblast-specific gene expression ensues only after their expression decreases. Therefore, an inverse correlation has been found between Twist expression and expression of osteoblast differentiation markers (Bialek et al., 2004). This has led investigators to propose that Runx2 action may be blocked in the very early stages of skeletogenesis and that Twist proteins may have a leading role in this Runx2 repression. Supporting this, it has been shown that Twist-1 and -2 deficiency unleashes premature osteoblast differentiation. Conversely, Twist-1 overexpression inhibits osteoblast differentiation. It was later discovered that twist proteins inhibit osteoblast differentiation by interacting with Runx2's DNA binding domain, thus abrogating Runx2´s DNA binding capacity and transactivating activity without affecting its expression levels (Bialek et al., 2004). This study reveals that osteoblast differentiation is a negatively regulated process early during skeletogenesis, despite the normal expression of Runx2, and that relief of inhibition by Twist proteins is a mandatory event preceding osteoblast differentiation. It is tempting to speculate that the action of Twist proteins permits the building up of enough cellular mass in the mesenchymal condensates by blocking premature onset of osteogenic differentiation. This will allow enough building-up of cellular mass that later will ensure that the appropriate bone density is attained by the forming skeleton. Therefore, Twist proteins block the premature onset of the osteogenic differentiation programme.

4.3 Regulation of osteogenic differentiation

While Runx2 and Osx provide a determinant major force in driving commitment to the osteoblastic cell lineage and together keep the cell differentiating along that pathway, its is clear that these transcription factors trigger differentiation-specific gene expression as a response to external osteogenic stimuli acting on pluripotent stem cells. Several well-studied external ligands with powerful osteogenic influence include Bone Morphogenetic Proteins (BMPs), Transforming Growth Factor-β (TGF-β), Glucocorticoids, Parathyroid Hormone (PH), Estrogen, Insulin-like growth factors (IGFs), Fibroblast Growth Factors (FGFs), Indian Hedgehog, Retinoic Acid (RA) and 1,25-dihydroxyvitamin D_3 (Canalis et al., 1993). While the osteogenic effect of these ligands have been established, the mechanisms that sensitize subpopulations of cells in the bone marrow to be responsive to some stimuli and not others are still under intense investigation. These osteogenic ligands exert their effects by acting through specific signaling pathways that most likely impinge upon Runx2 and/or Osx if they are to elicit an osteogenic response. Consistent with this, several intracellular signalling pathways have been identified in relation to osteogenic differentiation that serve as bridges linking the actions of these osteogenic ligands with Runx2 and Osterix regulation. Two of these are the Wnt/β-catenin signalling pathway and the Akt pathway. Each of these will be discussed in the following section and used to illustrate the mechanisms that integrate the action of osteogenic external stimuli to the regulation of Runx2 and Osx.

4.3.1 The Wnt pathway in osteogenic differentiation

The Wnt/β-catenin pathway has proved to be a very important signalling pathway controlling the embryonic patterning and morphogenesis of various tissues, including bone. Briefly described, the Wnt pathway is activated by several Wnt ligands that interact with Frizzled receptors in the surface of Wnt-responsive target cells. Activation of the Wnt pathway blocks the degradation of β-catenin, an adherens junction component that is normally targeted for proteasome-mediated degradation after detaching from the membrane. Blocking of β-catenin degradation by Wnt activity leads to its accumulation in the nucleus and subsequent binding to TCF/Lef Transcription factors. This β-catenin/TCF/Lef complex acts as a transcription factor that induces transcription of various target genes depending on the biological context (Logan and Nusse, 2004). As previously explained, chondrocytes and osteoblasts share a common bi-potential precursor within a subpopulation of mesenchymal stem cells, and therefore there must be mechanisms in place to ensure a balanced discrimination between osteogenesis and chondrogenesis during vertebrate skeletogenesis. Bi-potential progenitor cells within early mesenchymal condensations can differentiate into both osteoblasts and chondrocytes as they co-express Sox9 and Runx2. While the importance of Runx2 for osteogenic differentiation was described above, Sox9 is a transcription factor required for chondrocyte cell fate determination and marks early chondrogenic differentiation of mesenchymal progenitors (Akiyama et al., 2002). Inactivation of Sox9 blocks chondrocyte differentiation and leads to ectopic expression of osteoblast-specific genes in targeted progenitor cells (Akiyama et al., 2002). Conversely, cultured Runx2-/- calvarial cells differentiate into chondrocytes *in vitro* when treated with BMP-2 (Kobayashi et al., 2000). Therefore, there appears to be a competition or mutual suppression between the genetic pathways leading to osteoblastic and chondroblastic diferentiation in the common mesenchymal progenitors during both endochondral and intramembranous ossification. Interestingly, Wnt/β-catenin signalling has been implicated in the mutual exclusivity between these pathways, and appears to play a very important role in controlling the balance between the chondrogenic and osteogenic differentiation. The expression patterns of many Wnt ligands during skeletal development suggest the hypothesis that they may be actively signalling the mesenchymal condensations and affecting the balance between osteoblasts and chondrocyte differentiation within the condensations (Parr et al., 1993). Consistent with a role for Wnt/β-catenin in early specification, Wnt/β-catenin pathway activity was found to be upregulated in osteogenic mesenchymal condensations and in the differentiating osteoblasts (Day, et al., 2005). Furthermore, Wnt/β-catenin signalling prevented osteoblasts from differentiating into chondrocytes (Hill et al., 2005). Osteoblast precursors lacking β-catenin are blocked from differentiating into osteoblasts and develop into chondrocytes instead (Hill et al., 2005). *In vivo* ectopic Wnt/β-catenin signalling leads to the enhanced ossification and suppression of chondrocyte formation. Conversely, genetic inactivation of β-catenin causes ectopic formation of chondrocytes at the expense of osteoblast differentiation during both intramembranous and endochondral ossification, leading to disrupted normal skeletal development (Day et al., 2005). Moreover, inactivation of β-catenin in mesenchymal progenitor cells *in vitro* causes chondrocyte differentiation under conditions allowing only osteoblasts to form (Day et al., 2005). Taken together, these data show that Wnt/β-catenin is essential in determining whether mesenchymal progenitors will become osteoblasts or chondrocytes regardless of regional localization or ossification mechanisms (Day et al., 2005). Specifically, it inhibits chondrocyte differentiation, likely by suppressing Sox9 activity, and promotes osteogenic differentiation and bone formation, by enhancing Runx2 activity.

Interestingly, the Wnt/β-catenin pathway can also shed some light into the molecular mechanisms distinguishing endochondral from intramembranous ossification. It has been shown that β-catenin expression is transiently kept low in cells within the mesenchymal condensations that prefigure the future bones that arise by the endochondral mechanism, which requires the formation of a cartilage template that is later ossified (Day et al., 2005). This decreased β-catenin expression proportionally diminishes Wnt/β-catenin activity inside the mesenchymal condensations during endochondral bone formation in such a manner that at first only chondrocytes can form and osteoblast differentiation is repressed in the core of the mesenchymal condensations. Importantly, in this mechanism, osteoblast differentiation is later initiated at the periphery of the cartilaginous structure, where Wnt/β-catenin signalling is up-regulated. This agrees with the observation that several Wnt-activating ligands are expressed only at the periphery of the newly formed cartilage in the limb (Parr et al., 1993), while some Wnt antagonists, including Sfrp2 and Sfrp3, are expressed within the chondrogenic mesenchymal condensation (Day et al., 2005). In addition, it has been shown that Sox9 promotes the degradation of β-catenin (Akiyama et al., 2002), explaining the lack of Wnt/β-catenin activity in cartilage structures. The difference in Wnt/β-catenin signalling activity in the mesenchymal condensations during intramembranous and endochondral ossifications may be controlled by more upstream events. Further studies have shown that β-catenin and BMP-2 synergize to promote osteoblast differentiation and new bone formation (Mbalaviele et al., 2005). Thus, Wnt/β-catenin signalling may drive osteogenic lineage allocation by enhancing mesenchymal cell responsiveness to osteogenic factors such as BMP-2. Therefore, the function of Wnt/β-catenin during osteogenic differentiation is a dual one, consisting in the repression of chondrogenic differentiation in a subgroup of cells within the mesenchymal condensates, while making them more sensitive to the strong osteogenic influence of BMP-2.

4.3.2 The Akt-PI3K pathway in osteogenic differentiation

As explained above, some of the potent osteogenic ligands that act on mesenchymal cells include, among others, PDGF, IGF and VEGF. These external ligands impinge upon osteogenesis acting through different signalling mechanisms involving the Akt-PI3K pathways. Akt is a serine-threonine kinase activated by various ligands including IGFs through the phosphatidylinositol 3-kinase (PI3K) pathway (Scheid and Woodget, 2001). The Akt kinase is a key component of the signaling events elicited by potent bone anabolic factors. Akt enhances transcription factor-dependent osteoblast differentiation, acting specifically on Osx. As explained above, Runx2 exerts its effect on osteogenesis by requiring the downstream action of Osx. The interplay between external osteogenic stimuli and the activity of osteoblast-specific transcription factors is further illustrated by the observation that BMP-2, a potent osteogenic ligand, increases the levels of Osx in a manner that requires Akt activity. Akt phosphorylates and increases the osteogenic activity of Osx. It has been found that Akt phosphorylates Osx, increasing its stability, osteogenic activity and transactivation capacity. These results suggest that Akt activity enhances the osteogenic function of Osx, at least in part, through protein stabilization and that BMP-2 regulates the osteogenic function of Osx, at least in part, by activating Akt (Choi et al., 2011).

Akt activity is also required for Runx2 function. Interestingly, the interplay between Akt and Runx2 may be at the core of molecular mechanisms involved in the migration of mesenchymal stem cells that makes them to coalesce into mesenchymal condensations. As explained above, mesenchymal condensation of osteoblast precursors to form the anlagen that prefigure future bones is an essential pre-requisite for bone formation. Therefore, migration, segregation and arrangement of osteoblast precursors in relation to other pluripotent mesenchymal stem cells are important pre-requisites for skeletogenesis. Studies about the interaction between Runx2 and Akt may shed light into the question of how progenitor cells migrate and condensate to form the anlagen. These studies also point to chemiotaxis as a mechanism to direct migration of mesenchymal towards a common location. PDGF, IGF, and VEGF work as chemotactic factors through PI3K, and PI3K-Akt signalling is a major pathway for chemotaxis through tyrosine kinase receptors in fibroblasts. Akt likely mediates cell migration at least partly by activating Rho GTPases such as Rac1 and their effectors such as the p21-activated protein kinase, or Pak1 (Fujita et al., 2004; Ridley et al., 2003). It is tempting to speculate that this pathway is involved in migration and chemioattraction of mesenchymal stem cells, but further experimentations will have to be done to empirically establish this. Studies on Akt have shed some light in the mechanisms by which Runx2 may contribute to early commitment to an osteogenic lineage (Fujita et al., 2004). These studies have uncovered that at least some aspects of Runx2 function need Akt activity. For example, they showed that Runx 2 induces osteoblast migration by coupling with Akt-PI3K signalling. As expected, overexpression of Runx2 enhanced osteoblastic differentiation of C3H10T1/2 and MC3T3-E1 cell lines, but a novel finding was that Runx2 osteogenic effect was blocked by treatments that blocked Akt-mediated signalling, such as anti-IGF-1 antibodies, the drug LY294002 (a PI3K inhibitor) or adenoviral introduction of a dominant-negative Akt. In these studies, PI3K-Akt signalling enhanced Runx2´s DNA binding capacity and Runx2-dependent transcription. These results implicated Akt into the Runx2-mediated effect in inducing osteogenesis. Runx2 activation also induced cell migration, whereas the migratory enhancement produced by Runx2 was decreased by the Akt-abolishing treatments mentioned above. Furthermore, Runx2 up-regulated PI3K subunits (p85 and p110beta) and Akt (Fujita, et al., 20004).

In addition to a possible role for Runx2 in migration and condensation of mesenchymal cells to form the anlagens, Runx2-mediated migration may also play a role in bone remodelling by inducing the displacement of osteoblasts to the surface of bone that has undergone osteolysis by osteoclasts. This is supported by the fact that Runx2 expression is strongly induced in osteoblasts after bone fracture (Kawahata et al., 2003). This suggests that Runx2-mediated chemotaxis may be important for the migration of osteoblastic cells to the healing area. However, further investigation is required to confirm this, as well as to establish the involvement of Akt in osteoblast migration associated to bone healing.

4.3.3 Regulation of osteogenic differentiation by cell-to-cell adhesion

In addition to the external osteogenic ligands described in the previous section, cell-to-cell and cell-to-substrate adhesion is recognized as a major driving force of the osteogenic differentiation programme. That cell-to-cell and cell-to-substrate adhesion are integral components of bone formation and maintenance is widely accepted, and no discussion of osteogenic differentiation would be complete without this topic. Cell-to-cell adhesion plays an important role in the early mesenchymal condensation of osteoblast precursors that precedes ossification (Hall and Miyake, 2000). Embryonic bone development occurs by migration, aggregation, and condensation of immature mesenchymal progenitor cells to form the cartilaginous anlage. During these processes, pre-osteoblasts must be sorted from other mesenchymal cells, migrate and then align with neighboring osteoblasts (Kawaguchi et al., 2004). Cell-to-cell interactions permit cells to synchronize activity, equalize hormonal responses, and diffuse locally generated signals (Stains and Civitelli, 2005a, 2005b). These intercellular interactions also enable the establishment of concerted gene expression patterns among the cells that comprise the mesenchymal condensates.

Several lines of evidence highlight the importance of cell adhesion, whether it be to other cells or to the ECM, as an additional source of osteogenic cues that are at least as important for osteogenic differentiation as the ones provided by the soluble osteogenic factors mentioned above. For example, the maturation and organization of the ECM contributes to the shut down of proliferation, suggesting that attachment of osteoblasts to a well-organized matrix constitutes by itself a signal to stop proliferation. Culture conditions that enable the differentiation of primary calvaria osteoblasts necessarily involve high cell density with its consequent contact-dependent growth arrest. Therefore, induction of osteogenic differentiation *in vitro* only occurs at high cell density and is mediated by the establishment of cell-to-cell contacts. This is further supported by the observation that continuous passage of sub-confluent cultures, which avoids the attainment of high cellular densities, prevents osteogenic differentation. Formation of bone-nodules *in vitro* is also only achieved after osteoblast cultures have attained sufficient cellular density, suggesting that cooperativity among cells is required to form these structures (Aubin, 1999). This has been termed as a "community effect" in which the establishment of a group of differentiated osteoblasts may be dependent on cell-to-cell interactions that occur only when a critical number of cells is reached (Aubin, 1999). In summary, it can be truly said that osteogenic differentiation is a cell density dependent process.

Functional studies using neutralizing antibodies or anti sense oligonucleotides to disrupt the function of cadherins, which are one of the major protein components of the adherens junction that mediate cell-to-cell adhesion, show that cadherin-mediated cell-to-cell adhesion is involved in the control of osteoblast gene marker expression and differentiation (Marie, 2002). Hormonal and local soluble factors known to regulate osteoblast function also regulate N-cadherin expression and subsequent N-cadherin-mediated cell-to-cell adhesion associated with osteoblast differentiation and survival. Alterations of N-cadherin expression are associated with abnormal osteoblast differentiation and osteogenesis in pathological conditions (Marie, 2002).

Osteoblasts express various cadherins, the predominant and most closely associated with the osteoblast phenotype being OB- (also known as cadherin-11) and N- cadherin, although epithelial cadherin (E-cadherin) has been also found to be expressed in human bone marrow stromal cells (Turel and Rao, 1998), murine calvaria cells, rat osteosarcoma cells (Babich and

Foti, 1994; Tsutsumimoto et al., 1999), and human calvaria cells (Marie, 2002). During differentiation, progenitor cells express a changing repertoire of cadherins, which serves as a molecular fingerprint for identifying the differentiation stage and commitment of the progenitor (Stain and Civitelli, 2005a and 2005b). Thus, as cell-to-cell interactions are essential for cell aggregation and cell specification during embryogenesis, it can be said that cadherin mediated cell-to-cell interactions define if not direct, cell fate decisions in adult bone marrow mesenchymal stem cells (Stain and Civitelli, 2005a and 2005b). Each mesenchymal lineage has a characteristic cadherin expression profile, OB-cadherin being expressed constitutively in the osteoblast lineage while N-cadherin is expressed widely in mesenchymal lineage cells (Stain and Civitelli, 2005a and 2005b). The expression of N-cadherin in mesenchymal stem cells varies with cell differentiation towards the osteogenic, myogenic or adipogenic pathway. In mesenchyal stem cells, N-cadherin mRNA levels increase during osteogenic and myogenic differentiation while decreasing during adipogenic differentiation (Shin et al., 2000). OB-cadherin follows the same pattern (Kawaguchi et al., 2001; Shin et al., 2000). As adipogenesis proceeds, N-cad and OB-cadherin are further down regulated to the point that mature adypocytes do not express any of these cadherins (Kawaguchi et al., 2001; Shin et al., 2000). On the other hand, as mesenchymal cells progress towards myoblastic differentiation OB-cadherin decreases and M-cadherin becomes dominant (Shin et al., 2000). Therefore, OB-cadherin appears to be the only cadherin expressed exclusively in fully differentiated osteoblasts. Regarding the osteogenic lineage, N-cadherin is expressed at all stages of bone formation, although at various levels of expression, while OB-cadherin, although present in most stages of differentiation, seems to be significantly up-regulated in more mature osteoblasts. Osteoblasts also express R-cadherin/cadherin-4, but it is rapidly down regulated as differentiation advances (Stain and Civitelli, 2005a and 2005b), therefore its levels are negligible in mature osteoblasts. This suggests that R-cadherin may have an early role in lineage commitment, while being unnecessary during more advanced stages of differentiation, and fully dispensable in the mature osteoblast.

In osteogenic differentiation *in vitro*, N-cadherin mRNA levels increase at the stage of nodule formation and mineralization (Lin et al., 1999) and is further enhanced to accompany the later expression of Alkaline Phosphatase and Osteocalcin (Ferrari et al., 2000). The importance of N-cadherin for the expression of these markers of bone differentiation has been established *in vitro* by approaches such as culturing osteoblasts in the presence of N-cadherin inhibitory peptides (Cheng et al., 2000; Ferrari et al., 2000), neutralizing antibodies (Oberlander and Tuan, 1994), anti-sense oligonucleotides (Hay et al., 2000), and transfection with gene constructs encoding for mutant N-cadherins with dominant negative effects (Cheng et al., 2000; Ferrari et al., 2000). All of these treatments were shown to perturb cell-to-cell adhesion while adversely affecting osteogenic differentiation. As a consequence of these treatments, Alkaline Phosphatase expression in osteoblast cultures was down-regulated (Ferrari et al., 2000), expression of bone matrix proteins such as Bone Sialoprotein, Osteocalcin, and type I collagen, was reduced, and matrix mineralization was impaired (Cheng et al., 2000; Ferrari et al., 2000). Importantly, inhibition of N-cadherin function with one of the strategies mentioned above also lead to an impairment of BMP-2's osteogenic effect (Hay et al., 2000), again suggesting that BMP-2's osteogenic effect is cell density dependent and strongly linked to the establishment of intercellular contacts. According to these studies, treatment of cells with rhBMP-2 induced a rapid and transient increase in N- and E- cadherin mRNA and protein levels. It also induced cadherin-mediated adhesion which was blocked by anti E- and N- cadherin neutralizing antibodies. In addition, these antibodies decreased basal Alkaline Phosphatase activity as well as the rhBMP-2 induced activity. Treatment with cadherin neutralizing antibodies had the same detrimental effect on Runx2 function and Osteocalcin expression. As mentioned above, other local regulators of osteogenic differentiation are the FGFs. FGFs also appear to act at least in part by influencing cell-to-cell adhesion. FGF-2 transcriptionally increases N-cadherin mRNA levels in human calvaria osteoblasts. Specific anti-N-cadherin antibodies abolished FGF-2's capacity to promote cell aggregation (Debiais et al., 1998). N-cadherin expression has been shown to be regulated in osteoblasts by both BMPs and FGF. Regulation of the transcription of the N-cadherin gene is very complex and involves the PIP3 pathway downstream of FGF (Marie, 2002). Taken together, the studies summarized above show beyond doubt the strong interdependence that exists between external osteogenic signals and the establishment of intercellular adhesion. However, the details of the mechanisms explaining their mutual interdependence still await clarification.

There is evidence suggesting that elevated N-cadherin levels are necessary to maintain the osteoblastic differentiated state. For example, loss of N-cadherin expression with concomitant disruption of cell-to-cell adhesion allows osteoblasts to escape from their interactions with other osteoblasts and become embedded in the bone matrix thus becoming osteocytes (Ferrari et al., 2000; Kawaguchi et al., 2004). Therefore, loss of cellular adhesion due to downregulated N-cadherin levels may be related to the transformation of osteoblasts into osteocyte.

The exact roles of both OB- and N-cadherin in osteoblast differentiation and function, however, still remain elusive. It is possible, however, that they may have complementary or overlapping functions during osteogenic differentiation. Studies to distinguish their functions are made difficult by the fact that homozygous genetic deletion of N-cadherin in mice results in a lethal phenotype (Stains and Civitelli, 2005a and 2005b). This argues against the possibility that OB-cadherin can fully or partially compensate for N-cadherin deficiency. In contrast, genetic ablation of OB-cadherin in mice results in viable animals that appear normal at birth, despite slight reductions in calcification of the cranial sutures and femoral metaphysis (Stains and Civitelly, 2005a and 2005b; Kawaguchi et al., 2004). There is a modest osteopenia in OB-cadherin null mice by three months of age, characterized by diminished mineralizing surface and trabecular bone volume. This defect is cell autonomous since osteoblast function is impaired *in vitro*.

The difficulty of the embryonic lethality of N-cadherin deficiency has been overcome by using a conditional genetic knock-out approach (Castro et al., 2004). Mice expressing a conditional dominant negative N-cadherin mutant showed a delay in reaching peak bone mass as a result of impaired osteogenic differentiation. Bone formation rate in these mice is reduced 74% compared to wild type litter-mates controls. Consistent with an early role for cell adhesion molecules in lineage commitment, mice expressing the mutant N-cadherin also displayed an osteogenic to adipogenic shift, with 27% increase in the percent of body fat relative to controls. Bone marrow mesenchymal cells from these animals were skewed towards adipogenic commitment rather than osteogenic (Castro et al., 2004). Osteoblast differentiation was delayed in calvaria isolated from these transgenic mice (Castro et al., 2004). Nevertheless, further investigations need to be conducted in order to dissect the specific contribution of each cadherin to osteogenic differentiation and osteoblast function, as well as to clarify the specific mechanism and signalling pathways by which they act during these processes.

4.3.4 Regulation of osteogenic differentiation by epigenetic mechanisms and micro RNAs

The studies discussed above represent the foundation of our knowledge about osteogenic differentiation. Research on that area is still intense to this day, and recent findings add more levels of complexity to the regulation of osteogenic differentiation. Recent advances on bone research have uncovered the participation of epigenetic events in the regulation of osteogenic differentiation. Epigenetics encompasses all mechanisms that affect gene transcription without altering nucleotide sequence. These mechanisms invariably involve modifying either histones or the DNA itself by the addition of functional groups such as methyl and acetyl groups that will affect the interaction between DNA and chromatin proteins. The effect on gene expression can be either repressive or activating depending on the nature of the modification. Epigenetics these days is widely recognized as a major influence in the regulation of gene expression during development. On the other hand, several pathologies such as cancer, have been associated to abnormal epigenetic modifications (Cui et al., 2011). Recent investigations have focused on the role of epigenetic regulation in lineage-specific differentiation of mesenchymal stem cells, showing that unique patterns of DNA methylation and histone modifications play an important role in the induction of mesenchymal stem cell commitment and differentiation toward specific lineages (Teven et al., 2011). Epigenetic mechanisms may contribute to the up-regulation of osteoblast-specific genes during osteogenic differentiation. For example, it has been shown that CpG regions in promoters of Runx2 and Osterix, which are master transcription factors during osteogenic differentiation, are demethylated during the increase in gene expression associated with osteogenic differentiation. Conversely, enforced hypermethylation of these promoters by inactivation of Gdd45 suppressed the expression of osteoblast-specific genes with concomitant interruption of osteogenic differentiation (Zhang et al., 2011). These studies showed the important influence that epigenetic controls can exert over osteogenic differentiation, while pointing to Gadd45 as a possible player in the mechanisms involved in stem cell differentiation. Other studies have shown that acetylation of histones H3 and H4, as well as a decreased level of DNA methylation, increase accessibility of the Osteocalcin promoter to osteoinductive transcription factors (Teven et al., 2011). Furthermore, *in vitro* induced osteogenic differentiation of mesenchymal stem cells correlates with a decrease in Osteopontin promoter methylation together with increased Osteopontin expression (Teven et al., 2011).

While epigenetic mechanisms control gene expression by influencing chromatin condensation and thus the access of transcriptional complexes to gene promoters, micro RNAs, or miRNAs, silence gene expression by promoting the highly specific degradation of particular mRNAs via mechanisms that involve the actions of Risc and Dicer protein complexes. miRNAs are a diverse class of small non-coding RNA molecules that function as negative gene regulators (Ambros, 2004; Bartel, 2004), and they are now well-established silencers of gene expression during embryonic development. As in the case of epigenetic modifications, abnormal expression of miRNAs has been detected in several diseases (Maire et al., 2011; Mirabello et al., 2011). Recent studies have revealed the contribution of miRNAs to osteogenic differentiation (Zhang et al., 2011). It was recently discovered that a series of miRNAs controls osteogenic lineage progression by targeting Runx2. During both osteogenic and chondrogenic differentiation, these miRNAs were found to be inversely expressed relative to Runx2 in a lineage-related pattern in mesenchymal cell types (Zhang et al., 2011). Based on 3-UTR luciferase reporter, immunoblot, and mRNA stability assays, it was found that each miRNA directly attenuates Runx2 protein accumulation. miRNAs have also been implicated in the regulation of lineage commitment; it has been shown that a particular miRNA, designated as MiR-637, maintains the balance between adypocites and osteoblasts by directly targeting Osterix (Zhang et al., 2011). This miRNA suppressed the growth of mesenchymal stem cells and induced S-phase arrest. Expression of miR-637 was increased during adipocyte differentiation whereas it was decreased during osteoblast differentiation, which suggests that miR-637 could act as a mediator of adipo-osteogenic differentiation. Osterix was shown to be a direct target of miR-637 which significantly enhanced adipocyte formation and suppressed osteoblast differentiation in mesenchymal stem cells by directly suppressing Osx expression. Furthermore, miR-637 also significantly enhanced de-novo adipogenesis in nude mice (Zhang et al., 2011).

5. A role for pRb in osteogenic differentiation and osteosarcoma formation

There is strong evidence supporting a role for pRb in osteogenic differentiation and bone formation. A corollary of a role for pRb in osteogenic differentiation is that loss of pRb function will deviate osteoblast function away from the production of normal bone and redirect it towards the production of bone tumors or osteoasrcomas. Supporting this notion is the observation that pRb deletion seems to be a strong causative agent in the formation of osteosarcomas or bone tumors, and osteosarcomas are second only to retinoblastomas in people with inherited mutations in the *RB1* gene (Lueder et al., 1986).

Several observations strongly link pRb to osteogenic differentiation and osteosarcoma. First, the pocket family of proteins, to which pRb belongs together with p107 and p130, are already established regulators of the differentiation of mesenchymal lineages, specifically in chondrogenesis, myogenesis and adipogenesis (Chen et al., 1996; Gu et al., 1993; Novitch et al., 1999). Second, viral oncoproteins that target pRb prevent osteogenesis (Thomas et al., 2001). Third, and perhaps the strongest evidence linking pRb to osteogenic differentiation, is the observation that re-expression of pRb in the pRb-null Saos-2 human osteosarcoma cell line induces a senescence phenotype together with the expression of markers suggestive of bone differentiation (Sellers et al., 1998). These observations prompted several groups of researchers to investigate in more depth the exact mechanisms relating pRb to osteogenic differentiation. Several discoveries resulted from these investigations that further established a connection between pRb and bone. For example, it was shown that expression of HPV16-E7, a Human Papilloma Virus-encoded oncoprotein that binds and inactivates pRb, disrupted osteogenic differentiation (Thomas et al., 2001). In these studies, HPV16-E7 expression abolished most landmarks of osteogenic differentiation. Furthermore, pRb loss was able to abolish most aspects of the BMP-2-induced osteogenic differentiation, suggesting that BMP-2´s osteogenic action requires a functional pRb. Especially impaired by pRb deficiency were matrix mineralization and Osteocalcin expression, suggesting that pRb's intervention occurs in late differentiation inducing the expression of markers of the fully differentiated state and maintaining gene expression patterns associated with terminal differentiation. Interestingly, BMP-2 was still able to induce early markers of differentiation such as Runx2 and Alkaline Phosphatase expression even in the absence of pRb, suggesting a minimal impact of pRb loss the expression of early markers of differentiation. This is consistent with data obtained from human osteosarcoma tumors where Alkaline Phosphatase is expressed even in pRb-null tumor samples, while Osteocalcin is usually reduced or absent (Thomas et al., 2003). When the relevance of pRb for osteogenic differentiation was further probed, it was discovered that pRb forms a strong association with Runx2 and that pRb/Runx2 complexes bind to osteoblast specific promoters and induce their transcription. Furthermore, pRb was shown to significantly increase Runx2 transactivating capacity (Thomas et al., 2001). Interestingly, Runx2 is still being produced in the absence of pRb, but apparently lacks transactivation capacity. It is important to note, that naturally occurring pRb mutants, some presumed to confer sensitivity to osteosarcoma, are impaired in their capacity to bind and activate Runx2 (Thomas et al., 2003). Taken together, these studies have shown that pRb positively regulates Runx2's activity as a transcription factor. Given pRb's well-established role as a cell cycle repressor, these findings begged the question as to whether pRb's capacity to induce Runx2 activity and osteogenic differentiation is related to its capacity to arrest the cell cycle, or if these two functions are mechanistically distinct. Along these lines, all three pocket proteins were able to induce growth arrest in Saos-2, but only pRb increased activity of Runx2, suggesting that growth arrest per se does not increase Runx2 activity (Thomas et al., 2001). Furthermore, pRb mutants that fail to bind E2F and induce cell cycle arrest were nevertheless able to induce expression of osteoblast markers in Saos-2 cells (Sellers et al., 1998). From these studies it was concluded that although pRb engenders two tumor suppressive functions, one as a cell cycle repressor and the other as an inducer of differentiation, these two can nevertheless be mechanistically dissociated.

It is interesting to note that BMP-2 has been reported to increase the levels of the CKI p21 (Thomas et al., 2003; Yamato et al., 2000). Furthermore, in an *in vitro* model, p27, another CKI, has been observed to increase with osteogenic differentiation, specifically during matrix formation and mineralization stages (Drissi et al., 1999). The mechanisms by which BMP-2 increases p21 await further clarification. However, it is tempting to propose a model in which BMP-2 activates Runx2 function by increasing CKI levels with consequent inactivation of the Cyclin/Cdk complexes that phosphorylate pRb. In such a scenario, active, hypophosphorylated pRb will be able to, first, bind and inactivate E2F thus promoting cell cycle exit, and second, bind to Runx2 and enhance its capacity to initiate osteoblast-specific gene expression. Such a mechanism not only would explain BMP-2's strong osteogenic effect, but would also explain pRb/Runx2 activation in response to BMP-2.

The experiments discussed above in which pRb deletion abrogates predominantly markers of late osteogenic differentiation such as Osteocalcin and matrix mineralization (Thomas et al., 2001) suggest a role for pRb in the latest stages of osteogenic differentiation and in the maintenance of the osteoblast differentiated phenotype. However, the possibility that BMP-2 may activate pRb, and consequently Runx2, by increasing CKI expression, opens the door for an intervention of pRb earlier in osteogenic differentiation, particularly in the earlier stages involving proliferative arrest and commitment to an osteoblastic lineage. Therefore, pRb's strongest influence on osteogenic differentiation could be first during early commitment, and then later during the attainment of the fully mature osteoblastic phenotype, and subsequently for the maintenance of such a state. In fact, recent evidence supports a role for pRb in the earlier commitment stages of osteogenic differentiation. Conditional deletion of pRb in osteoprogenitor cells in mice resulted in an increased pool of mesenchymal progenitor cells in calvaria of pRb-deficient mice. These pRb-deficient progenitors showed clear adipogenic ability with increased multipotency (Calo et al., 2010; Gutierrez et al., 2008), suggesting that pRb loss resulted in an inability to irreversibly enter the osteogenic differentiation pathway. Interestingly, the ossification defects observed in pRb deficient mice can be suppressed by deletion of E2F1 (Berman et al., 2008), suggesting that the impaired osteogenesis observed upon pRb loss could be a consequence of over-proliferating osteoprogenitors that are unable to undergo irreversible cell cycle withdrawal in order to commit to a specific cell lineage. Therefore, pRb's role in the early commitment stages of osteogenic differentiation clearly depends on pRb's capacity to induce terminal cell cycle withdrawal. On the other hand, pRb's involvement in the induction of the expression of late markers of differentiation such as Osteocalcin, appears to be independent of pRb's capacity to repress cell cycle progression by inactivating E2F, since, as discussed above, pRb mutants that are unable to bind E2F and induce a proliferative arrest are nevertheless capable of inducing the expression of late markers of osteogenic differentiation (Sellers et al., 1998).

Work done in our laboratory has also contributed to the elucidation of pRb's role in osteoblast differentiation and function. We have uncovered a role for pRb as a regulator of osteoblast cell adhesion, and our data suggest that promoting the proper cell-to-cell contacts is another mechanism by which pRb regulates osteoblast differentiation and function. This function could synergize with the previously reported pRb function of enhancing Runx2 mediated transcription of osteoblast-specific genes. Our data show that pRb regulates the expression of a wide repertoire of cell adhesion genes in osteoblasts and also regulates the assembly of adherens junctions, which are membrane-associated complexes involved in cell adhesion (Sosa-García et al., 2010). We generated pRb knock-out mice in which the *RB*1 gene was excised specifically in osteoblasts using the cre-lox P system and found that osteoblasts from pRb knock out mice did not assemble adherens junction at their membranes. pRb depletion in wild type osteoblasts using RNAi also disrupted adherens junctions. Microarrays comparing pRb-expressing and pRb-deficient osteoblasts showed that pRb controls the expression of a number of genes coding for cell adhesion proteins, including cadherins. Furthermore, pRb knock-out mice showed bone abnormalities consistent with osteoblast adhesion defects. Importantly, we found that deleting pRb led to a decrease in the expression of OB-cadherin, which is a cadherin type expressed exclusively in osteoblasts. This decrease in OB-cadherin was accompanied by an increase of comparable magnitude in the expression of N-cadherin, probably compensatory in nature (Sosa-García et al., 2010). Therefore, pRb loss in osteoblasts can lead to a dramatic disarray in the expression of cell adhesion molecules which in turn may negatively affect osteogenic differentiation. Taken together, our data suggest that pRb is required to temporally regulate changes in the expressions of cadherins during osteogenic differentiation, such that expression of specific cadherins is triggered with the right timing during differentiation. pRb loss, by promoting unregulated cadherin expression, could hamper the proper homotypical intercellular contacts, resulting in defective osteoblast differentiation and function with consequent disruption of bone integrity or formation of bone tumors.

5.1 pRb loss in osteosarcomas

Osteosarcomas are relatively rare forms of pediatric cancers, with approximately 1000 new cases diagnosed yearly in the USA (Sandberg and Bridge, 2003). They are, however, a particularly common non-hematologic malignancy in children (Sandberg and Bridge, 2003). Osteosarcomas typically arise in the metaphyseal regions of long bones, within the medullary cavity, and penetrate the cortex of the bone to involve the surrounding soft tissues (Sandberg and Bridge, 2003). The distal femur, proximal tibia, and proximal humerus represent the three most common sites of tumor formation. It is noteworthy that almost all osteoarcomas are of high grade, are poorly differentiated, and have a poor prognosis, with 10-20% of diagnosed cases having detectable metastases at diagnosis (Dahlin, 1975). Pulmonary metatases are the most common cause of death (Broadhead et al., 2011). Further indicating the aggressive and malignant nature of this tumor type, only approximately 10% of patients with osteosarcomas achieve long-term disease free intervals (Sandberg and Bridge, 2003). Given the important role of pRb for osteogenic differentiation, it is not surprising that there is abundant evidence pointing to pRb loss as a strong causative factor for osteosarcomas. The incidence of osteosarcoma is increased 1000-fold in patients who inherit mutations in the *RB1* gene, relative to the general population (Lueder et al., 1986). Also, pRb loss occurs in about 70% of sporadic osteosarcomas (Araki et al., 1991). Loss of heterozygocity at the *RB1* gene is present in 60-70% of tumors and it has been proposed as a poor prognostic factor in osteosarcomas (Araki et al., 1991). Patients with hereditary retinoblastomas, which as discussed previously arise after homozygous loss of the *RB1* gene, have a high risk of second cancers, 50% of which are osteosarcomas (Lueder et al., 1996). Therefore, the strong association between pRb loss and osteosarcoma formation has been well established. From these observations, and consistent with pRb's role in osteogenic differentiation, it is apparent that bone tissue is particularly sensitive to the loss of pRb's tumor suppressive function. It is important to note that existing data indicate that osteosarcoma tumors display a broad range of genetic and molecular alterations, including the gains, losses, or arrangements of chromosomal regions, which in turn could result in the inactivation of tumor suppressor genes and in the deregulation of major signaling pathways. However, except for p53 and pRb mutations, no consensus changes have been identified in all osteosarcoma tumors (Tang et al., 2008). To determine if pRb and p53 losses are sufficient for osteosarcoma formation, attempts to generate a mouse model of osteosarcomas were done using conditional and transgenic mouse strains to inactivate pRb and p53 specifically in osteoblast precursors (Berman et al., 2008). Consistent with the available tumor data, and suggesting that abrogation of p53 and pRb function suffices to trigger the events associated with osteosarcoma formation, the resulting pRb; p53 double mutant animals, although viable, developed early onset osteosarcomas with complete penetrance. These mice tumors displayed many of the characteristics of their human counterparts, including being highly metastatic (Berman et al., 2008).

Emerging evidence suggests osteosarcoma should be regarded as a differentiation disease, thus establishing a potential link between defective osteogenic differentiation and bone tumorigenesis. Pathologic and molecular features of most osteosarcoma tumors strongly suggest that they may be caused by genetic and epigenetic disruptions of osteoblast differentiation pathways (Haydon et al., 2007). Potential cancer stem cells responsible for osteosarcoma development have yet to be identified, lending further credence to the notion that osteosarcomas may arise from progenitors with impaired differentiation capacity. This view is further supported by the observation that osteosarcoma tumors are comprised of cells that exhibit characteristics of undifferentiated osteoblasts (Haydon et al., 2007; Thomas et al., 2004; Zenmyo et al., 2001). In one study, 81% of osteosarcomas were either poorly differentiated or undifferentiated (Thomas et al., 2004), and the late marker of osteogenic differentiation, Osteocalcin, was undetectable in >75% of osteosarcomas (Hopyan et al., 1999). *In vitro* studies further support this view by showing that terminal osteoblast differentiation, mediated by Runx2 and p27, is disrupted in osteosarcoma (Thomas et al., 2004). The appreciation of osteosarcomas as arising due to differentiation defects comes as no surprise given that it is now widely recognized that pRb loss is one of its causative factors. By being incapable of irreversibly withdrawing from the cell cycle, osteoprogenitor cells that have undergone pRb loss will continue their proliferation while being unable to initiate their differentiation pathways. In the absence of pRb, Runx2 transactivating capacity will be severely diminished, as it has indeed been shown to occur (Thomas et al., 2001), with the consequent loss of expression of bone markers. This may explain the commonly observed absence of Osteocalcin expression in osteosarcoma tumors, as well as their poorly differentiated state. The increased pool of poorly differentiated and rapidly dividing osteoprogenitors may also be susceptible to additional transforming events that could cooperate with pRb loss to further advance the genesis of osteosarcomas (Gutierrez et al., 2008). In addition, as described above, pRb expression has been shown to be important for the expression of OB-cadherin, which is the cadherin type that is unique to the fully mature and differentiated osteoblast, as well as for the establishment of the cell-to-cell adhesion that is so important for osteoblast differentiation and function (Sosa-García et al., 2010). pRb loss could cause major disruption of cell-to-cell adhesion, and this could in turn promote later stages of tumorigenesis in which osteosarcoma cells spread, invade and colonize other tissues. Therefore, pRb loss facilitates various stages of osteosarcoma formation, from the early disruption of proper lineage commitment with a consequent disruption of osteogenic differentiation, to facilitating later stages of metastasis by disrupting intercellular adhesion.

6. Summary

Over two decades of research on pRb have demonstrated this protein to be a truly potent tumor suppressor. Its potency as a tumor suppressor stems from the fact that it has been implicated in a wide range of cellular process that go way beyond cell cycle repression, and that range from tissue differentiation to intercellular adhesion. Due to the involvement of pRb in such a diverse variety of cellular processes it is only natural that its absence or inactivation, such as is observed in most human cancers, leads to a major disarray in cellular homeostasis. Cells whose physiology is disrupted at many levels by pRb loss are fertile ground for the accumulation of additional genetic alterations, which in turn could cooperate with pRb loss to drive tumorigenesis. pRb's role as a cell cycle repressor is a complement to its role as an inducer of differentiation. By blocking the former and inducing the later, pRb's function may be at the center of the mechanisms that ensure that proliferation and differentiation remain mutually exclusive cellular behaviors. In terms of osteogenic differentiation, pRb function is now recognized as being essential for this process. pRb's roles in osteogenic differentiation are summarized in Figure 2. BMP-2, a potent osteogenic inductor, may exert its osteogenic influence, at least in part, by acting through pRb, specifically by increasing the p21 levels that will in turn block phosphorylation and inactivation of pRb. As described above, increased levels of p27 have also been demonstrated during osteogenic differentiation (Drissi et al., 1999), and this may also contribute to pRb activation by collaborating with p21 in the repression of Cyclin/Cdk complexes. Once active, pRb represses the E2F-mediated expression of proliferation genes, thus leading to the cell cycle arrest necessary for commitment and initiation of differentiation. Concomitantly, excess hypophosphorylated pRb binds and enhances the activity of Runx2, the main transcription factor driving osteoblast-specific gene expression.

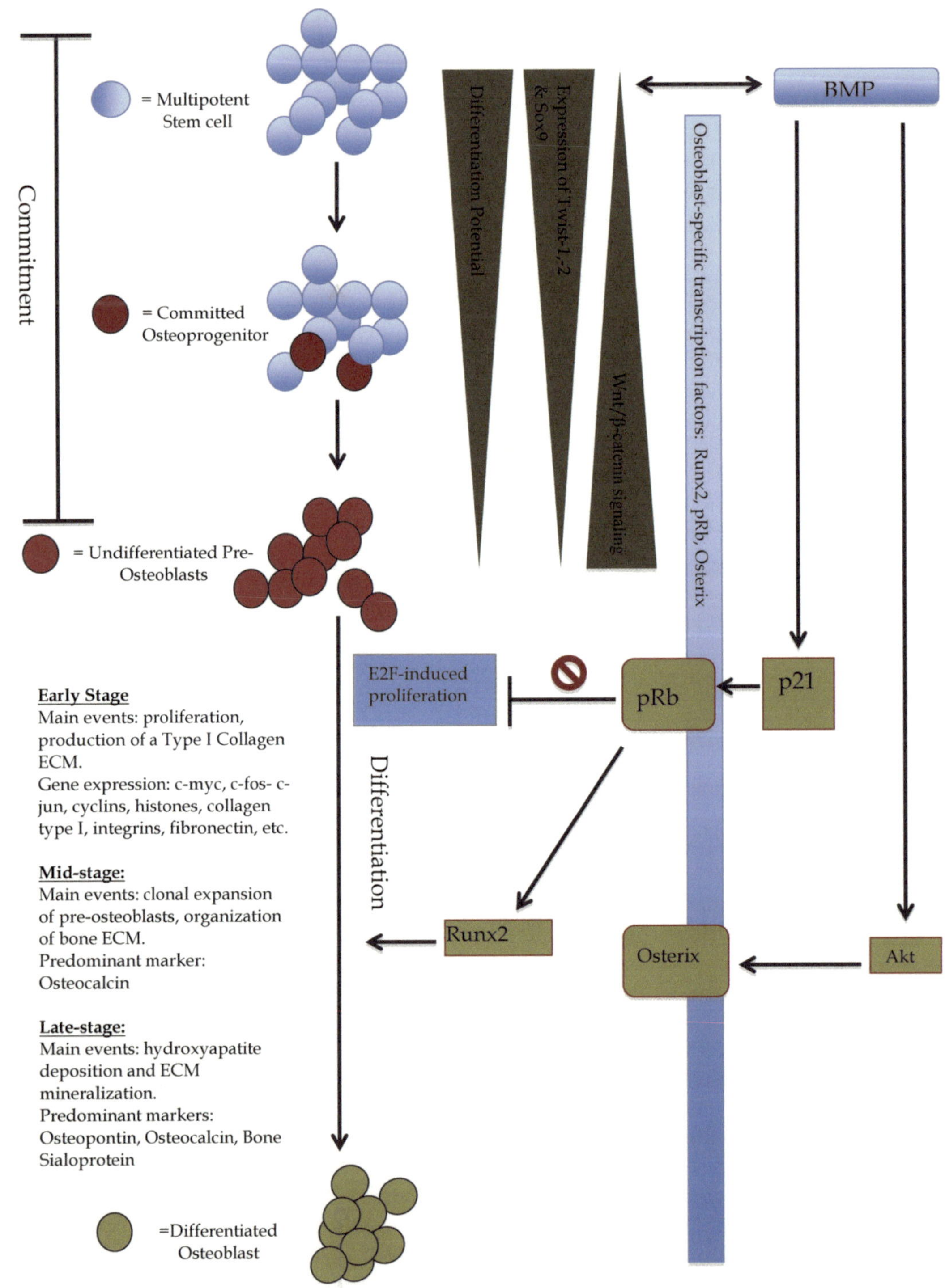

Fig. 2. The process of osteogenic differentiation starting from the commitment of multipotent stem to the osteoblastic lineage and culminating with the production of fully

mature osteoblasts (shown in the figure from top to bottom). Commitment to the osteoblastic lineage results in the progressive restriction of differentiation potential, possibly due to decreased expression of inducers of chondroblastic differentiation (Sox9) together with decrease in repressors of the osteoblastic lineage (Twist-1 and -2). This in turn allows the activation of the Wnt/beta-catenin pathway, which furthers strengthens osteogenic commitment possibly by sensitizing cells to the effect of BMP-2. In addition to synergizing with the Wnt/beta-catenin pathway, BMP-2 leads to increased p21 levels, which by inactivating Cyclin/Cdk complexes, promotes pRb activation. Increased levels of p27 have also been demonstrated (not shown in the figure), and may also contribute to pRb activation by collaborating with p21 in the repression of Cyclin/Cdk complexes. Once active, pRb represses the E2F-mediated expression of proliferation genes, thus leading to the cell cycle arrest necessary for the initiation of differentiation. Concomitantly, hypophosphorylated pRb binds and enhances the activity of Runx2, the main transcription factor driving osteoblast-specific gene expression. Commitment and differentiation are further strengthened by Osterix, which acts downstream of Runx2 and is also activated by BMP-2 acting through Akt. Once cells are irreversibly committed and become growth arrested, differentiation proceeds through the three main stages shown in the figure, each of them characterized by a predominant event and a specific gene expression pattern.

7. Acknowledgements

The author wishes to thank past and present members of his laboratory, as well as Drs. W. Douglas Cress and Phillip W. Hinds for helpful discussions about the topics discussed in this review. The author apologizes to the countless researchers who have made significant contributions to the pRb and osteogenesis fields, and whose work could not be cited due solely to space constrains.

8. References

Akiyama H, Chaboissier MC, Martin JF, Schedl A & de Crombrugghe B. 2002. The transcription factor Sox9 has essential roles in successive steps of the chondrocyte differentiation pathway and is required for expression of Sox5 and Sox6. *Genes Dev.* Nov 1;16(21): 2813-28.

Ambros, V. 2004. The functions of animal microRNAs. *Nature.* 431: 350–355.

Araki N, Uchida A, Kimura T, Yoshikawa H, Aoki Y, Ueda T, Takai S, Miki T & Ono K. 1991. Involvement of the retinoblastoma gene in primary osteosarcomas and other bone and soft-tissue tumors. Clin Orthop Relat Res. 1991 Sep;(270):271-7.

Aubin JE. 1999. Osteoprogenitor cell frequency in rat bone marrow stromal populations: role for heterotypic cell-cell interactions in osteoblast differentiation. *J Cell Biochem.* Mar 1;72(3):396-410.

Babich M & Foti LR. 1994. E-cadherins identified in osteoblastic cells: effects of parathyroid hormone and extracellular calcium on localization. *Life Sci.* 54(11): PL201-8.

Banerjee C, McCabe LR, Choi JY, Hiebert SW, Stein JL, Stein GS & Lian JB. 1997. Runt homology domain proteins in osteoblast differentiation: AML3/CBFA1 is a major component of a bone-specific complex. *J Cell Biochem.* Jul 1;66(1): 1-8.

Bartel, D.P. 2004. MicroRNAs: genomics, biogenesis, mechanism, and function. *Cell.* 116: 281–297.

Berman SD, Calo E, Landman AS, Danielian PS, Miller ES, West JC, Fonhoue BD, Caron A, Bronson R, Bouxsein ML, Mukherjee S, & Lees JA. 2008. Metastatic osteosarcoma induced by inactivation of Rb and p53 in the osteoblast lineage. *Proc Natl Acad Sci U S A.* Aug 19;105(33): 11851-6.

Berman SD, Yuan TL, Miller ES, Lee EY, Caron A & Lees JA. 2008. The retinoblastoma protein tumor suppressor is important for appropriate osteoblast differentiation and bone development. *Mol Cancer Res.* Sep;6(9):1440-51.

Bialek P, Kern B, Yang X, Schrock M, Sosic D, Hong N, Wu H, Yu K, Ornitz DM, Olson EN, Justice MJ & Karsenty G. 2004. A twist code determines the onset of osteoblast differentiation. *Dev Cell.* Mar;6(3): 423-35.

Bianco P, Fisher LW, Young MF, Termine JD & Robey PG.1991. Expression of bone sialoprotein (BSP) in developing human tissues. *Calcif Tissue Int.* Dec;49(6): 421-6.

Braig M & Schmitt CA. 2006. Oncogene-induced senescence: putting the brakes on tumor development. *Cancer Res.* Mar 15;66(6): 2881-4.

Broadhead ML, Clark JC, Myers DE, Dass CR & Choong PF. 2011. The molecular pathogenesis of osteosarcoma: a review. *Sarcoma.* 2011;2011: 959248.

Buchkovich K, Duffy LA & Harlow E. 1989. The retinoblastoma protein is phosphorylated during specific phases of the cell cycle. *Cell.* Sep 22;58(6): 1097-105.

Calo E, Quintero-Estades JA, Danielian PS, Nedelcu S, Berman SD & Lees JA. 2010. Rb regulates fate choice and lineage commitment in vivo. *Nature.* Aug 26;466(7310): 1110-4.

Campisi J. 2001. Cellular senescence as a tumor-suppressor mechanism. *TRENDS in Cell Biology.* Nov;11(11): S27-S31.

Canalis E, Pash J & Varghese S. 1993. Skeletal growth factors. *Crit Rev Eukaryot Gene Expr.* 3(3): 155-66.

Castro CH, Shin CS, Stains JP, Cheng SL, Sheikh S, Mbalaviele G, Szejnfeld VL & Civitelli R. 2004. Targeted expression of a dominant-negative N-cadherin in vivo delays peak bone mass and increases adipogenesis. *J Cell Sci.* Jun 1;117(Pt 13): 2853-64.

Cavenee WK, Dryja TP, Phillips RA, Benedict WF, Godbout R, Gallie BL, Murphree AL, Strong LC & White RL. 1983. Expression of recessive alleles by chromosomal mechanisms in retinoblastoma. *Nature.* Oct 27-Nov 2;305(5937): 779-84.

Chen PL, Riley DJ, Chen-Kiang S & Lee WH. 1996. Retinoblastoma protein directly interacts with and activates the transcription factor NF-IL6. *Proc Natl Acad Sci U S A.* Jan 9;93(1): 465-9.

Cheng SL, Shin CS, Towler DA & Civitelli R. 2000. A dominant negative cadherin inhibits osteoblast differentiation. *J Bone Miner Res.* Dec;15(12): 2362-70.

Choi YH, Jeong HM, Jin YH, Li H, Yeo CY & Lee KY. 2011. Akt phosphorylates and regulates the osteogenic activity of Osterix. *Biochem Biophys Res Commun.* Aug 5;411(3): 637-41.

Classon M, Kennedy BK, Mulloy R & Harlow E. 2000. Opposing roles of pRB and p107 in adipocyte differentiation.*Proc Natl Acad Sci U S A.* Sep 26;97(20): 10826-31.

Cobrinik D. 2005. Pocket proteins and cell cycle control. *Oncogene.* Apr 18;24(17): 2796-809.

Cui J, Wang W, Li Z, Zhang Z, Wu B & Zeng L. 2011. Epigenetic changes in osteosarcoma. *Bull Cancer.* Jul;98(7): E62-8.

Dahlin DC. 1975. Pathology of Osteosarcoma. Clin Orthop Relat Res. 1975 Sep;(111):23-32.

Day TF, Guo X, Garrett-Beal L & Yang Y. 2005. Wnt/beta-catenin signaling in mesenchymal progenitors controls osteoblast and chondrocyte differentiation during vertebrate skeletogenesis. *Dev Cell.* May;8(5): 739-50.

Debiais F, Hott M, Graulet AM & Marie PJ. 1998. The effects of fibroblast growth factor-2 on human neonatal calvaria osteoblastic cells are differentiation stage specific. *J Bone Miner Res.* Apr;13(4): 645-54.

DeGregori J, Leone G, Miron A, Jakoi L, & Nevins JR. 1997. Distinct roles for E2F proteins in cell growth control and apoptosis. *Proc Natl Acad Sci U S A.* Jul 8;94(14): 7245-50.

Drissi H, Hushka D, Aslam F, Nguyen Q, Buffone E, Koff A, van Wijnen A, Lian JB, Stein JL & Stein GS. 1999. The cell cycle regulator p27kip1 contributes to growth and differentiation of osteoblasts. *Cancer Res.* Aug 1;59(15): 3705-11.

Du W, Vidal M, Xie JE & Dyson N. 1996. RBF, a novel RB-related gene that regulates E2F activity and interacts with cyclin E in Drosophila. *Genes Dev.* May 15;10(10): 1206-18.

Ducy P. 2000. Cbfa1: a molecular switch in osteoblast biology. *Dev Dyn.* Dec;219(4): 461-71.

Durfee T, Becherer K, Chen PL, Yeh SH, Yang Y, Kilburn AE, Lee WH & Elledge SJ. 1993. The retinoblastoma protein associates with the protein phosphatase type 1 catalytic subunit. *Genes Dev.* Apr;7(4): 555-69.

Dyson N. 1998. The regulation of E2F by pRB-family proteins. *Genes Dev.* Aug 1;12(15): 2245-62.

Ferrari SL, Traianedes K, Thorne M, Lafage-Proust MH, Genever P, Cecchini MG, Behar V, Bisello A, Chorev M, Rosenblatt M & Suva LJ. 2000. A role for N-cadherin in the development of the differentiated osteoblastic phenotype. *J Bone Miner Res.* Feb;15(2): 198-208.

Friend SH, Bernards R, Rogelj S, Weinberg RA, Rapaport JM, Albert DM & Dryja TP. 1986. A human DNA segment with properties of the gene that predisposes to retinoblastoma and osteosarcoma. *Nature.* Oct 16-22;323(6089): 643-6.

Fujita T, Azuma Y, Fukuyama R, Hattori Y, Yoshida C, Koida M, Ogita K & Komori T. 2004. Runx2 induces osteoblast and chondrocyte differentiation and enhances their migration by coupling with PI3K-Akt signaling. *J Cell Biol.* Jul 5;166(1): 85-95.

Godbout R, Dryja TP, Squire J, Gallie BL & Phillips RA. 1983. Somatic inactivation of genes on chromosome 13 is a common event in retinoblastoma. *Nature.* Aug 4-10;304(5925): 451-3.

Gu W, Schneider JW, Condorelli G, Kaushal S, Mahdavi V & Nadal-Ginard B. 1993. Interaction of myogenic factors and the retinoblastoma protein mediates muscle cell commitment and differentiation. *Cell.* Feb 12;72(3): 309-24.

Gutierrez GM, Kong E, Sabbagh Y, Brown NE, Lee JS, Demay MB, Thomas DM & Hinds PW. 2008. Impaired bone development and increased mesenchymal progenitor cells in calvaria of RB1-/- mice. *Proc Natl Acad Sci U S A.* Nov 25;105(47): 18402-7.

Hall BK & Miyake T. 1992. The membranous skeleton: the role of cell condensations in vertebrate skeletogenesis. *Anat Embryol (Berl).* Jul;186(2):107-24.

Hall BK & Miyake T. 2000. All for one and one for all: condensations and the initiation of skeletal development. *Bioessays.* Feb;22(2): 138-47.

Hanahan D & Weinberg RA. 2000. The hallmarks of cancer. *Cell.* Jan 7;100(1): 57-70.

Hanahan D & Weinberg RA. 2011. Hallmarks of cancer: the next generation. *Cell.* Mar 4;144(5): 646-74.

Harbour JW & Dean DC. 2000. The Rb/E2F pathway: expanding roles and emerging paradigms. *Genes Dev.* Oct 1;14(19): 2393-409.

Haÿ E, Lemonnier J, Modrowski D, Lomri A, Lasmoles F & Marie PJ. 2000. N- and E-cadherin mediate early human calvaria osteoblast differentiation promoted by bone morphogenetic protein-2. *J Cell Physiol.* Apr;183(1): 117-28.

Haydon RC, Luu HH & He TC. 2007. Osteosarcoma and osteoblastic differentiation: a new perspective on oncogenesis. *Clin Orthop Relat Res.* Jan;454: 237-46.

Hill TP, Später D, Taketo MM, Birchmeier W & Hartmann C. 2005. Canonical Wnt/beta-catenin signaling prevents osteoblasts from differentiating into chondrocytes. *Dev Cell.* 2005 May;8(5): 727-38.

Hopyan S, Gokgoz N, Bell RS, Andrulis IL, Alman BA & Wunder JS. 1999. Expression of osteocalcin and its transcriptional regulators core-binding factor alpha 1 and MSX2 in osteoid-forming tumours. *J Orthop Res.* Sep;17(5): 633-8.

Horowitz JM, Park SH, Bogenmann E, Cheng JC, Yandell DW, Kaye FJ, Minna JD, Dryja TP & Weinberg RA. 1990. Frequent inactivation of the retinoblastoma anti-oncogene is restricted to a subset of human tumor cells._Proc Natl Acad Sci U S A. 1990 Apr;87(7):2775-9.

Hussussian CJ, Struewing JP, Goldstein AM, Higgins PA, Ally DS, Sheahan MD, Clark WH Jr, Tucker MA & Dracopoli NC. 1994. Germline p16 mutations in familial melanoma. *Nat Genet.* Sep;8(1): 15-21.

Kawaguchi J, Kii I, Sugiyama Y, Takeshita S & Kudo A. 2001. The transition of cadherin expression in osteoblast differentiation from mesenchymal cells: consistent expression of cadherin-11 in osteoblast lineage. *J Bone Miner Res.* Feb;16(2): 260.

Kawahata H, Kikkawa T, Higashibata Y, Sakuma T, Huening M, Sato M, Sugimoto M, Kuriyama K, Terai K, Kitamura Y & Nomura S. 2003. Enhanced expression of Runx2/PEBP2alphaA/CBFA1/AML3 during fracture healing. *J Orthop Sci.* 8(1): 102-8.

Kaye FJ. 2002. RB and cyclin dependent kinase pathways: defining a distinction between RB and p16 loss in lung cancer. *Oncogene.* Oct 7;21(45): 6908-14.

Knudsen ES & Knudsen KE. 2006. Retinoblastoma tumor suppressor: where cancer meets the cell cycle.*Exp Biol Med (Maywood).* Jul;231(7): 1271-81.

Knudsen ES & Wang JY. 1996. Differential regulation of retinoblastoma protein function by specific Cdk phosphorylation sites. *J Biol Chem.* Apr 5;271(14): 8313-20.

Kobayashi H, Gao Y, Ueta C, Yamaguchi A & Komori T. 2000. Multilineage differentiation of Cbfa1-deficient calvarial cells in vitro. *Biochem Biophys Res Commun.* Jul 5;273(2): 630-6.

Komori T, Yagi H, Nomura S, Yamaguchi A, Sasaki K, Deguchi K, Shimizu Y, Bronson RT, Gao YH, Inada M, Sato M, Okamoto R, Kitamura Y, Yoshiki S & Kishimoto T. 1997. Targeted disruption of Cbfa1 results in a complete lack of bone formation owing to maturational arrest of osteoblasts. *Cell.* May 30;89(5): 755-64.

Komori T. 2002. Runx2, a multifunctional transcription factor in skeletal development. *J Cell Biochem.* 2002;87(1): 1-8.

Landsberg RL, Sero JE, Danielian PS, Yuan TL, Lee EY & Lees JA. 2003. The role of E2F4 in adipogenesis is independent of its cell cycle regulatory activity. *Proc Natl Acad Sci U S A.* Mar 4;100(5): 2456-61.

Lee EY, Chang CY, Hu N, Wang YC, Lai CC, Herrup K, Lee WH & Bradley A. 1992. Mice deficient for Rb are nonviable and show defects in neurogenesis and haematopoiesis. *Nature.* Sep 24;359(6393):v288-94.

Lee WH, Bookstein R, Hong F, Young LJ, Shew JY & Lee EY. 1987. Human retinoblastoma susceptibility gene: cloning, identification, and sequence. *Science.* Mar 13;235(4794): 1394-9.

Lengner CJ, Hassan MQ, Serra RW, Lepper C, van Wijnen AJ, Stein JL, Lian JB, & Stein GS. 2005. Nkx3.2-mediated repression of Runx2 promotes chondrogenic differentiation. *J Biol Chem.* Apr 22;280(16): 15872-9.

Lin WL, Chien HH & Cho MI. 1999. N-cadherin expression during periodontal ligament cell differentiation in vitro. *J Periodontol.* Sep;70(9): 1039-45.

Lipinski MM & Jacks T. 1999. The retinoblastoma gene family in differentiation and development. *Oncogene.* Dec 20;18(55): 7873-82.

Liu H, Dibling B, Spike B, Dirlam A & Macleod K. 2004. New roles for the RB tumor suppressor protein. *Curr Opin Genet Dev.* Feb; 14(1): 55-64.

Logan CY & Nusse R. 2004. The Wnt signaling pathway in development and disease. *Annu Rev Cell Dev Biol.* 20: 781-810.

Lopez-Kostner F, Alvarez K, de la Fuente M, Wielandt AM, Orellana P & Hurtado C. 2010. Novel human pathological mutations. Gene symbol: APC. Disease: adenomatous polyposis coli. *Hum Genet.* Apr;127(4): 480.

Lu X & Horvitz HR. 1998. lin-35 and lin-53, two genes that antagonize a C. elegans Ras pathway, encode proteins similar to Rb and its binding protein RbAp48. *Cell.* Dec 23;95(7): 981-91.

Ludlow JW, DeCaprio JA, Huang CM, Lee WH, Paucha E & Livingston DM. 1989. SV40 large T antigen binds preferentially to an underphosphorylated member of the retinoblastoma susceptibility gene product family. *Cell.* Jan 13;56(1): 57-65.

Ludlow JW, Glendening CL, Livingston DM & DeCarprio JA. 1993. Specific enzymatic dephosphorylation of the retinoblastoma protein. *Mol Cell Biol.* Jan;13(1): 367-72.

Lueder GT, Judisch F & O'Gorman TW. 1986. Second nonocular tumors in survivors of heritable retinoblastoma. Arch Ophthalmol. 1986 Mar;104(3):372-3.

Lundberg AS, Hahn WC, Gupta P & Weinberg RA. 2000. Genes involved in senescence and immortalization. *Curr Opin Cell Biol.* Dec;12(6): 705-9.

Maire G, Martin JW, Yoshimoto M, Chilton-MacNeill S, Zielenska M & Squire JA. 2011. Analysis of miRNA-gene expression-genomic profiles reveals complex mechanisms of microRNA deregulation in osteosarcoma. *Cancer Genet.* Mar;204(3): 138-46.

Marie PJ. 2002. Role of N-cadherin in bone formation. *J Cell Physiol.* Mar;190(3): 297-305.

Marino S, Hoogervoorst D, Brandner S & Berns A. 2003. Rb and p107 are required for normal cerebellar development and granule cell survival but not for Purkinje cell persistence. *Development.* Aug;130(15): 3359-68.

Marom R, Shur I, Solomon R & Benayahu D. 2005. Characterization of adhesion and differentiation markers of osteogenic marrow stromal cells. *J Cell Physiol.* Jan;202(1): 41-8.

Mbalaviele G, Sheikh S, Stains JP, Salazar VS, Cheng SL, Chen D & Civitelli R. 2005. Beta-catenin and BMP-2 synergize to promote osteoblast differentiation and new bone formation. *J Cell Biochem.* Feb 1;94(2): 403-18.

Mirabello L, Yu K, Berndt SI, Burdett L, Wang Z, Chowdhury S, Teshome K, Uzoka A, Hutchinson A, Grotmol T, Douglass C, Hayes RB, Hoover RN & Savage SA. 2011. A comprehensive candidate gene approach identifies genetic variation associated with osteosarcoma. *BMC Cancer*. May 29; 11: 209.

Narita M, Nũnez S, Heard E, Narita M, Lin AW, Hearn SA, Spector DL, Hannon GJ & Lowe SW. 2003. Rb-mediated heterochromatin formation and silencing of E2F target genes during cellular senescence. *Cell*. Jun 13;113(6): 703-1

Nguyen DX & McCance DJ. 2005. Role of the retinoblastoma tumor suppressor protein in cellular differentiation. *J Cell Biochem*. Apr 1;94(5): 870-9.

Novitch BG, Spicer DB, Kim PS, Cheung WL & Lassar AB. 1999. pRb is required for MEF2-dependent gene expression as well as cell-cycle arrest during skeletal muscle differentiation. *Curr Biol*. May 6;9(9): 449-59.

Oberlender SA & Tuan RS. 1994. Spatiotemporal profile of N-cadherin expression in the developing limb mesenchyme. *Cell Adhes Commun*. Dec;2(6):521-37.

Otto F, Thornell AP, Crompton T, Denzel A, Gilmour KC, Rosewell IR, Stamp GW, Beddington RS, Mundlos S, Olsen BR, Selby PB & Owen MJ. 1997. Cbfa1, a candidate gene for cleidocranial dysplasia syndrome, is essential for osteoblast differentiation and bone development. *Cell*. May 30;89(5): 765-71.

Parr BA, Shea MJ, Vassileva G & McMahon AP. 1993. Mouse Wnt genes exhibit discrete domains of expression in the early embryonic CNS and limb buds. *Development*. Sep;119(1): 247-61.

Ridley AJ, Schwartz MA, Burridge K, Firtel RA, Ginsberg MH, Borisy G, Parsons JT & Horwitz AR. 2003. Cell migration: integrating signals from front to back. *Science*. Dec 5;302(5651): 1704-9.

Ross JF, Liu X & Dynlacht BD. 1999. Mechanism of transcriptional repression of E2F by the retinoblastoma tumor suppressor protein. *Mol Cell*. Feb;3(2): 195-205.

Sandberg AA & Bridge JA. 2003. Updates on the cytogenetics and molecular genetics of bone and soft tissue tumors: osteosarcoma and related tumors. *Cancer Genet Cytogenet*. Aug;145(1): 1-30.

Scheid MP & Woodgett JR. 2001. PKB/AKT: functional insights from genetic models. *Nat Rev Mol Cell Biol*. Oct;2(10): 760-8.

Sellers WR, Novitch BG, Miyake S, Heith A, Otterson GA, Kaye FJ, Lassar AB & Kaelin WG Jr. 1998. Stable binding to E2F is not required for the retinoblastoma protein to activate transcription, promote differentiation, and suppress tumor cell growth. *Genes Dev*. Jan 1;12(1):95-106.

Sherr CJ & McCormick F. 2002. The RB and p53 pathways in cancer. *Cancer Cell*. Aug;2(2): 103-12.

Sherr CJ & Roberts JM. 1999. CDK inhibitors: positive and negative regulators of G1-phase progression. *Genes Dev*. Jun 15;13(12): 1501-12.

Shin CS, Lecanda F, Sheikh S, Weitzmann L, Cheng SL & Civitelli R. 2000. Relative abundance of different cadherins defines differentiation of mesenchymal precursors into osteogenic, myogenic, or adipogenic pathways. *J Cell Biochem*. Jun 12;78(4): 566-77.

Sosa-García B, Gunduz V, Vázquez-Rivera V, Cress WD, Wright G, Bian H, Hinds PW & Santiago-Cardona PG. 2010. A role for the retinoblastoma protein as a regulator of mouse osteoblast cell adhesion: implications for osteogenesis and osteosarcoma formation. *PLoS One*. Nov 11;5(11): e13954.

Stains JP & Civitelli R. 2005. Cell-cell interactions in regulating osteogenesis and osteoblast function. *Birth Defects Res C Embryo Today*. Mar;75(1): 72-80.

Stains JP & Civitelli R. 2005. Cell-to-cell interactions in bone. *Biochem Biophys Res Commun*. Mar 18;328(3): 721-7.

Stevaux O & Dyson NJ. 2002. A revised picture of the E2F transcriptional network and RB function. *Curr Opin Cell Biol*. Dec;14(6): 684-91.

Tang N, Song WX, Luo J, Haydon RC & He TC. 2008. Osteosarcoma development and stem cell differentiation. *Clin Orthop Relat Res*. Sep;466(9): 2114-30.

Teven CM, Liu X, Hu N, Tang N, Kim SH, Huang E, Yang K, Li M, Gao JL, Liu H, Natale RB, Luther G, Luo Q, Wang L, Rames R, Bi Y, Luo J, Luu HH, Haydon RC, Reid RR & He TC. 2011. Epigenetic regulation of mesenchymal stem cells: a focus on osteogenic and adipogenic differentiation. *Stem Cells Int*. 2011:201371.

Thomas DM, Carty SA, Piscopo DM, Lee JS, Wang WF, Forrester WC & Hinds PW. 2001. The retinoblastoma protein acts as a transcriptional coactivator required for osteogenic differentiation. *Mol Cell*. 2001 Aug;8(2): 303-16.

Thomas DM, Johnson SA, Sims NA, Trivett MK, Slavin JL, Rubin BP, Waring P, McArthur GA, Walkley CR, Holloway AJ, Diyagama D, Grim JE, Clurman BE, Bowtell DD, Lee JS, Gutierrez GM, Piscopo DM, Carty SA & Hinds PW. 2004. Terminal osteoblast differentiation, mediated by runx2 and p27KIP1, is disrupted in osteosarcoma. *J Cell Biol*. Dec 6;167(5): 925-34.

Thomas DM, Yang HS, Alexander K & Hinds PW. 2003. Role of the retinoblastoma protein in differentiation and senescence. *Cancer Biol Ther*. Mar-Apr;2(2): 124-30.

Tsutsumimoto T, Kawasaki S, Ebara S & Takaoka K. 1999. TNF-alpha and IL-1beta suppress N-cadherin expression in MC3T3-E1 cells. *J Bone Miner Res*. Oct;14(10): 1751-60.

Turel KR & Rao SG. 1998. Expression of the cell adhesion molecule E-cadherin by the human bone marrow stromal cells and its probable role in CD34(+) stem cell adhesion. *Cell Biol Int*. 22(9-10): 641-8.

Vooijs M & Berns A. 1999. Developmental defects and tumor predisposition in Rb mutant mice. *Oncogene*. Sep 20;18(38): 5293-303.

Wu L, de Bruin A, Saavedra HI, Starovic M, Trimboli A, Yang Y, Opavska J, Wilson P, Thompson JC, Ostrowski MC, Rosol TJ, Woollett LA, Weinstein M, Cross JC, Robinson ML & Leone G. 2003. Extra-embryonic function of Rb is essential for embryonic development and viability. *Nature*. Feb 27;421(6926):942-7.

Wyndford-Thomas D. 1999. Cellular senescence and cancer. *J. Pathol*. 187: 100-111

Xu HJ, Zhou Y, Ji W, Perng GS, Kruzelock R, Kong CT, Bast RC, Mills GB, Li J & Hu SX. 1997. Reexpression of the retinoblastoma protein in tumor cells induces senescence and telomerase inhibition. *Oncogene*. Nov 20;15(21): 2589-96.

Yamato K, Hashimoto S, Okahashi N, Ishisaki A, Nonaka K, Koseki T, Kizaki M, Ikeda Y & Nishihara T. 2000. Dissociation of bone morphogenetic protein-mediated growth arrest and apoptosis of mouse B cells by HPV-16 E6/E7. *Exp Cell Res*. May 25;257(1): 198-205.

Zenmyo M, Komiya S, Hamada T, Hiraoka K, Kato S, Fujii T, Yano H, Irie K & Nagata K. 2001. Transcriptional activation of p21 by vitamin D(3) or vitamin K(2) leads to differentiation of p53-deficient MG-63 osteosarcoma cells. *Hum Pathol.* Apr;32(4): 410-6.

Zhang JF, Fu WM, He ML, Wang H, Wang WM, Yu SC, Bian XW, Zhou J, Lin MC, Lu G, Poon WS & Kung HF. 2011. MiR-637 Maintains the Balance between Adipocytes and Osteoblasts by Directly Targeting Osterix. *Mol Biol Cell.* 2011 Aug 31.

Zhang RP, Shao JZ & Xiang LX. 2011. Gadd45a plays an essential role in active DNA demethylation during terminal osteogenic differentiation of adipose-derived mesenchymal stem cells. *J Biol Chem.* Sep 14.

Zhang Y, Xie RL, Croce CM, Stein JL, Lian JB, van Wijnen AJ & Stein GS. 2011. A program of microRNAs controls osteogenic lineage progression by targeting transcription factor Runx2. *Proc Natl Acad Sci U S A.* Jun 14;108(24):9863-8.

Zheng L & Lee WH. 2001. The retinoblastoma gene: a prototypic and multifunctional tumor suppressor. *Exp Cell Res.* Mar 10;264(1): 2-18.

11

Vascularization in the Bone Repair

Jian Zhou and Jian Dong*
Department of Orthopedic Surgery, Zhongshan Hospital, Fudan University, Shanghai, China

1. Introduction

The repair of critical-size bone defects resulted from severe traumatic injury, infection, surgery for bone cancer or congenital malformation remains a continuous challenge for orthopedists. Currently, autogenous bone grafting is a clinical gold standard for bone repair, and provides excellent osteoconduction, osteoinduction, high-healing rate and absence of immunogenic reaction after surgery. However, autogenous bone grafts are associated with the morbidity of donors, additional surgical procedures for harvest, and limitations in the quantity and available bone size. Bone tissue engineering has become a new and promising alternative approach for the repair of bone defects. Moreover, the clinical application of these advanced technologies in the field of tissue engineering seldom leads to satisfactory results. Increasing evidences have demonstrated that the key factor for the poor repair with tissue-engineered bone is poor vascularization (Nakasa et al. 2005; Kawamura et al. 2006). Bone is a highly vascularized tissue that relies on the supply of essential nutrients and oxygen from blood vessels for maintaining skeletal integrity (Kanczler and Oreffo 2008). Under the circumstance of a well-developed vascular network, the osteoblasts can produce osteoid tissues, differentiate to osteocytes, and form healthy bone. In order to provide sufficient oxygen for survival, osteoblasts must reside within 150-200 mm of a capillary lumen and no cells are greater than 0.2 mm from a blood vessel (Kannan et al. 2005). Without the perfusion of blood supply, the osteoblasts in the middle of tissue-engineered constructs will be necrosis due to ineffective transportation of oxygen, nutrients and metabolites (Smith et al. 2004; Rouwkema et al. 2008). Insufficient vascularization can often restrain the formation of new bones and delay the healing of bones. Therefore, vascularization plays a key role in bone regeneration. The rate and range of vascular growth are the determinants of the efficiency and consequence of new bone formation.

2. The role of angiogenesis in bone development

Besides providing nutrients and removing waste products, intraosseous vasculature also can accomplish other important functions including bone development and remodeling. Bone formation and development occurs through two distinct processes: intramembraneous and endochondral ossification. The vascularization is the prerequisite of two different processes of ossification (Clarkin et al. 2008). In intramembranous bone formation, mesenchymal stem cells (MSCs) can be transported through capillaries and differentiate

* Corresponding Author

directly into mature osteoblasts. These osteoblasts then deposit bone matrix and lead to bone formation. On the other hand, during the endochondral ossification, the chondrocytes secret angiogenic growth factors promoting the invasion of blood vessels, which then bring along a number of highly specialized cells and replace the cartilage mold with bone and bone marrow (Chung et al. 2004). Vasculature also plays a key role in bone formation by the production of growth factors that control the recruitment, proliferation, differentiation and function of various cells including osteoblasts and osteoclasts. These growth factors are secreted by endothelial cells (ECs) (Red-Horse et al. 2007).

During the bone remodeling, the osteoblasts play an important role in the balance of resorption and bone deposition by secreting osteoprotegerin that is an inhibitor of osteoclast activity. However, the mature osteocytes lose the capability to produce this molecule (Marx et al. 2007). Blood vessels transport osteoprogenitor cells for the deposition of new bones (Barou et al. 2002). The invading vasculature, thus, serves as both a reservoir and a conduit for the recruitment of essential cells involved in bone remodeling, and provides critical signals necessary for bone morphogenesis (Brandi et al. 2006).

3. Interaction between osteoblasts and endothelial cells

The intercellular signaling between vessel-forming cells and bone-forming cells plays a critical role in bone integrity. The cell-to-cell communication is crucial to coordinate cell behavior, which is necessary for the development and remodeling of bones (Rivron et al. 2008). Several models have been established for studying cellular interactions between osteoblasts (OBs) and ECs in two-dimensional culture dishes (Guillotin et al. 2008 and Grellier et al. 2009), three-dimensional (3D) scaffolds (Choong et al. 2006 and Unger et al. 2007), or 3D spheroids (Wenger et al. 2004 and Stahl et al. 2005). The OBs and ECs can communicate through a couple of mechanisms such as indirect cell contact (Guillotin et al. 2004) through the secretion of diffusible factors with paracrine and autocrine action, and gap junction communication mediating direct cytoplasmic connections between adjacent cells (Villars et al. 2002).

Many diffusible factors released from ECs and OBs that affect the growth and differentiation of both cell types has been identified. Some diffusible factors secreted by ECs include platelet-derived growth factor AB (PDGF-AB), transforming growth factor β_1 (TGF-β_1), transforming growth factor β_2 (TGF-β_2), fibroblast growth factors-2 (FGF-2), epidermal growth factor (EGF), osteoprotegerin (OPG), and bone morphogenetic protein 2 (BMP-2) (Bouletreau et al. 2002), which can affect the migration and proliferation of OBs and the differentiation of osteoprogenitor cells. In contrast, vascular endothelial growth factor (VEGF) secreted by OBs can promote the proliferation of ECs, and stimulate the differentiation and angiogenesis through the activation of specific receptors (Clarkin et al. 2008 and Clarkin et al 2008).

Gap junction is another mechanism for direct cell-to-cell communications. Some special membrane domains composed of aqueous intracellular channels provide direct cytoplasmic connections between cells, and allow for the passage of ions or small molecules between adjacent cells, thus ECs and OBs can communicate and exchange information (Dbouk et al. 2009). Several predominant gap junction proteins including Cx43, Cx37 and Cx40 have been identified to express in ECs and OBs (Yeh et al. 2006). Similarly, the communication via Cx43 gap junctions can promote the expression of osteoblastic differentiation markers such as alkaline phosphatase (ALP), osteocalcin (OC) and bone sialoprotein in OBs (Guillotin et al. 2008).

4. Strategies for improving vascularization

Several strategies for improving vascularization have been proposed. These strategies include the modification of scaffold design, the delivery of angiogenic factors, cell-based techniques, and microsurgery strategies (Rouwkema et al. 2008; Phelps et al. 2010).

4.1 Modification of scaffold design

Biomaterial scaffold, a key component in the bone tissue engineering, serves as a template for cell interactions and the formation of extracellular matrix in bones. The scaffolds should match certain criteria including biocompatibility, biodegradability and mechanical properties similar to the bone repair site. However, the scaffold itself should also be engineered to promote rapid and effective vascularization, and the architecture and design of a scaffold is the key factor for controlling the rate of vascularization after implantation. Currently, the effect of pore size and interpore distance on the scaffolds during the growth of endothelial cells has been evaluated (Narayan and Venkatraman 2008). The growth of endothelial cells can be improved by a smaller pore size (5-20 μm) and lower interpore distance. However, the growth of blood vessels is more extensive in scaffolds with larger pore size (> 250 μm) than those with smaller pore size (Druecke et al. 2004). Other *in vivo* studies have also confirmed that a higher porosity and pore size can result in extensive osteogenesis and sufficient vascularization (Bonfield, 2006), which can be explained by the fact that large pores facilitate vascular ingrowth and osteoblastic cell migration into the scaffold and promote the vascularization and osteogenesis. Porosity also plays an important role in the vascularization of scaffolds. The high porosity allows for the maximum space of vascularization, osteoblast migration and bone deposition (Karageorgiou and Kaplan 2005). In addition, high porosity has a beneficial effect on the diffusion of nutrients and oxygen, transportation and vascularization (Park et al. 2009). The scaffold for bone tissue engineering must possess interconnecting open pores for the maximum potential of vascularization; otherwise, it will be inhibited (Karageorgiou and Kaplan 2005). The interconnected pores facilitate cell migration and vascularization (Jovanovic et al. 2010). This strategy for promoting vascularization still relies on the vessel ingrowth from the host. Limited benefits can be achieved due to the single use. Therefore, it is strongly recommended to combine the scaffold design with other strategies.

4.2 Delivery of angiogenic factors

It is well understood that the local and controlled release of growth factors from a tissue-engineered scaffold can effectively enhance the vascularization of engineered tissues (De Laporte et al. 2010; Zhu et al. 2008). Many angiogenic factors such as vascular endothelial growth factor (VEGF) (des Rieux et al. 2011; Anderson et al. 2011), fibroblast growth factor (FGF) (Kim et al. 2010; Zhu et al. 2008), TGF-β (Lee et al. 2006) and angiopoietin 1 (Ang1) (Chiu and Radisic 2010) have been used for promoting the vascularization of scaffolds. VEGF has gained considerable attention due to its central role in physiology and neovascularization of endothelial cells. The VEGF diffused from the scaffolds or released as the scaffold degrades can stimulate local vessels to sprout towards the implanted tissue-engineered constructs. Current reports have demonstrated that the controlled release of FGF-1 from alginate microbeads can result in an increase of initial vessel invasion into the collagen scaffolds and a longer persistence of vascular network formation (Moya et al. 2010; Uriel et al. 2006). However, the dosage must be tightly controlled because excessive amounts of VEGF and FGF can cause high permeability and poor long-term stability (Ozawa et al. 2004; Zisch et al. 2003). Growth factors including TGF-β and Ang1 for the stabilization of new vessels are also important because subsequent stabilization of newly-formed vessels is critical for the generation of functional vascular networks within tissue-engineered constructs. TGF-β can stimulate the mobilization and recruitment of endothelial cells, and thus accelerating vascularization. Ang 1 plays a key role in regulating vessel homeostasis and stabilization of newly-generated capillaries (Fiedler et al. 2006; Zisch et al. 2003). The neovascularization requires the temporal and spatial expression of multiple angiogenic growth factors, which stimulates different stages of blood-vessel formation to enhance the vascularization of tissue-engineered bones. More and more researchers are investigating the delivery of two sets of factors to mimics under *in vivo* conditions (Tengood et al. 2010; Sun et al. 2011). The combinatorial application of angiogenic factors for stimulating new blood-vessel formation and maturation is highly necessary for the optimal vascularization of tissue-engineered constructs.

4.3 Cell-based techniques

Regardless of the approach adopted to improve vascularization, all of these strategies include endothelia cells. Previous studies have shown that the addition of endothelial cells to tissue cultures can result in the formation of vascular structures *in vitro* and can anastomose to the vessels of the host after implantation (Tremblay et al. 2005; Levenberg et al. 2005). Another approach to accelerate the vascularization of tissue-engineered graft is the co-culture with endothelial cells based on the principle that the transplanted ECs will interact with host ECs and vasculature to establish faster blood supply. The sources of ECs used in the promotion of vascularization in bone tissue engineering included mature ECs, endothelial progenitor cells (EPCs) and MSCs-derived ECs.

Mature ECs can be isolated from a wide variety of sources such as umbilical cords, kidney vasculars, fat tissues and saphenous veins. Previous studies have revealed the 3D pre-vascular network formation when the human umbilical vein endothelia cells are co-cultured with human mesenchymal stem cells in a spheroid co-culture model. After implantation, the pre-vascular network can be developed further and the structures containing lumen can be observed regularly (Rouwkema et al. 2006). The co-culture of rat bone marrow MSCs with kidney vascular ECs on 3D scaffolds exhibits a pre-vascular network-like structure after *in vivo* implantation and results in the increased amount and size of new bone formation when compared with the control group (Sun et al. 2007). These results suggest that mature ECs can efficiently enhance the vascularization of the tissue-engineered grafts. However, the low availability and proliferation capability will severely restrict its large-scale applications (Kim and Von Recum, 2008).

An alternative source of ECs to promote vascularization in tissue engineering is endothelial progenitor cells. The EPCs are enriched in bone marrow, peripheral blood and umbilical cord blood. EPCs have greater proliferation capability than mature ECs (Lin et al. 2000) and can differentiate into ECs *in vitro*, thus contributing to the formation of vascular networks (Rafii and Lyden 2003). Physical and biochemical interactions between EPCs derived from bone marrow and MSCs in a co-culture system *in vitro*. These studies suggest the co-culture of EPCs derived from bone marrow and MSCs can induce endothelial phenotype and angiogenesis without the addition of exogenous growth factors (Aguirre et al. 2010). The co-culture of MSCs and peripheral blood EPCs in Matrigel with 2-3 mm of biphasic calcium phosphate particles for the analysis of bone formation at 6 weeks after implantation in nude mice has demonstrated that co-implantation of EPCs isolated from peripheral blood can significantly enhance osteogenic differentiation *in vitro* and support bone formation *in vivo* (Fedorovich et al. 2010). The influence of EPCs combined with mesenchymal stem cells on early vascularization and bone healing in critical-size defect *in vivo* has also been evaluated to reveal an improvement of early vascularization in the combinatorial group of EPCs and MSCs. Meanwhile, more bony bridges also can be observed in the combinatorial group between EPCs and MSCs at 8 weeks after implantation. These studies suggest that the combinatorial delivery of MSCs and EPCs can support early vascularization and accelerate bone healing.

Similarly, previous studies have been proved that MSCs can be induced to differentiate into ECs and these ECs have more proliferation potential than the terminally-differentiated ECs (Oswald et al. 2004). The MSCs-derived ECS should be ideal for pre-vascularized bone tissue engineering and the pre-vascularized bone tissue engineering construct can be prepared by a single, easily accessible, bone marrow biopsy. ECs and osteogenic cells derived from bone marrow have been seeded in an apatite-coated poly(lactide-co-glycolide)/hydroxyapatite composite scaffolds and then transplanted into critical-size calvarial defects in mmunodeficient mice (Kim et al. 2010). The bone regeneration reveals a significant enhancement due to the addition of ECs derived from bone marrow. Critical-size ulnar defects in the rabbits have also been repaired through vascularized tissue-engineered bone (Zhou et al. 2010). The vascularized tissue-engineered bone is constructed with MSCs and MSC-derived ECs and then co-cultured in porous β-tricalcium phosphate ceramic. The rabbits treated with vascularized tissue-engineered bone exhibit more extensive osteogenesis and better vascularization. Therefore, the ECs derived from bone marrow can be used as a source for pre-vascularized bone tissue engineering with multiple advantages. First, bone marrow aspiration is less invasive. Second, the use of autologous bone marrow cell grafts can avoid immune rejection.

4.4 Microsurgery strategies

Another promising approach for enhancing vascularization in tissue engineering is the hybrid strategy coupled with microsurgery approaches with bone tissue-engineered constructs such as flap fabrication and arteriovenous (AV) loop (Kneser et al. 2006). The vascularization of tissue-engineered grafts basically consists of a two-stage surgical procedure. In the first stage, the scaffolds loaded with cells and/or growth factors are implanted into a site of rich vascularization, usually a muscle or the forearm. Then the capillaries are grown into the scaffold to form a microvascular network in the engineered graft at the initial implantation site after several weeks (Kneser et al. 2006). In the second stage, the tissue-engineered construct with microvascular network is harvested and then re-implanted at the defect site. The microvascular network in the tissue-engineered grafts will anastomose with the host vessels and result in instantaneous perfusion of the entire construct (Kneser et al. 2006). For example, the studies have been conducted the in situ implantation of prefabricated tissue-engineered bone flaps and recombinant human bone morphogenetic protein-2 (rhBMP-2) to accomplish the mandible reconstruction (Zhou et al. 2010). The AV-loop model provides a new approach for the fabrication of axially vascularized tissue so that the vascularization of tissue-engineered grafts can be emanated from internal vascular pedicle independent of local conditions. This AV-loop approach has applied to induce axial vascularization in a bovine cancellous bone matrix (Beier et al. 2011). The micro-CT scans and histomorphometry have showed a significant increase of axial vascularization in bovine cancellous bone matrix constructs, and immunohistochemistry has confirmed the endothelial linking of newly-formed vessels. Similarly, a vascularized tissue-engineered bone graft composed of implanted MSCs and a vascular bundle into the xenogeneic deproteinized cancellous bone (XDCB) scaffold has also constructed (Zhao et al. 2011). The histological and biomechanical examinations have showed that the combination of MSCs and a vascular bundle implantation can result in the promotion of vascularization and osteogenesis in the XDCB graft, and the improvement of new bone formation and mechanical properties during the repair of radius defects. These studies suggest that the vascular bundle implantation is a promising strategy for promoting vascularization in the tissue-engineered grafts.

5. Conclusion and future directions

Insufficient vascularization remains one of the major problems in bone tissue engineering. The critical factor for the limitation of clinical application of tissue-engineered bone is poor vascularization. Multiple approaches such as scaffold design, angiogenic factor delivery, cell-based technique and microsurgery strategy have been explored to promote the vascularization in the field of tissue engineering. These approaches may generate capillary-like structures within the tissue-engineered graft, however, the best method for successful application *in vivo* is still uncertain because there is no convincing evidence. Therefore, the integration of several strategies for enhancing the repair of bone defects is highly desired in the future.

6. References

Anderson, S.M.; Siegman, S.N.; Segura, T. (2011) The effect of vascular endothelial growth factor (VEGF) presentation within fibrin matrices on endothelial cell branching. Biomaterials, 32 (30): 7432-7443.

Aguirre, A.; Planell, J.A.; Engel, E. (2010) Dynamics of bone marrow-derived endothelial progenitor cell/mesenchymal stem cell interaction in co-culture and its implications in angiogenesis. Biochem Bioph Res Co, 400(2): 284-291.

Barou, O.; Mekraldi, S.; Vico, L.; Boivin, G.; Alexandre, C.; Lafage-Proust, M.H. (2002) Relationships between trabecular bone remodeling and bone vascularization: A quantitative study. Bone, 30(4): 604-612.

Beier, J. P.; Hess, A.; Loew, J.; Heinrich, J.; Boos, A. M.; Arkudas, A.; Polykandriotis, E.; Bleiziffer, O.; Horch, R. E.; Kneser, U. (2011) De novo Generation of an Axially Vascularized Processed Bovine Cancellous-Bone Substitute in the Sheep Arteriovenous-Loop Model. Eur Surg Res, 46 (3): 148-155.

Bonfield, W. (2006) Designing porous scaffolds for tissue engineering. Philos Trans A: Math Phys Eng Sci, 364: 227-232.

Brandi, M.L.; Collin-Osdoby, P. (2006) Vascular biology and the skeleton. J Bone Miner Res, 21(2): 183-192.

Bouletreau, P.J.; Warren, S.M.; Spector, J.A.; Peled, Z.M; Gerrets, R.P.; Greenwald, J.A.; Longaker, M.T. (2002) Hypoxia and VEGF up-regulate BMP-2 mRNA and protein expression in microvascular endothelial cells: implications for fracture healing. Plast Reconstr Surg, 109(7): 2384–2397.

Chiu, L.L.Y.; Radisic, M. (2010) Scaffolds with covalently immobilized VEGF and Angiopoietin-1 for vascularization of engineered tissues. Biomaterials, 31 (2): 226-241.

Choong, C.S.; Hutmacher, D.W.; Triffitt J.T. (2006) Co-culture of bone marrow fibroblasts and endothelial cells on modified polycaprolactone substrates for enhanced potentials in bone tissue engineering. Tissue Eng. 12(9): 2521-2531.

Chung, U.I.; Kawaguchi, H.; Takato, T.; Nakamura, K. (2004) Distinct osteogenic mechanisms of bones of distinct origins. J Orthop Sci, 9 (4): 410-414.

Clarkin, C.E.; Emery, R.J.; Pitsillides, A.A.; Wheeler-Jones, C.P.D. (2008) Evaluation of VEGF-Mediated signaling in primary human cells reveals a paracrine action for VEGF in osteoblast-mediated crosstalk to endothelial cells. J Cell Physiol, 214 (2): 537-544.

Clarkin, C.E.; Garonna, E.; Pitsillides, A.A.; Weeler-Jones, C.P.D. (2008) Heterotypic contact reveals a COX-2-mediated suppression of osteoblast differentiation by endothelial cells: A negative modulatory role for prostanoids in VEGF-mediated cell: cell communication? Exp Cell Res, 314(17): 3152–3161.

Dbouk, H.A.; Mroue, R.M.; El-Sabban, M.E.; Talhouk, R.S. (2009) Connexins: a myriad of functions extending beyond assembly of gap junction channels. Cell Commun Signal, 7, 4.

De Laporte, L.; des Rieux, A.; Tuinstra, H.M.; Zelivyanskaya, M.L.; De Clerck, N.M.; Postnov, A.A.; Preat, V.; Shea, L.D. (2011) Vascular endothelial growth factor and fibroblast growth factor 2 delivery from spinal cord bridges to enhance angiogenesis following injury. J Biomed Mater Res A, 98A (3): 372-382.

Des Rieux, A.; Ucakar, B.; Mupendwa, B.P.K.; Colau, D.; Feron, O.; Carmeliet, P.; Preat, V. (2011) 3D systems delivering VEGF to promote angiogenesis for tissue engineering. J Control Release, 150(3): 272-278.

Druecke, D.; Langer, S.; Lamme, E.; Pieper, J.; Ugarkovic, M.; Steinau, H.U.; Homann, H.H. (2004) Neovascularization of poly(ether ester) blockcopolymer scaffolds in vivo: long-term investigations using intravital fluorescent microscopy. J Biomed Mater Res A, 68A (1): 10–18.

Fedorovich, N.E.; Haverslag, R.T.; Dhert, W.J.A.; Alblas, J. (2010) The Role of Endothelial Progenitor Cells in Prevascularized Bone Tissue Engineering: Development of Heterogeneous Constructs. Tissue Eng A, 16 (7): 2355-2367.

Fiedler, U.; Augustin, H.G. (2006) Angiopoietins: a link between angiogenesis and inflammation. Trends Immunol, 27 (12): 552-558.

Grellier, M.; Ferreira-Tojais, N. Bourget, C.; Bareille, R.; Guillemot, F.; Amedee, J. (2009) Role of vascular endothelial growth factor in the communication between human osteoprogenitors and endothelial cells. J Cell Biochem, 106(3): 390–398.

Guillotin, B.; Bareille, R.; Bourget, C.; Bordenave, L.; Amedee, J. (2008) Interaction between human umbilical vein endothelial cells and human osteoprogenitors triggers pleiotropic effect that may support osteoblastic function. Bone 42(6): 1080–1091.

Guillotin, B.; Bourget, C.; Remy-Zolgadri, M.; Bareille, R.; Fernandez, P.; Conrad, V.; Amedee-Vilamitjana, J. (2004) Human primary endothelial cells stimulate human osteoprogenitor cell differentiation Cell Physiol Biochem, 14(4-6): 325-332.

Jovanovic, D.; Engels, G.E.; Plantinga, J.A.; Bruinsma, M.; van Oeveren, W.; Schouten, A.J.; van Luyn, M.J.A.; Harmsen, M.C. (2010) Novel polyurethanes with interconnected porous structure induce in vivo tissue remodeling and accompanied vascularization. J Biomed Mater Res A, 95A (1): 198-208.Kanczler, J.M. & Oreffo, R.O. (2008). Osteogenesis and angiogenesis: the potential for engineering bone. Eur Cell Mater, 15: 100-114.

Kannan, R.Y.; Salacinski, H.J.; Sales, K.; Butler, P. & Seifalian, A.M. (2005). The roles of tissue engineering and vascularisation in the development of micro-vascular networks: a review. Biomaterials, 26 (14): 1857-1875.

Karageorgiou, V.; Kaplan, D. (2005) Porosity of 3D biomaterial scaffolds and osteogenesis. Biomaterials, 26(27): 5474-5491.

Kawamura, K.; Yajima, H.; Ohgushi, H.; Tomita, Y.; Kobata, Y., Shigematsu, K. & Takakura, Y. (2006). Experimental study of vascularized tissue-engineered bone grafts. Plastic and Reconstructive Surgery, 117 (5): 1471-1479.

Kneser, U.; Polykandriotis, E.; Ohnolz, J.; Heidner, K.; Grabinger, L.; Euler, S.; Amann, K.U.; Hess, A.; Brune, K.; Greil, P.; Sturzl, M.; Horch, R.E. (2006) Engineering of vascularized transplantable bone tissues: induction of axial vascularization in an osteoconductive matrix using an arteriovenous loop. Tissue Eng, 12 (7), 1721–1731.

Kneser, U.; Schaefer, D.J.; Polykandriotis, E.; Horch, R.E. (2006) Tissue engineering of bone: the reconstructive surgeon's point of view. Cell. Mol. Med, 10 (1): 7-11.

Kim, M.S.; Bhang, S.H.; Yang, H.S.; Rim, N.G.; Jun, I.; Kim, S.I.; Kim, B.S.; Shin, H. (2010) Development of Functional Fibrous Matrices for the Controlled Release of Basic Fibroblast Growth Factor to Improve Therapeutic Angiogenesis. Tissue Eng A, 16 (10): 2999-3010.

Kim, S.S.; Park, M.S.; Cho, S.W.; Kang, S.W.; Ahn, K.M.; Lee, J.H.; Kim, B.S. (2010) Enhanced bone formation by marrow-derived endothelial and osteogenic cell transplantation. J Biomed Mater Res A, 92A (1): 246-253.

Kim, S.; Von Recum, H. (2008) Endothelial stem cells and precursors for tissue engineering: Cell source, differentiation, selection, and application. Tissue Eng B, 14 (1): 133-147.

Lee, J.Y.; Kim, K.H.; Shin, S.Y.; Rhyu, I.C.; Lee, Y.M.; Park, Y.J.; Chung, C.P.; Lee, S.J. (2006) Enhanced bone formation by transforming growth factor-beta 1-releasing collagen/chitosan microgranules. J Biomed Mater Res A, 76A (3): 530-539.

Levenberg, S.; Rouwkema, J.; Macdonald, M.; Garfein, E.S.; Kohane, D.S.; Darland, D.C.; Marini, R.; van Blitterswijk, C.A.; Mulligan, R.C.; D'Amore, P.A.; Langer, R. (2005) Engineering vascularized skeletal muscle tissue. Nat Biotechnol 23 (7): 879-884.

Lin, Y.; Weisdorf, D.J.; Solovey, A.; Hebbel, R.P. (2000) Origins of circulating endothelial cells and endothelial outgrowth from blood. J Clin Invest, 105 (1): 71-77.

Marx, R.E. (2007) Bone and bone graft healing. Oral Maxillofac Surg Clin. North Am. 19(4): 455-466.

Moya, M.L.; Garfinkel, M.R.; Liu, X.; Lucas, S.; Opara, E.C.; Greisler, H.P.; Brey, E.M. (2010) Fibroblast growth factor-1 (FGF-1) loaded microbeads enhance local capillary neovascularization. J Surg Res, 160(2): 208-212.

Nakasa, T.; Ishida, O.; Sunagawa, T.; Nakamae, A.; Yasunaga, Y.; Agung, M. & Ochi, M. (2005). Prefabrication of vascularized bone graft using a combination of fibroblast growth factor-2 and vascular bundle implantation into a novel interconnected porous calcium hydroxyapatite ceramic. Journal of Biomedical Materials Research Part A, 75A (2): 350-355.

Narayan, D.; Venkatraman, S. S. (2008) Effect of pore size and interpore distance on endothelial cell growth on polymers. J Biomed Mater Res A, 87A (3): 710-718.

Oswald, J.; Boxberger, S.; Jorgensen, B.; Feldmann, S.; Ehninger, G.; Bornhauser, M.; Werner, C. (2004) Mesenchymal stem cells can be differentiated into endothelial cells in vitro. Stem Cells. 22 (3): 377-384.

Ozawa, C.R.; Banfi, A.; Glazer, N.L.; Thurston, G.; Springer, M.L.; Kraft, P.E.; McDonald, D.M.; Blau, H.M. (2004) Microenvironmental VEGF concentration, not total dose, determines a threshold between normal and aberrant angiogenesis. J Clin Invest, 113 (4): 516-527.

Park, S.; Kim, G.; Jeon, Y.C.; Koh, Y.; Kim, W. (2009) 3D polycaprolactone scaffolds with controlled pore structure using a rapid prototyping system. J Mater Scti-Mater M, 20 (1): 229-234.

Phelps EA, García AJ. (2010) Engineering more than a cell: vascularization strategies in tissue engineering. Current Opinion in Biotechnology, 21: 704–709.

Rafii, S.; Lyden, D. (2003) Therapeutic stem and progenitor cell transplantation for organ vascularization and regeneration. Nat Med, 9 (6): 702-712.

Red-Horse, K.; Crawford, Y.; Shojaei, F.; Ferrara, N. (2007) Endothelium-microenvironment interactions in the developing embryo and in the adult. Dev Cell, 12 (2): 181-194.

Rivron, N.C.; Liu, J.; Rouwkema, J.; de Boer, J.; van Blitterswijk, C.A. (2008) Engineering vascularised tissues in vitro. Eur Cell Mater, 15: 27–40.

Rouwkema, J.; De Boer, J.; Van Blitterswijk, C.A. (2006) Endothelial cells assemble into a 3-dimensional prevascular network in a bone tissue engineering construct. Tissue. Eng. 12 (9): 2685-2693.

Rouwkema J, Rivron NC, van Blitterswijk CA. (2008) Vascularization in tissue engineering. Trends in Biotechnology, 26(8): 434–441.

Seebach, C.; Henrich, D.; Kahling, C.; Wilhelm, K.; Tami, A.E.; Alini, M.; Marzi, I. (2010) Endothelial Progenitor Cells and Mesenchymal Stem Cells Seeded onto b-TCP Granules Enhance Early Vascularization and Bone Healing in a Critical-Sized Bone Defect in Rats. Tissue Eng A, 16 (6): 1961-1970.

Smith, M.K.; Peters, M.C.; Richardson, T.P.; Garbern, J.C. & Mooney, D.J. (2004) Locally enhanced angiogenesis promotes transplanted cell survival. Tissue Engineering, 10(1-2): 63–71.

Stahl, A.; Wu, X.; Wenger, A.; Klagsburn, M.; Kurschat, P. (2005) Endothelial progenitor cell sprouting in spheroid cultures is resistant to inhibition by osteoblasts: a model for bone replacement grafts. FEBS Lett, 579(24): 5338–5342.

Sun, H.C.; Qu, Z.; Guo, Y.; Zang, G.X.; Yang, B. (2007) In vitro and in vivo effects of rat kidney vascular endothelial cells on osteogenesis of rat bone marrow mesenchymal stem cells growing on polylactide-glycoli acid (PLGA) scaffolds. Biomed. Eng. Online. 6: 41.

Sun, G.; Shen, Y.I.; Kusuma, S.; Fox-Talbot, K.; Steenbergen, C.J.; Gerecht, S. (2011) Functional neovascularization of biodegradable dextran hydrogels with multiple angiogenic growth factors. Biomaterials, 32(1): 95-106.

Tengood, J.E.; Kovach, K.M.; Vescovi, P.E.; Russell, A.J.; Little, S.R. (2010) Sequential delivery of vascular endothelial growth factor and sphingosine 1-phosphate for angiogenesis. Biomaterials, 31 (30): 7805-7812.

Tremblay, P.L.; Hudon, V.; Berthod, F.; Germain, L.; Auger, F.A. (2005) Inosculation of tissue-engineered capillaries with the host's vasculature in a reconstructed skin transplanted on mice. Am J Transplant, 5 (5): 1002-1010.

Unger, R.E.; Sartoris, A.; Peters, K.; Motta, A.; Migliaresi, C.; Kunkel, M.; Bulnheim, U.; Rychly, J.; Kirkpatrick, C.J. (2007) Tissue-like self-assembly in cocultures of endothelial cells and osteoblasts and the formation of microcapillary-like structures on three-dimensional porous biomaterials Biomaterials, 28(27): 3965-3976.

Uriel, S.; Brey, E.M.; Greisler, H.P. (2006) Sustained low levels of fibroblast growth factor-1 promote persistent microvascular network formation. Am J Surg, 192(5): 604-609.

Villars, F.; Guillotin, B.; Amedee, T.; Dutoya, S.; Bordenave, L.; Bareille, R.; Amedee, J. (2002) Effect of HUVEC on human osteoprogenitor cell differentiation needs heterotypic gap junction communication Am J Physiol Cell Physiol. 282(4): C775-C785.

Wenger, A.; Stahl, A.; Weber, H.; Finkenzeller, G.; Augustin, H.G.; Stark, G.B.; Kneser, U. (2004) Modulation of in vitro angiogenesis in a three dimensional spheroidal coculture model for bone tissue engineering. Tissue eng, 10(9-10): 1536-1547.

Yeh, H.I.; Lee, P.Y.; Su, C.H.; Tian, T.Y.; Ko, Y.S.; Tsai, C.H. (2006) Reduced expression of endothelial connexins 43 and 37 in hypertensive rats is rectified after 7-day carvedilol treatment. Am J Hypertens, 19(2): 129–135.

Zhu, X.H.; Tabata, Y.; Wang, C.H.; Tong, Y.W. (2008) Delivery of Basic Fibroblast Growth Factor from Gelatin Microsphere Scaffold for the Growth of Human Umbilical Vein Endothelial Cells. Tissue Eng A, 14(12): 1939-1947.

Zhao, M.D.; Zhou, J.; Li, X.L.; Fang, T.L.; Dai, W.D.; Yin, W.P.; Dong, J. (2011) Repair of Bone Defect with Vascularized Tissue Engineered Bone Graft Seeded with Mesenchymal Stem Cells in Rabbits. Microsurgery, 31 (2): 130-137.

Zhou, J.; Lin, H.; Fang, T.L.; Li, X.L.; Dai, W.D.; Uemura, T.; Dong, J. (2010) The repair of large segmental bone defects in the rabbit with vascularized tissue engineered bone. Biomaterials, 31 (6): 1171-1179.

Zhou, M.; Peng, X.; Mao, C.; Xu, F.; Hu, M.; Yu, G.Y. (2010) Primate mandibular reconstruction with prefabricated, vascularized tissue-engineered bone flaps and recombinant human bone morphogenetic protein-2 implanted in situ. Biomaterials, 31 (18): 4935-4943.

Zisch, A.H.; Lutolf, M.P.; Hubbell, J.A. (2003) Biopolymeric delivery matrices for angiogenic growth factors. Cardiovasc. Pathol. 12 (6): 295–310.